Biological, Chemical, and Radiological Terrorism

Alan L. Melnick

Biological, Chemical, and Radiological Terrorism

Emergency Preparedness and Response for the Primary Care Physician

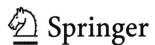 Springer

Alan L. Melnick, MD, MPH
Health Officer
Clark County, Washington
Associate Professor
Department of Family Medicine
Oregon Health Science University
Portland, Oregon 97201
USA

ISBN: 978-0-387-47231-7   e-ISBN: 978-0-387-47232-4

Library of Congress Control Number: 2007940366

Selection from *An Autobiography: The Story of My Experiments with Truth* by Mohandas Ghandi, copyright © 1957 by Beacon Press.

Portions of this book were previously presented in Melnick A. The Family Physician's Role in Responding to Biological, Chemical and Radiological Terrorism. In: Taylor, R (Ed.). Family Medicine: Principles and Practice, 6th ed. New York: Springer, 2003:1107–1127. Reprinted with permission.

Printed on acid-free paper.

9 8 7 6 5 4 3 2 1

springer.com

You must not lose faith in humanity.
Humanity is an ocean; if a few drops of the
ocean are dirty, the ocean does not become
dirty.

Mahatma Gandhi
An Autobiography: The Story of
My Experiments with Truth

For Kelly and Martin, and for the families of primary healthcare and public health workers worldwide.

Preface

The intentional use of biological or chemical agents to cause disease or destroy food and water supplies for political or economic reasons dates to antiquity. The turn of the twentieth century heralded the development of lethal biological and chemical weapons capable of mass destruction. By the final two decades of the twentieth century, individuals and small groups learned how to obtain and use these weapons effectively. The events of the past few decades, including the World Trade Center and anthrax attacks in 2001, have shown that small groups of individuals, as well as nations, have the resources to coordinate attacks using chemical, biological and radiological agents.

Given the long history of biological and chemical warfare, and given that that many of these agents are relatively easy to obtain and use, future attacks are possible. If they occur, primary care clinicians will have key roles to play in protecting their patients and the public. The illnesses that biological, chemical and radiological weapons cause can be difficult to distinguish from naturally occurring illness. Clearly, clinicians will need a basic understanding of diseases caused by these agents, including their associated epidemiology, and an understanding on how to work with public health officials to protect their patients and the public.

This book is written for primary care clinicians – family physicians, pediatricians, internists, nurse practitioners and physician assistants – who will be the front-line responders to patients suffering from or concerned about exposure to biological, chemical and radiological agents. Although the book has a public health perspective, it does not require detailed knowledge of public health programs and principles. Knowledge of the basic concepts of epidemiology, communicable disease, chemical and radiological exposures, obtained through training and practical experience, should suffice.

The first five chapters provide a background of the epidemiology and clinical aspects of diseases caused by biological, chemical and radiological weapons. Chapter 1 provides a brief introduction to the role clinicians might play in responding to attacks involving weapons of mass destruction. Chapter 2 discusses the general features of biological terrorism and the diseases caused by pathogens terrorists are most likely to use, including their epidemiology, clinical diagnosis, treatment and prevention. The prevention discussion includes infection control and mass prophylaxis. Chapter 3 describes the basic features of chemical attacks, general precautions in triaging and treating patients exposed to chemical agents, and a description of diseases caused by chemical agents terrorists are most likely to use, including diagnosis, treatment, and prevention.

Chapter 4 discusses the general features of radiological terrorism, including the types of radiological weapons terrorists are likely to use, general precautions in triaging and treating patients exposed to radiological agents and a description of radiological illness, including diagnosis and treatment. Whether or not individuals suffer from direct exposure, many will approach their physicians with concerns, fears, anxieties, and stress symptoms following terrorist events. Chapter 5 describes the epidemiology of mental health conditions associated with mass disasters, followed by treatment and prevention recommendations for primary care clinicians.

Recent events, including the Salmonella attacks in Oregon and the 2001 Anthrax attacks in Florida, New Jersey, New York City, and Washington, DC, have taught us that primary care clinicians need more than an understanding of the clinical presentation, treatment and prophylaxis of disease caused by biological, chemical, and radiological agents. To protect their communities as well as their patients, primary care clinicians must know how to work with public health officials (1). Early warnings to local health officials, who work closely with law enforcement, can be successful in preventing additional casualties. Chapter 6 describes how primary care physicians and other clinicians can participate in early detection and community wide prevention and treatment of biological, chemical, and radiological disasters. Potential roles for primary care clinicians include participating in surveillance activities, reporting suspected cases to public health officials, and responding to the surge of affected patients.

Although the purpose of this book is to prepare primary care clinicians and students to respond to the intentional use of biological, chemical, and radiological weapons, the lessons in this book should be applicable to accidental disasters, such as chemical spills, and natural disasters, such as earthquakes and floods, for several reasons. By disrupting food and water distribution systems and by disrupting waste disposal systems, accidental and natural disasters can increase the risk for communicable disease. Intentional and natural communicable disease outbreaks, such as pandemic flu, are likely to create similar management challenges for primary care clinicians and public health departments. The presentation of disease due to chemical and radiological agents is similar whether exposure is accidental or intentional. Any mass disaster is likely to cause some degree of fear, anxiety, and stress for some people regardless of whether they are directly injured. Regardless of the cause, primary care clinicians can be most helpful in any disaster if they know how to work with public health officials and if they are part of a coordinated response. Not surprisingly, many public health officials, at local, state, and federal levels, are developing all hazard plans. This book will be successful if it encourages primary care clinicians to develop closer working relationships with their public health colleagues. When faced with a disaster, we will work together to protect the health of our patients and our communities.

Alan L. Melnick

Reference

Gerberding, JL, Hughes, JM, Koplan, JP. Bioterrorism Preparedness and Response. Clinicians and Public Health Agencies as Essential Partners. JAMA, 287(7):898–900, 2002

Acknowledgments

Shortly after the Anthrax attacks in the fall of 2001, Robert Taylor, MD, Professor Emeritus, Department of Family Medicine, Oregon Health & Science University, had the wisdom and foresight to include a chapter on the Family Physician's Role in Responding to Biologic and Chemical Terrorism in the Sixth Edition of his Textbook, *Family Medicine, Principles and Practice*. I am thankful to Dr. Taylor, who graciously asked me to write the chapter.

Robert Albano, Senior Editor, Springer, immediately recognized the need for an entire book devoted to the topic of biological, chemical, and radiological terrorism preparedness for primary care physicians. He offered me the opportunity to write this book, and his enthusiasm and commitment to the project helped me get started.

Margaret Burns, Development Editor, provided support throughout the project. She kept me on track, she provided insightful editorial comments and improvements, and her humor and patience with me helped me turn the idea for this book into a reality. I could not have completed this book without her support.

Nearly 20 years ago, Harold Osterud, MD, MPH, Former Chair of the Oregon Health & Science University Department of Public Health & General Preventive Medicine, provided incredible mentorship in introducing me to the world of preventive medicine and public health. Since then, I have been fortunate to work in two rewarding professional environments: family medicine and public health. My colleagues at the Oregon Health & Science University Department of Family Medicine have shown me how to serve on the front lines of primary care as a family physician. My Public Health colleagues in the Oregon Conference of Local Public Health Officials (CLHO), the Oregon Public Health Division, the National Association of County and City Health Officials (NACCHO) and the Public Health Leadership Society (PHLS) have shown me how to be a public health official. I am thankful to all of them for showing me how primary care clinicians and public health officials can work together to protect and promote health for everyone.

Contents

Chapter 1
Emergency Preparedness for the Primary Care Physician

Brief History of Biological and Chemical Warfare

Biological and chemical warfare date to biblical times. The Old Testament describes a series of plagues, some involving biologic agents, that convinced the Pharaoh to let the Jews escape slavery in Egypt, and Judges 9:45 has a reference to the use of salt to destroy crops (1). As early as 300 BC, Persian, Greek, and Roman literature discussed using animal and human cadavers to contaminate drinking water. In the middle ages, Tatar troops catapulted plague victims over their enemy's city walls (1–3). Aerosolized weapons appeared in the in the mid-seventeenth century, when a Polish infantryman suggested creating hollowed bombs filled with rabid dog saliva and other materials that could cause disease (1,3). In 1763, bioterrorism arrived in the New World, when British troops supplied smallpox contaminated blankets to Indian tribes during the French and Indian War (1–3).

The turn of the twentieth century heralded the development of more effective, lethal weapons of mass destruction. During World War I, the use of chlorine, phosgene and mustard gas killed or injured more than a million troops and civilians (1,4). Recognizing the actual and potential consequences of these weapons, world leaders approved the 1925 Geneva Protocol of the Prohibition of the Use in War of Asphyxiating, Poisonous or Other Gases and of Bacteriological Methods of Warfare (1). However, the protocol fell short in several areas: it did not prevent countries from asserting their right to respond in kind when attacked with these weapons, it did not prohibit research and development of these agents, it did not prohibit the production and stockpiling of agents and delivery systems, and participation was not universal (1). For example, the United States did not ratify the Geneva Protocol until 1975, 50 years after its inception (1).

The development and use of biologic and chemical agents accelerated after World War I, when Japan began extensive biological weapon research, eventually exposing over 10,000 prisoners to a wide range of chemical and biologic agents (1,3). In Europe, the Nazi party recruited physicians to support the development and use of biological and chemical agents. Besides contributing to the murder of six million Jews with Zyclon B, Nazi physicians exposed concentration camp

A. L. Melnick (ed.), *Biological, Chemical, and Radiological Terrorism.*
© Springer 2008

victims to biologic agents, such as Rickettsia species, Plasmodia species, and Hepatitis A, as well as experimental drugs and vaccines (1,2).

The Axis partners were not alone in developing, testing and using chemical and biological agents. In the early 1940s, the United States began research in the use of chemical and biological agents, such as Anthrax, Botulinum toxin, and herbicides through its Chemical Warfare Service, later changing the name to the War Research Service. American leaders considered using chemical and biological weapons against the Japanese if the war had continued past August 1945 (1). Over the ensuing 30 years, warring nations accused each other of using chemical and biologic agents. For example, during the Korean War, North Korea and China accused the United States and United Nations troops of using chemical and biological agents, and during the Vietnam War, the United States accused North Vietnam of using mycotoxins in Laos (1,2).

Throughout the Cold War, the Soviet Union and the United States engaged in considerable research and development of biological and chemical weapons. In 1949, without consent of those who might become exposed, the United States intentionally attacked itself by spraying *Serratia marcescens* into the Pentagon's ventilation system. The Serratia spread effectively throughout the facility, convincing the military that the incredible threat these weapons posed justified continuation of this type of research (1). Documents obtained through the Freedom of Information Act revealed that the military exposed unknowing and nonconsenting civilian populations in Virginia, San Francisco, New York, and elsewhere to *Serratia marcescens* and Bacillus globigii from 1949 to 1960 (1–3). *Serratia* studies continued until 1969 (1).

Soviet Union research began earlier, in 1928 with typhus. Following World War II, the Soviet Union expanded its research efforts after obtaining Japanese biological and chemical weapon research data (1). At its peak, the Soviet military biological research division, the "Biopreparat," employed up to 55,000 microbiologists, physicians, engineers and nontechnical personnel (1,2).

In 1969, at President Nixon's direction, the United States unilaterally decided to ban offensive biological research and destroy its offensive arsenal (1). While critics complained that the distinction between offensive and defensive biological weapons research was spurious, the United States and the Soviet Union continued to engage in biological weapons research (3). A few years later, in 1972, the multinational Biological Weapons convention banned the production of biological weapons and their toxins (1). However, the Soviet Union continued research and development, culminating in the accidental release of Anthrax spores from a research facility in Sverdlovsk in 1979. The resulting outbreak, causing 66 deaths, was the largest documented outbreak of inhalational Anthrax (1–3,5).

By the final two decades of the twentieth century, individuals and small groups learned how to obtain and use biological and chemical weapons effectively. The tamper resistant pharmaceutical packaging we are familiar with today is a consequence of the intentional contamination of Extra Strength Tylenol capsules with cyanide (1). The first documented case of domestic biological terrorism occurred in Oregon in 1984, when a religious cult, the Rajneesh commune, sprinkled

Salmonella typhimurium into salad bars in an attempt to influence a local election (1–3,6). As a result, 751 people developed enteritis and at least 45 patients required hospitalization (2,6). In the mid-1990s, the Japanese cult Aum Shinrikyo sprayed Sarin gas in the Tokyo subway system, causing nearly 3,800 injuries and 12 deaths (7). The ensuing investigation revealed that the cult had planned other attacks with a variety of biological and chemical agents (1,2,7). In 1996, a disgruntled laboratory worker infected 12 of her co-workers to *Shigella dysenteriae* (1,3,8). Mass poisoning events involving arsenic, cyanide, sodium azide, and cresol have caused illness in several Japanese cities (1). Stolen radioactive sources, specifically ^{60}Co (radioactive cobalt) ^{137}Cs (radioactive cesium) have led to injuries in Brazil, Mexico, and Thailand (9).

The events of the past few decades, have shown that small groups of individuals, as well as nations, have the resources to coordinate attacks using chemical, biological, and radiological agents. Given the long history of biological and chemical warfare, and given that that many of these agents are relatively easy to obtain and use, future attacks are possible. If they occur, primary care clinicians will have key roles to play in protecting their patients and the public. The illnesses that biological, chemical, and radiological weapons cause can be difficult to distinguish from naturally occurring illness. Clearly, clinicians will need a basic understanding of diseases caused by these agents, including their associated epidemiology, and an understanding on how to work with public health officials to protect their patients and the public.

Recent Events

In April 2000, the centers for disease control and prevention (CDC) warned physicians and public health officials against ignoring the possibility of chemical and biological terrorism (10). The CDC based its warning on terrorist activities over the previous 10 years, including the Sarin gas attack in the Tokyo subway and the discovery of military bio-weapons programs in Iraq and the former Soviet Union. While noting these events, the report stated that the public health system must be prepared to detect covert biological and chemical attacks and prevent the accompanying illness and injury. In addition, the CDC reminded primary health-care providers throughout the United States to be "vigilant because they will probably be the first to observe and report unusual illnesses or injuries."

In spite of this and other warnings, most primary care physicians have spent little time planning for terrorism. One reason may be the rarity of these events, especially on US soil. Until recently, the only reported case of bioterrorism in the United States was the 1984 salmonella attack in Oregon. It is unlikely that authors of family medicine textbooks written before September 2001 considered devoting significant space for discussions about how family physicians should respond to terrorist attacks.

The September 11, 2001 events in New York City and Washington DC abruptly changed our perspectives about the likelihood that terrorists could direct weapons of mass destruction against civilian communities in the United States. The public, including physicians, suddenly began to recognize the consequences of being unprepared for such terrorist attacks, especially those associated with chemical and biological weapons. Shortly after the September attacks, the CDC recommended heightened surveillance for any unusual disease occurrence or increased numbers of illnesses that might be associated with terrorist attacks.

On October 4, 2001, the CDC and their state and local partners reported a case of inhalational anthrax in Florida (11). Over the following several weeks, public health authorities reported additional cases from Florida and New York City. Investigations revealed that the intentional release of *Bacillus anthracis* was responsible for these cases (12). By November 9, 22 cases (17 confirmed and five suspected) of bioterrorism-related anthrax were reported from Washington DC, Florida, New Jersey, and New York City (13). Ten of these cases were the inhalational form, resulting in four deaths; the other 12 cases were cutaneous anthrax. Of the ten inhalation cases, most were people who had processed, handled, or received letters containing *B. anthracis* spores.

The association of anthrax with mail increased the level of public alarm. State and territorial public health officials responding to a CDC survey from September 11 through October 17 estimated their health departments had received 7,000 reports of potential bioterrorist threats. Potential threats included suspicious packages, letters containing powder, and potential dispersal devices. Nearly 5,000 of these reports required telephone follow-up and about 1,000 of the reports led to testing of suspicious materials at a public health laboratory (14). Public health officials were not alone. Patients deluged physicians' offices with concerns about suspicious envelopes and packages and concerns about anthrax symptoms. Although only four areas of the United States had identified bioterrorism-associated anthrax infections, physicians and public health officials across the nation were obliged to respond to bioterrorist hoaxes and threats, as well as anxious patients.

These events illustrate how family physicians and other primary care clinicians have been and will be on the front line in detecting and responding to terrorist threats and events. We can summarize their roles:

- Addressing patient concerns about their risk of terrorist-caused illness
- Reporting credible risks to law enforcement and public health authorities
- Detecting terrorist-caused illness
- Providing effective prophylactic therapy to exposed patients
- Providing effective treatment for patients with terrorist-caused illness
- Recommending actions families can take to protect themselves from future risks
- Providing counseling to families traumatized by terrorist threats and activities

This book provides information useful for primary care clinicians in performing these roles including:

- The features of terrorist attacks distinguishing them from other forms of disasters
- The types of biologic, chemical, or radiological agents terrorists are likely to use
- The clinical manifestations of these agents, including the routes of exposure
- How to provide effective preventive treatment for those exposed
- How to treat terrorist-caused illness
- How to identify patients at risk of exposure
- How to care for common mental health problems associated with disasters
- Understanding how to work with public health officials in detecting and responding to terrorist attacks

References

1. Malloy, CD. A History of Biological and Chemical Warfare and Terrorism. Public Health Issues in Disaster Preparedness. Focus on Bioterrorism. Journal of Public Health Management and Practice, 6(4). Aspen Publishers, Gaithersburg Maryland. Pps 85–92, 2001
2. Christopher, GW, Cieslak, TJ, Pavlin, JA, Eitzen, EM. Biological Warfare: A Historical Perspective. Journal of the American Medical Association, 278(5):412–417, 1997
3. Lesho, E, Dorsey, D, Bunner, D. Feces, Dead Horses and Fleas. Evolution of the Hostile Use of Biological Agents. Western Journal of Medicine, 168(6):512–516, 1998
4. Blanc, PD. The Legacy of War Gas. The American Journal of Medicine, 106:689–690, 1999
5. Meselson, M, Guillemin, J, Hugh-Jones, M, Langmuir, A, Popova, I, Shelokov, A, Yampolskaya, O. The Sverdlovsk Anthrax Outbreak of 1979. Science, 266(5188):1202–1208, 1994
6. Torok, T, Tauxe, RV, Wise, RP, Livengood, JR, Sokolow, R, Mauvais, S, Birkness, KA, Skeels, MR, Horan, JM, Foster, LR. A Large Community Outbreak of Salmonellosis Caused by Intentional Contamination of Restaurant Salad Bars. Journal of the American Medical Association, 278(5):389–395, 1997
7. Olson, KB. Aum Shinrikyo: Once and Future Threat? Emerging Infectious Disease, 5(4):513–516, 1999
8. Kolavic, S, Kimura, A, Simons, S, Slutsker, L, Barth, S, Haley, CE. An Outbreak of Shigella Dysenteriae Type 2 Among Laboratory Workers Due to Intentional Food Contamination. Journal of the American Medical Association, 278(5):396–398, 1997
9. Leikin, JB, McFee, RB, Walter, FG, Edsall, K. A Primer for Nuclear Terrorism. Disease-a-Month, 49(8):485–516
10. Centers for Disease Control and Prevention. Biological and Chemical Terrorism: Strategic Plan for Preparedness and Response. Recommendations of the CDC Strategic Planning Workgroup. Morbidity and Mortality Weekly Report 49, no. RR04 (April 21, 2000): 1–14
11. Centers for Disease Control and Prevention. Ongoing investigation of anthrax – Florida, October 2001. Morbidity and Mortality Weekly Report 50, 40:877, 2001
12. Centers for Disease Control and Prevention. Update: Investigation of Anthrax Associated with Intentional Exposure and Interim Public Health Guidelines. Morbidity and Mortality Weekly Report 50, 41:889–893, 2001

13. Centers for Disease Control and Prevention. Update: Investigation of Bioterrorism-Related Anthrax and Adverse Events from Antimicrobial Prophylaxis. Morbidity and Mortality Weekly Report 50, 44:973–976, 2001
14. Centers for Disease Control and Prevention. Update: Investigation of Bioterrorism-Related Anthrax and Interim Guidelines for Clinical Evaluation of Persons with Possible Anthrax. Morbidity and Mortality Weekly Report 50, 43:941–948, 2001

Chapter 2
Biological Terrorism

Features of Biological Terrorist Attacks

Historically, most planning for an emergency response to terrorism has focused on overt attacks such as bombings and attacks using chemicals. Chemical events are also likely to be overt because inhalation or skin/mucous membrane absorption of chemicals produces effects that are usually immediate and obvious. For obvious reasons, explosive and chemical attacks elicit an immediate response by law enforcement, fire and Emergency Medical Services personnel. In comparison to chemicals and explosives, the impact of biologic agents is more likely to be covert and delayed. As the recent anthrax events demonstrated, biologic agents do not have an immediate impact due to the interval between exposure and the onset of illness (the incubation period) (1). Consequently, the most likely responders to future biologic attacks will be family physicians and other primary health care providers. For example, after an intentional, covert release of Variola virus, some infected patients would arrive at their doctors' offices and local emergency rooms 1–2 weeks later. Other infected people may have traveled, and they would probably show up at emergency rooms distant from their homes. Their symptoms would appear at first to be an ordinary viral infection, including fever, back pain, headache, and nausea. As the disease progressed, many physicians would not recognize the characteristic early stage papular rash of smallpox. After the rash became pustular and patients began dying, the terrorists could be continents away, and patients would be disseminating the disease further through person-to-person contact. Soon after, secondary cases would begin to occur, resulting in dissemination throughout the world.

Table 2.1 summarizes the distinguishing features between explosive, chemical and biologic attacks, pointing out why early detection and response to biologic terrorism are critical. Without adequate preparation, a large-scale attack could overwhelm the public health and health care system. Large numbers of infected patients would seek medical care, resulting in a corresponding need for medical supplies, equipment, diagnostic tests, and hospital beds. The October 2001 anthrax events revealed that the "worried-well" would also seek medical attention, causing additional strain on physician and public health resources. First responders and medical

A. L. Melnick (ed.), *Biological, Chemical, and Radiological Terrorism.*
© Springer 2008

Table 2.1 Features distinguishing biological attacks from chemical and explosive attacks

Chemical/explosive agents	Biological agents
Overt	Covert
Immediate	Delayed (incubation period)
Police/fire/EMS detection and response	Medical/public health detection and response
Injuries occur at once	Continuing new cases due to transmission
Cases at location of event	Cases at multiple locations

Source: Melnick A. The family physician's role in responding to biologic and chemical terrorism. In: Family medicine: principles and practice. Taylor R (Ed.). Springer: New York, 2003. Reprinted with permission.

personnel could also be at risk of exposure, and widespread panic and fear of contagion would disrupt everyday life (1).

Terrorists could deliver biologic pathogens by several routes of exposure, including inhalation, oral ingestion (contamination of food or water), or percutaneous absorption. However, the inhalation route is the most efficient and effective. Although these agents have vastly different characteristics, terrorists could use readily available technology to incorporate them into aerosolized particles 1–10 μm in size, capable of penetrating into distal bronchioles and alveoli. Hand held industrial sprayers, used indoors or outdoors, are capable of exposing large numbers of people, and small particles can remain suspended for hours, depending on the meteorological conditions (2).

The accidental contamination of chicken feed with dioxin contaminated fat in Europe shows how food exposure could occur. Because dioxin does not cause immediate symptoms, authorities did not discover the contamination for months in 1999, and Europeans probably consumed the dioxin in chicken meat and eggs sold that year. One lesson learned from this event is that physicians and public health officials need to recognize and report unusual or suspicious health problems in animals as well as humans (1). The 1999 West Nile virus epidemic in birds and humans in New York City reinforced this lesson. Fortunately, biological and chemical contamination of public water supplies will usually pose little risk due to dilution by the large volume of water.

Primary care clinicians must be vigilant for indications that terrorists have released a biologic agent. These indications include (3):

1. An unusual temporal or geographic cluster of illness. For example, the occurrence of similar symptoms in people who attended the same public event or gathering or patients presenting with clinical signs and symptoms suggestive of an infectious disease outbreak should raise suspicion. One indication may be two or more patients presenting with an unexplained febrile illness associated with sepsis, pneumonia, respiratory failure, rash, or a botulism-like syndrome with flaccid muscle paralysis. Suspicion should be heightened if these symptoms occurred in previously healthy persons.
2. An unusual age distribution for common diseases. For example, an increase in what looks like chickenpox in adult patients could be smallpox.

3. A large number of cases of acute flaccid paralysis with prominent bulbar palsies, suggestive of a release of botulinum toxin.

Biological Agents Terrorists Are Likely to Use

Terrorists can choose from countless biological agents and the list can seem overwhelming. However, to best protect our patients and their families, primary care clinicians should focus their attention on the agents that terrorists are most likely to use and that have the greatest potential for mass casualties. The CDC has defined three categories of agents, "A," "B," and "C" with potential as weapons, based on several criteria (1) (see Table 2.2):

–   Ease of dissemination or transmission
–   Potential for major public health impact such as high mortality
–   Potential for public panic and social disruption
–   Requirements for public health preparedness

Category C agents are the third highest priority. These agents include emerging pathogens such as Nipah virus and Hanta virus that terrorists could develop as weapons in the future based on their availability, their ease of production and dissemination and their potential for high morbidity and mortality rates and major health impact.

Based on these criteria, Category A contains seven agents of highest concern for the CDC:

–   *Bacillus anthracis* (Anthrax)
–   *Yersinia pestis* (Plague)
–   *Variola major* (Smallpox)
–   *Clostridium botulinum toxin* (Botulism)
–   *Francisella tularensis* (Tularemia)
–   Filoviruses (Ebola hemorrhagic fever, Marburg hemorrhagic fever)
–   Arenaviruses (Lassa (Lassa fever), Junin (Argentine hemorrhagic fever), and related viruses)

Table 2.2 CDC Categories A and B for biological agents with potential as weapons

	Category A (high priority)	Category B (second highest priority)
Ease of dissemination	Easily disseminated or transmitted person to person	Moderately easy to disseminate
Potential public health impact	High mortality rates and potential for major public health impact	Moderate morbidity rates and low mortality
Potential for panic and disruption	Might cause public panic and social disruption	
Requirements for Preparedness	Require special action for public health preparedness	Require specific enhancements of CDC's diagnostic capacity and enhanced disease surveillance

Source: CDC Public Domain (http://www.bt.cdc.gov/agent/agentlist-category.asp)

This chapter focuses on the biologic agents in category A. Those interested in additional information on agents not covered in this chapter, including those in categories B and C, should visit the CDC web site at http://www.bt.cdc.gov.

Anthrax

The Working Group on Civilian Biodefense, composed of 23 representatives from academic medical centers, research organizations and government, military, public health and emergency management institutions and agencies, considered potential scenarios and developed the recommendations for anthrax diagnosis, treatment and prevention outlined in this chapter. These recommendations, based on a literature review and professional expertise, are subject to change based on new information (4).

Microbiology and Epidemiology

Bacillus anthracis, the organism responsible for anthrax, is an anaerobic, gram positive, spore-forming rod. Anthrax bacilli cannot survive long outside of a human or animal host. Instead, the bacilli form spores in situations where nutrients are unavailable, such as when infected body fluids are exposed to the air. Anthrax spores are incredibly hardy, capable of surviving for decades in the environment, making them relatively easy to store and transport as a biological weapon. When exposed to nutrient-rich environments, such as human or animal blood or tissues, the spores germinate into the bacillus form (5).

Anthrax spores, commonly found in the soil throughout the world (5), can cause infection when ingested by herbivore animals. Naturally occurring human infections follow exposure to the infected animals or infected animal products. Occupational exposure has been the most common cause of anthrax, with industrial mill wool sorters at greatest risk. From 1900 to 1978, there were 18 reported human cases in the United States, all in occupations associated with specific exposure, such as goat hair mill workers, tannery workers, and laboratory workers. Widespread animal vaccination programs have reduced animal mortality from anthrax and naturally occurring human anthrax is now a very rare disease (5).

Anthrax can present as one of three types of infection in humans: inhalational, cutaneous and gastrointestinal. Cutaneous anthrax is the most common naturally occurring form, with about 224 cases reported between 1944 and 1994 in the United Sates. Inhalational anthrax, the most likely form of anthrax to follow a biologic attack, is incredibly rare. Until the 2001 terrorist attacks, the last reported inhalational anthrax case in the United States occurred over 20 years earlier in 1978. Naturally occurring gastrointestinal anthrax is uncommon, with outbreaks occasionally reported in Africa and Asia (4). It is unlikely that gastrointestinal illness would result from a terrorist attack. Experiments on primates have revealed that ingesting spores is unlikely to cause illness. Instead, gastrointestinal anthrax follows ingestion of insufficiently cooked meat from animals with active infection with the vegetative, bacillus form of anthrax.

Anthrax as a Biological Weapon

Research on anthrax as a biological weapon began 80 years ago, long before the October 2001 attacks. In 1979, a Soviet Union military facility developing bio-weapons experienced an accidental release of anthrax spores. The accident caused 79 cases of anthrax with 68 deaths, demonstrating the potential lethal effectiveness of anthrax aerosols. In 1995, the same Japanese terrorist group responsible for the release of Sarin gas in a Tokyo subway released aerosols containing anthrax and botulism throughout Tokyo eight different times. The release did not cause any illness, perhaps because the anthrax used came from a strain used for animal vaccinations that was not a significant risk for humans (4).

In the 2001 anthrax attacks, terrorists contaminated five letters with powder containing anthrax spores, and sent the letters from Trenton, New Jersey to Florida, New York City, and Washington DC. Three years after the attack, authorities had not yet discovered the source of the anthrax used to contaminate the letters. One of the letters, sent to Senator Daschle's office, contained 2 g of the powder. Although the source of the report is unclear, a New York Daily News article reported that the powder contained between 100 billion and 1 trillion spores per gram (4).

The 2001 anthrax attacks resulted in 22 human anthrax cases. However, the method used in the attack – contaminating mail and relying on sorting machines to create aerosols when processing the mail – was a relatively inefficient way of exposing large numbers of people to anthrax. Perhaps a more effective way to expose large numbers of people would be to disperse aerosols either inside buildings where large numbers of people gather, such as concert halls or sports arenas, or outside over similar gatherings, such as sports stadiums. This release could easily be surreptitious, because the powder is odorless and invisible when dispersed through the air. The former Soviet Union and Iraq (4,6) have created an aerosolized preparation of anthrax and have tested it as a weapon. In addition, in the 1960s, the United States weapons tested an aerosolized form of anthrax over the Pacific Ocean.

Two different reports, one by the World Health Organization (WHO) and one by the US Congressional Office of Technology (OTA), predicted large numbers of casualties following outdoor dispersal of anthrax aerosols. The 1970 WHO report estimated that an aerosol release of 50 kg of anthrax over an urban area of 5 million people would cause 250,000 casualties, with 100,000 people dying without treatment. The 1993 OTA report estimated 130,000 to 3 million deaths following the release of a 100 kg aerosol upwind of Washington DC. Although the October 2001 attacks caused far fewer casualties, the amount of anthrax, as reflected in the Daschle letter, was much smaller.

Clinical Presentation and Diagnosis

Cutaneous Anthrax

Topical exposure to anthrax spores can result in cutaneous anthrax, especially in areas with previous cuts or abrasions. Uncovered areas, such as the arms, hands, face, and neck are the most likely sites for cutaneous anthrax. Unlike inhalational anthrax, experience does not reflect a prolonged latency period, and in Sverdlovsk, no cutaneous cases occurred more than 12 days after the aerosol release (4,5).

The germinating spores produce toxins resulting in local edema. The first sign of cutaneous anthrax is an initial pruritic macule or papule, which enlarges into an ulcer by day two. Next, 1–3 mm vesicles may appear, releasing clear or serosanguinous fluid. Gram stain of the fluid may reveal numerous organisms. The hallmark of cutaneous anthrax, a painless, depressed, black eschar follows, and is frequently associated with extensive local edema. The black eschar is what gives *B. anthracis* its name: anthrakis is the Greek word for coal. Over the next 1–2 weeks, the eschar dries, loosens, and falls off, most often leaving no permanent scar. Patients with cutaneous anthrax may also develop lymphangitis and painful lymphadenopathy, often with associated systemic symptoms. Antibiotic therapy does not change the course of the skin manifestations, but it does reduce the likelihood of systemic disease, reducing the mortality rate from 20% to near zero. Figure 2.1 summarizes the clinical evaluation of persons with possible cutaneous anthrax (5,7).

Clinicians suspecting cutaneous anthrax should order a Gram stain and culture of the vesicular fluid, as well as blood cultures. Previous antibiotics will reduce the sensitivity of the Gram stain and cultures. If the Gram stain and cultures are negative, especially if the patient is already on antibiotics, a punch biopsy is helpful in making the diagnosis. Only a laboratory capable of performing immunohistochemical staining or polymerase chain reactions (PCRs) assays should process the specimen (4). Physicians sending such specimens should alert the lab that they suspect cutaneous anthrax. Physicians suspecting cutaneous anthrax must also report the case immediately to their local public health department.

Gastrointestinal Anthrax

Infection in the upper gastrointestinal tract causes the oral-pharyngeal form, with development of an oral or esophageal ulcer and accompanying regional lymphadenopathy, edema and sepsis. Lower tract infections cause intestinal lesions predominantly in the terminal ileum or cecum. These infections present initially with malaise, nausea, and vomiting, progressing rapidly to hematochezia, acute abdomen, or sepsis. Some patients develop massive ascites. The mortality rate is high, given the difficulty of early diagnosis (5).

Given the rapid transit of food through the gastrointestinal system, it is unlikely that exposure to spores could cause gastrointestinal anthrax. Instead, gastrointestinal

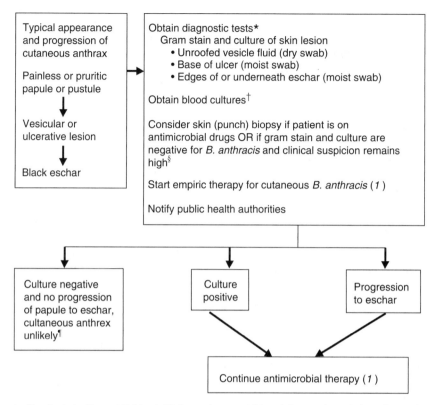

* Serologic testing available at CDC may be an additional diagnostic technique for confirmation of cases of cutaneous anthrax.

† If blood cultures are positive for *B. anthracis*, treat with antimicrobials as for inhalational antrax (*1*).

§ Punch biopsy should be submitted in formalin to CDC. Polymerase chain reaction can also be done on formalin-fixed specimen. Gram stain and culture are frequently negative for *B. anthracis* after initiation of antimicrobials.

¶ Continued antimicrobial prophylaxis for inhalational anthrax for 60 days if aerosol exposure to *B. anthracis* is known or suspected (*2*).

Reference

1. CDC. Update: investigation of bioterrorism-related anthrax and interim guidelines for exposure management and antimicrobial therapy, October 2001. MMWR 2001;50:909–19.

2. CDC. Update: investigation of anthrax associated with intentional exposure and interim public health guidelines, October 2001. MMWR 2001;50:889–93.

Fig. 2.1 Clinical evaluation of persons with possible cutaneous anthrax. (From (7), public domain, from Morbidity and Mortality Weekly Report.)

anthrax probably results from ingestion of poorly cooked meat contaminated with the germinated bacillus form of anthrax. Unlike the hardy anthrax spores, the germinated form of anthrax is difficult to store and transport. Therefore, gastrointestinal anthrax is unlikely to result from a terrorist attack. There were no cases of gastrointestinal anthrax following the Sverdlovsk release or the October 2001 attacks.

Inhalational Anthrax

Inhalational anthrax results from the deposition of spores into the alveolar spaces. Spores not ingested by macrophages in the alveoli travel by lymphatics to mediastinal lymph nodes, where they can germinate into the vegetative form and reproduce rapidly. The time from deposition to germination is variable, with cases occurring 2–43 days after exposure in Sverdlovsk (4). Exposed monkeys have developed disease up to 98 days after exposure (4), and one monkey had spores in the mediastinal nodes capable of germinating 100 days after exposure (4). The estimated LD50 (lethal dose sufficient to kill 50% of exposed persons) is 2,500–55,000 inhaled spores (5). However, recent primate studies suggest that one to three spores are capable of causing some cases if large numbers of people are exposed (8).

Inhalational anthrax does not cause a typical bronchopneumonia, so the term anthrax pneumonia is misleading. The organisms germinating in the mediastinal nodes release toxins resulting in hemorrhage, edema, and necrosis. Postmortem study of those who died following the 1979 accidental release of anthrax spores in Sverdlovsk (in the former Soviet Union) revealed hemorrhagic thoracic lymphadenitis and hemorrhagic mediastinitis in all patients. About half of the patients had hemorrhagic meningitis as well.

Early diagnosis is difficult and requires a high index of suspicion. Based on information from cases occurring before 2001, the clinical presentation of inhalational anthrax occurs in two stages. At first, symptoms are nonspecific, including fever, dyspnea, cough, headache, vomiting, chills, weakness, abdominal pain, and chest pain. Laboratory studies are not specific during the first stage, which could last from hours to a few days. The second stage develops abruptly, with sudden

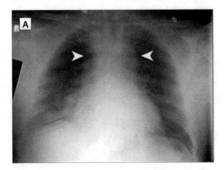

Fig. 2.2 Widened mediastinum on chest X-ray in patient with inhalational anthrax following the October 2001 Attacks. (From Inglesby et al. (4). Copyright© 2002 American Medical Association. All rights reserved.)

fever, dyspnea, diaphoresis, and shock. Stridor may result from massive lymphadenopathy and expansion of the mediastinum. A chest radiograph most often shows a
widened mediastinum consistent with lymphadenopathy (4) (Fig. 2.2).

Data on symptoms and signs from the October 2001 attack are available for the first
ten of the eleven inhalational cases. All ten patients first presented with malaise and
fever. Prominent symptoms included cough, nausea, and vomiting. In addition, most of
the patients had drenching seats, not previously described, and dyspnea, chest pain and
headaches. Fever and tachycardia were the presenting physical findings in the majority
of patients. Early laboratory findings included hypoxemia and transaminase elevations
(4). All ten cases had abnormal chest X-ray results, including seven with mediastinal
widening, seven with infiltrates and eight with pleural effusions (4). Chest computerized
tomography results were available for eight patients, and all were abnormal. Seven had
mediastinal widening, six had infiltrates and eight had pleural effusions (4). Table 2.3
identifies the symptoms presented by the first ten patients with inhalational anthrax, and
Table 2.4 identifies their clinical signs, laboratory, and diagnostic findings.

The mortality rate of occupationally acquired inhalational anthrax cases in the
United States had been 89%, but most of these cases occurred before the development
of critical care units, and in some cases, before the advent of antibiotics. In the October
2001 attacks, five of 11 patients with inhalational anthrax died. This recent experience
suggests that early diagnosis and treatment is critical to improving survival.

The incubation period is known for six of the cases associated with the October
2001 attacks. The median incubation period, based on the known time of exposure
and the onset of symptoms, was 4 days, with a range of 4–6 days. Patients sought
medical care after a median time of 3.5 days after symptom onset, with a range of 1–7
days. Eight of the first ten patients with inhalational anthrax were in the early stages
of the disease when they first presented for care. Of these eight patients, six received
antibiotics with activity against anthrax the day they presented, and all six of these
patients survived. All four of the patients who received antibiotics active against
anthrax after they developed fulminant illness died (9).

Table 2.3 Symptoms for ten patients with inhalational anthrax, fall 2001

Symptoms	$N = 10$
Fever, chills	10
Fatigue, malaise, lethargy	10
Cough (minimal or nonproductive)	9
Nausea or vomiting	9
Dyspnea	8
Sweats, often drenching	7
Chest discomfort or pleuritic pain	7
Myalgias	6
Headache	5
Confusion	4
Abdominal pain	3
Sore throat	2
Rhinorrhea	1

Table 2.4 Physical, laboratory and diagnostic findings, first ten patients with inhalational anthrax, fall 2001

Physical findings	
Fever (>37.8°C.)	7/10
Tachycardia (heart rate >100 min⁻¹)	8/10
Hypotension (systolic blood pressure <110 mmHg)	1/10
Laboratory results	
White blood cell count (medium range)	9.8×10^3 mm³
Differential–neutrophilia (>70%)	7/10
Neutrophil band forms (>5%)	4/5
Elevated transaminases (SGOT or SGPT >40)	9/10
Hypoxemia (alveolar-arterial oxygen gradient >30 mmHg on room air saturation <94%)	6/10
Metabolic acidosis	2/10
Elevated creatinine (>1.5 mg dL⁻¹)	1/10
Chest X-ray findings	
Any abnormality	10/10
Mediastinal widening	7/10
Infiltrates/consolidation	7/10
Pleural effusion	8/10
Chest computed tomography findings	
Any abnormality	8/8
Mediastinal widening, lymphadenopathy	7/8
Pleural effusion	8/8
Infiltrates/consolidation	6/8

Source: Reprinted with permission from Inglesby et al. (4). Copyright © 2002 American Medical Association. All Rights reserved.

SGOT serum glutamic oxalocetic transminase, *SGPT* serum glutamic pyruvic transaminase

Early Diagnosis of Inhalational Anthrax: Differentiating Anthrax from Influenza-like Illness

Given the generic symptoms and findings in the early stage of inhalational anthrax, the key to early diagnosis relies on clinicians being able to differentiate inhalational anthrax from influenza-like illness (ILI). To do so, clinicians evaluating patients with ILI must carefully consider epidemiologic, clinical and if indicated, laboratory and radiographic findings (10). ILI is a nonspecific respiratory illness characterized by fever, fatigue, cough, and other symptoms (10). Besides influenza, ILI has many other causes including other viruses, such as rhinoviruses, respiratory syncytial virus (RSV), adenoviruses, and parainfluenza virus. Other, less common causes of ILI are bacterial, such as *Legionella spp*, *Chlamydia pneumoniae*, *Mycoplasma pneumoniae*, and *Streptococcus pneumoniae*. Each year, adults can average three and children can average six episodes of ILI. Some causes of ILI, specifically influenza, RSV and some bacterial infections can lead to serious complications requiring hospitalization, making them particularly difficult to differentiate from inhalational anthrax.

The ten cases of inhalational anthrax following the October 2001 terrorist event provide epidemiologic clues helping clinicians differentiate inhalational anthrax from ILI. Nine of the ten cases occurred among postal workers, persons exposed to letters or areas known contaminated with anthrax spores, and media employees. Inhalational anthrax is not transmissible from person to person. Consequently, nine of the ten cases were located in only a few communities. In comparison, viral causes of ILI are spread person to person, causing millions of cases each year across all communities. In addition, nonanthrax causes of ILI have a typical seasonal pattern. Pneumococcal disease, influenza and RSV infection generally peak in the winter, mycoplasma and legionellosis are more common in the summer and fall, rhinoviruses and parainfluenza virus infections usually peak during the fall and spring, and adenoviruses circulate throughout the year.

Table 2.5 shows how clinical signs and symptoms identified in the October 2001 cases can help clinicians distinguish other causes of ILI from inhalational anthrax. Most cases of nonanthrax ILI are associated with nasal congestion and rhinorrhea. In comparison, only one of the ten patients in the October 2001 outbreak complained of rhinorrhea.

A history of influenza vaccination does not help differentiate inhalational anthrax from other causes of ILI. The vaccine does not prevent ILI caused by infectious agents other than influenza, and many persons vaccinated against influenza will still get ILI. Therefore, a history of receipt of vaccine does not increase the probability of inhalational anthrax as a cause of ILI, especially among persons who have no probable exposure to anthrax.

Chest radiograph findings can help differentiate nonanthrax ILI from inhalational anthrax. In the October 2001 outbreak, all ten inhalational anthrax patients presented with abnormal chest radiographs. The radiographic findings were easier to discern with posteroanterior and lateral views, compared to portable anteroposterior views. In comparison, most cases of ILI are not associated with radiographic

Table 2.5 Clinical findings of inhalational anthrax, laboratory confirmed influenza, and other causes of influenza-like illness

Symptom/sign	Inhalational anthrax ($n = 10$) (%)	Laboratory-confirmed influenza (%)	ILI from other causes (%)
Elevated temperature	70	68–77	40–73
Fever or chills	100	83–90	75–89
Fatigue/malaise	100	75–94	62–94
Cough (minimal or nonproductive)	90	84–93	72–80
Shortness of breath	80	6	6
Chest discomfort or pleuritic chest pain	60	35	23
Headache	50	84–91	74–89
Myalgias	50	67–94	73–94
Sore throat	20	64–84	64–84
Rhinorrhea	10	79	68
Nausea or vomiting	80	12	12
Abdominal pain	30	22	22

Source: From (10), public domain, Morbidity and Mortality Weekly Report

findings of pneumonia, which occurs most often among the very young, the elderly or those with chronic pulmonary disease (10).

Because pneumonia is not a prominent feature of inhalational anthrax, sputum gram stains and cultures are not likely to be helpful (4). Nasal swabs are not useful as a diagnostic test, and negative nasal swabs do not rule out inhalational anthrax.

The most useful microbiologic test for anthrax is a standard blood culture, which should show growth within 6–24 h. Blood cultures are likely to be positive early in the course of illness. In the October 2001 inhalational anthrax cases, all patients who had not received antibiotic therapy had blood cultures positive for *B. anthracis*. However, blood rapidly becomes sterile after initiation of antibiotic therapy, so the sensitivity of blood cultures declines significantly for patients with prior antibiotic therapy (9). Clinicians should order blood cultures only for patients in situations where they suspect bacteremia and not routinely on all patients with ILI symptoms who have no probable exposure to anthrax. When ordering blood cultures, clinicians must alert the laboratory to the possibility of anthrax, so that the lab performs appropriate biochemical testing and species identification.

Rapid diagnostic tests for anthrax are not available, so clinicians need to be vigilant about recognizing unusual radiologic findings. Even without blood cultures, a chest radiograph showing a widened mediastinum in a previously healthy person with evidence of severe flu-like symptoms is essentially pathognomonic of advanced inhalational anthrax. Although the patient's prognosis may be poor even with treatment, immediate reporting may lead to earlier diagnosis in others. Clinicians evaluating a previously healthy patient with symptoms and signs consistent with those experienced by patients in the October 2001 attacks (Table 2.6), must immediately notify their local public health department about a suspected case.

Exposure Evaluation

After the October 2001 terrorist release of anthrax, thousands of patients called physician's offices with concerns about possible anthrax. Some were asymptomatic, while others were experiencing upper respiratory or other symptoms suggestive of a viral ILI. Concern about recent exposure to suspicious mail was a theme common to many of these calls. Given the small number of actual anthrax cases, the "worried well" generated the vast majority of these calls, taxing the resources of physicians and other health care providers.

Figures 2.1 and 2.3 summarize the recommended clinical evaluation for patients with possible cutaneous anthrax and inhalational anthrax, respectively (7). Clearly, taking a history is the most essential step in the clinical evaluation. When taking a history, primary care clinicians should ask questions regarding the patient's concern about exposure with two goals in mind:

–   First, assess the probability of exposure. By doing so, clinicians can determine whether the patient is at risk for anthrax disease, whether to notify public health officials and law enforcement agencies and whether to begin preventive or curative

Table 2.6 Epidemiology and clinical presentation of inhalational anthrax

Epidemiology	Incubation period	Clinical syndrome	Diagnostic studies	Microbiology	Pathology
Sudden appearance of multiple cases of severe flu-like illness with fulminant course and high mortality or acute febrile illness in persons identified at risk following a specific attack	Average: 1–7 days Range: 2–60 days	Nonspecific viral syndrome followed in 2–5 days by severe respiratory distress, mediastinitis, shock and death	CXR: widened mediastinum, infiltrates, pleural effusion Chest CT scan: hyperdense hilar and mediastinal nodes, mediastinal edema, infiltrates, pleural effusion Thoracentesis: hemorrhagic pleural effusions	Peripheral blood smear: gram + bacilli on unspun smear Blood culture: growth of large gram + bacilli with preliminary identification of Bacillus species	Hemorrhagic mediastinitis, hemorrhagic thoracic lymphadenitis, hemorrhagic meningitis

Source: Data from (4,5,11)

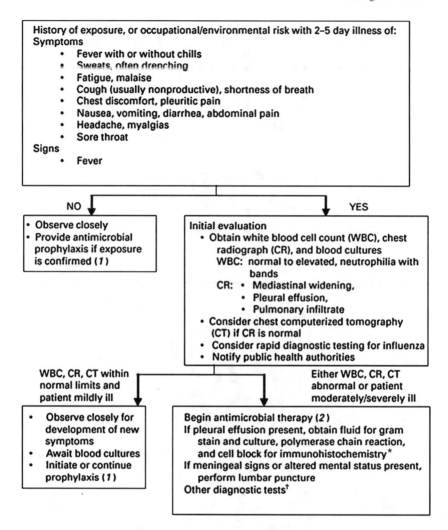

History of exposure, or occupational/environmental risk with 2–5 day illness of:
Symptoms
- Fever with or without chills
- Sweats, often drenching
- Fatigue, malaise
- Cough (usually nonproductive), shortness of breath
- Chest discomfort, pleuritic pain
- Nausea, vomiting, diarrhea, abdominal pain
- Headache, myalgias
- Sore throat
Signs
- Fever

NO

YES

- Observe closely
- Provide antimicrobial prophylaxis if exposure is confirmed (1)

Initial evaluation
- Obtain white blood cell count (WBC), chest radiograph (CR), and blood cultures
  WBC: normal to elevated, neutrophilia with bands
  CR: • Mediastinal widening,
      • Pleural effusion,
      • Pulmonary infiltrate
- Consider chest computerized tomography (CT) if CR is normal
- Consider rapid diagnostic testing for influenza
- Notify public health authorities

WBC, CR, CT within normal limits and patient mildly ill

Either WBC, CR, CT abnormal or patient moderately/severely ill

- Observe closely for development of new symptoms
- Await blood cultures
- Initiate or continue prophylaxis (1)

Begin antimicrobial therapy (2)
If pleural effusion present, obtain fluid for gram stain and culture, polymerase chain reaction, and cell block for immunohistochemistry*
If meningeal signs or altered mental status present, perform lumbar puncture
Other diagnostic tests†

* Available through CDC or LRN. Cell block obtained by centrifugation of pleural fluid.
† Serologic testing available at CDC may be an additional diagnostic technique.

References
1. CDC. Update: investigation of anthrax associated with intentional exposure and interim public health guidelines, October 2001. MMWR 2001;50:889–93.
2. CDC. Update: investigation of bioterrorism-related anthrax and interim guidelines for exposure management and antimicrobial therapy, October 2001. MMWR 2001;50:909–19.

Fig. 2.3 Recommended clinical evaluation for patients with possible inhalational anthrax. (From (7), public domain, of Morbidity and Mortality Weekly Report, 50: 43:941, 2001.)

treatment. Given the volume of patient telephone calls, physicians should consider training their nursing staff to triage the calls to reduce the number of patients requiring evaluation that is more extensive.
– Second, review with the patient his/her level of risk. If patients come to the office for further evaluation, the visit provides opportunities to educate patients and the public on how to evaluate their risk and how to take reasonable measures to protect themselves and their families

Over a telephone call or during an office visit, questions physicians and their staff should ask their patients include:

– Have you been exposed to a situation where anthrax transmission has been confirmed or under investigation?
– Have you had any contact with a substance believed to be contaminated with anthrax?
– When, where and under what circumstances did the contact occur?
– What was the nature of the contact (skin, inhalation, ingestion)?
– Was any powder suspended in the air?
– Did other people come into contact with the substance?
– Were you exposed to a suspicious package/mail item? If so, why was it suspicious?
– Were you exposed to something else, why do you believe it was contaminated?
– Where is the substance/package? Is it contained safely (e.g., in a plastic zip-lock bag)?

To assist physicians and other responders in evaluating exposure, local, state, and federal law enforcement authorities have released guidelines on identification of packages/envelopes potentially contaminated with anthrax. Characteristics of suspicious packages include (http://www.oregon.gov/DHS/ph/acd/bioterrorism/cdc1018.pdf):

– Inappropriate or unusual labeling
– Excessive postage
– Handwritten or poorly typed addresses
– Misspellings of common words
– Strange return address or no return address
– Incorrect titles or title without a name
– Not addressed to a specific person
– Marked with restrictions, such as "Personal," "Confidential," or "Do not X-ray"
– Marked with any threatening language
– Postmarked from a city or state that does not match the return address
– Powdery substance felt through or appearing on the package or envelope
– Oily stains, discoloration, or odor
– Lopsided or uneven envelope
– Excessive packaging material such as masking tape, string, etc.
– Other suspicious signs

– Excessive weight
– Ticking sound
– Protruding wires or aluminum foil

If the clinical evaluation and the exposure evaluation reveal a credible threat of anthrax exposure, clinicians must immediately report the case to the local health department and local law enforcement agency.

Treatment

A high index of suspicion, prompt diagnosis, and immediate initiation of effective antimicrobial treatment are critical for treating inhalational anthrax. Clinicians must report suspected or confirmed cases of anthrax to local and state public health authorities immediately to prompt an epidemiologic investigation. Because of the rarity of the disease, neither adequate clinical experience nor controlled trials are available to validate current recommendations for treatment. Because of the high-associated mortality, the CDC and the Working Group for Civilian Biodefense recommend two or more known effective antibiotics.

Table 2.7 summarizes their recommendations for a contained casualty situation, similar to the October 2001 attacks, in which relatively small numbers of victims require treatment. The recommendations could change as we gather more experience with treating anthrax. Ciprofloxacin or doxycycline is recommended for initial intravenous therapy until susceptibility results are available. Other antibiotics suggested for use in combination with ciprofloxacin or doxycycline include rifampin, vancomycin, imipenem, chloramphenicol, penicillin and ampicillin, clindamycin and clarithromycin. Cephalosporins and trimethroprim–sulfamethoxazole are not recommended as therapy (11). Although penicillin is labeled for use to treat inhalational anthrax, data from the October 2001 outbreak revealed the presence of beta-lactamases in *B. anthracis* isolates form Florida, New York City, and Washington DC. Therefore, penicillin or amoxicillin alone are not recommended for treatment of systemic anthrax infection (11). The recommendations for gastrointestinal anthrax, including oropharyngeal anthrax, are the same as those for inhalational anthrax.

Neither doxycycline nor a fluoroquinolone may reach therapeutic levels in the cerebrospinal fluid. Therefore, ciprofloxacin augmented with chloramphenicol, rifampin, or penicillin is the treatment of choice for suspected or confirmed anthrax meningitis (4).

The toxin produced by *B. anthracis* is a major cause of the morbidity associated with the disease. One study suggested corticosteroids as adjunct therapy for inhalational anthrax associated with extensive edema, respiratory failure and meningitis (11,12).

In an attack resulting in mass casualties, resources may be insufficient to provide the intravenous treatment outlined in Table 2.7. Instead, only oral antibiotics may be available. Table 2.8 outlines the recommendations for mass treatment with oral antibiotics. These recommendations are the same as those for postexposure prophylaxis for people without active disease.

Table 2.7 Inhalational treatment protocol for contained casualty situation, similar to that associated with the October 2001 bioterrorism attack

Category	Initial therapy (intravenous)[a]	Duration
Adults	Ciprofloxacin, 400 mg every 12 h[b] or Doxycycline 100 mg every 12 h[c,d] and one or two additional antimicrobials[e]	IV treatment initially.[f] Switch to oral antimicrobial therapy when clinically appropriate: Ciprofloxacin 500 mg po BID or Doxycycline 100 mg po BID. Continue for 60 days (IV and po combined)[g]
Children	Ciprofloxacin 10–15 mg kg^{-1} every 12 h,[h] or Doxycycline	IV treatment initially.[f] Switch to oral antimicrobial therapy when clinically appropriate: Ciprofloxacin 10–15 mg kg^{-1} po every 12 h.[i] or Doxycycline[j]
	>8 years and >45 kg: 100 mg every 12 h	>8 years and >45 kg: 100 mg po BID
	>8 years and ≤45 kg: 2.2 mg kg^{-1} every 12 h	>8 years and ≤45 kg: 2.2 mg kg^{-1} po BID
	≤8 years: 2.2 mg kg^{-1} every 12 h and one or two additional antimicrobials[e]	≤8 years: 2.2 mg kg^{-1} po BID. Continue for 60 days (IV and po combined)[g]
Pregnant women[k]	Same for nonpregnant adults (the high death rate from the infection outweighs the risk posed by the antimicrobial agent)	IV treatment initially. Switch to oral antimicrobial therapy when clinically appropriate.[b] Oral therapy regimens same for nonpregnant adults
Immuncompromised persons	Same for nonimmunocompromised persons and children	Same for nonimmunocompromised persons and children

Source: Reprinted with permission from Inglesby et al. (4). Copyright© 2002 American Medical Association. All rights reserved

[a]For gastrointestinal and or oropharyngeal anthrax, use regimens recommended for inhalational anthrax

[b]Ciprofloxacin or doxycycline should be considered an essential part of first-line therapy for inhalational anthrax

[c]If meningitis is suspected, doxycycline may be less optimal because of poor central nervous penetration

[d]Steroids may be considered as an adjunct therapy for patients with severe edema and for meningitis based on experience with bacterial meningitis of other etiologies

[e]Other agents with in vitro activity include rifampin, vancomycin, penicillin, ampicillin, chloramphenicol, imipenem, clindamycin, and clarithromycin. Because of concerns of constitutive and inducible beta-lactamases in *B. anthracis,* penicillin and ampicillin should not be used alone. Consultation with an infectious disease specialist is advised

[f]Initial therapy may be altered based on clinical course of the patient; one or two antimicrobial agents (e.g., ciprofloxacin or doxycycline) may be adequate as the patient improves

[g]Because of the potential persistence of spores after an aerosol exposure, antimicrobial therapy should be continued for 60 days

[h]If intravenous ciprofloxacin is not available, oral ciprofloxacin may be acceptable because it is rapidly and well absorbed from the gastrointestinal tract with no substantial loss by first pass metabolism. Maximum serum concentrations are attained 1–2 h after oral dosing but may not be achieved if vomiting or ileus are present

[i]In children, ciprofloxacin dosage should not exceed 1 g d^{-1}

[j]The American Academy of Pediatrics recommends treatment of young children with tetracyclines for serious infections (e.g., Rocky Mountain spotted fever)

[k]Although tetracyclines are not recommended during pregnancy, their use may be indicated for life-threatening illness. Adverse effects on developing teeth and bones are dose related; therefore, doxycycline might be used for a short time (7–14 days) before 6 months of gestation

Table 2.8 Recommendations for treatment in mass casualty situation or postexposure prophylaxis for prevention of inhalational anthrax after intentional exposure to *B. anthracis*

Category	Initial oral therapy[a]	Alternative therapy if strain proven susceptible	Duration
Adults	Ciprofloxacin 500 mg po BID	Doxycycline 100 mg po q 12 h[b] or Amoxicillin, 500 mg po q 8 h	60 days
Pregnant women	Ciprofloxacin 500 mg po BID	Amoxicillin 500 mg po q 8 h[c]	60 days
Children	Ciprofloxacin 10–15 mg kg^{-1} po Q 12 h (maximum 1 g d^{-1}) or Doxycycline[d] ≥45 kg – use adult doses <45 kg–2.5 mg kg^{-1} po q 12 h	Weight ≥20 kg: amoxicillin 500 mg po q 8 h[c] Weight <20 kg: amoxicillin 40 mg kg^{-1} po q 8 h[c]	60 days
Immunocompromised persons	Same as for nonimmunosuppressed adults and children		

Source: Reprinted with permission from Inglesby et al. (4). Copyright© 2002 American Medical Association. All rights reserved.

[a]Studies suggest ofloxacin (400 mg po q 12 h or levofloxacin, 500 mg po q 24 h could be substituted for ciprofloxacin

[b]Studies suggest that 500 mg of tetracycline po q 6 h could be substituted for doxycycline. In addition, 400 mg of gatifloxicin or monifloxacin, po daily could be substituted

[c]If antibiotic susceptibility testing, lack of resources or adverse reactions preclude use of ciprofloxacin

[d]According to the CDC, use amoxicillin only after 10–14 days of fluoroquinolones or doxycycline treatment and only then if there are contraindications to fluoroquinolones or tetracyclines such as pregnancy, lactation, age <18 years or intolerance

Ciprofloxacin and doxycycline are also the drugs of choice for cutaneous anthrax (see Table 2.9). For patients with signs of systemic involvement, such as extensive edema or head and neck lesions, the CDC and the Working Group recommend intravenous therapy with multiple antibiotics. Although treatment causes skin lesions to become culture negative within 24 h, the lesions still develop into eschars. Corticosteroids may be helpful for toxin mediated morbidity associated with extensive edema or swelling of the head and neck areas. A 7–10 day course of antibiotics is typically effective for cutaneous anthrax. However, the CDC recommends 60 days of treatment for patients with bioterrorist induced cutaneous anthrax, because many of these patients are also at risk for aerosol exposure and could harbor spores within their lungs (11).

Preventive Therapy

There are three regimens available to protect people from anthrax: Preexposure vaccine, postexposure prophylactic therapy with antibiotics, and postexposure

Table 2.9 Cutaneous anthrax treatment protocol

Category	Initial therapy (oral)[a]	Duration
Adults[b]	Ciprofloxacin 500 mg BID or Doxycycline 100 mg BID	60 days[c]
Children[b]	Ciprofloxacin 10–15 mg kg^{-1} every 12 h (not to exceed 1 g d^{-1})[a] or Doxyclycline	60 days[c]
	>8 years and >45 kg: 100 mg every 12 h	
	>8 years and ≤45 kg: 2.2 mg kg^{-1} every 12 h ≤8 years: 2.2 mg kg^{-1} every 12 h	
Pregnant women[d,e]	Ciprofloxacin 500 mg BID or Doxycycline 100 mg BID	60 days[c]
Immunocompromised persons[b]	Same for nonimmunocompromised persons and children	60 days[c]

Source: Reprinted with permission from Inglesby et al. (4). Copyright© 2002 American Medical Association. All rights reserved.

[a]Ciprofloxacin or doxycycline should be considered first-line therapy. Amoxicillin 500 mg PO TID for adults or 80 mg kg^{-1} d^{-1} divided every 8 h for children is an option for completion of therapy after clinical improvement. Oral amoxicillin dose is based on the need to achieve appropriate minimum inhibitory concentration levels

[b]Cutaneous anthrax with signs of systemic involvement, extensive edema, or lesions on the head or neck require intravenous therapy, and a multidrug approach is recommended

[c]Previous guidelines have suggested treating cutaneous anthrax for 7–10 days, but 60 days is recommended in the setting of this attack, given the likelihood of exposure to aerosolized *B. anthracis*

[d]The American Academy of Pediatrics recommends treatment of young children with tetracyclines for serious infections (e.g., Rocky Mountain spotted fever)

[e]Although tetracyclines are not recommended during pregnancy, their use may be indicated for life-threatening illness. Adverse effects on developing teeth and bones are dose related; therefore, doxycycline might be used for a short time (7–14 days) before 6 months of gestation

prophylactic therapy with a combination of antibiotics and vaccine. The vaccine alone is not effective postexposure.

Preexposure Anthrax Vaccination

The observation that inoculating animals with attenuated strains of *B. anthracis* protected them from anthrax led to the modern anthrax vaccine. Unfortunately, the veterinary version of the vaccine, an avirulent variant of *B. anthracis*, while effective, is associated with occasional casualties and is therefore unacceptable for human use.

A 1904 study demonstrating that extracts from edema fluid from anthrax lesions provided protection in animals led to the eventual development of a safer, cell-free vaccine for humans. Anthrax vaccine now used in the United States, BioThrax (formerly anthrax vaccine absorbed or AVA), is an inactivated cell-free filtrate prepared from an attenuated strain of *B. anthracis*. The vaccine contains no live or dead bacteria. Primary vaccination requires three subcutaneous injections at 0, 2, and 4 weeks, followed by three booster injections at 6, 12, and 18 months. An annual booster injection is required to maintain immunity. The evidence for this particular schedule is not clear (13,14). Studies comparing alternative routes of administration (intramuscular vs. subcutaneous) and alternative schedules are ongoing. There is no evidence indicating that increased spacing reduces effectiveness or safety. Therefore, any interruption of the vaccination schedule should not require restarting the series or adding additional doses (13,14).

Animal studies have demonstrated that the human cell-free anthrax vaccine is probably effective for preexposure prophylaxis. The vaccine is not effective alone for postexposure prophylaxis. Unfortunately, the animal studies employed several different species, routes of administration, vaccination preparations, and vaccination schedules. A study involving macaque monkeys that most closely reflected human conditions revealed that the vaccine is effective in preventing inhalation anthrax. One human study, a 1962 randomized clinical trial involving over 1,000 mill workers, using the precursor to the current anthrax vaccine, demonstrated a vaccine efficacy of 92.5% for protection against anthrax, cutaneous and inhalational. During the study, an anthrax outbreak resulted in five cases of inhalation anthrax in mill workers who received placebo or did not participate compared to no cases in the vaccinated population. Given that the only human study is an occupational cohort, there are no data on the effectiveness of the vaccine for children under 18 or adults greater than 65. The duration of vaccine efficacy is also unknown (13,14).

Data on vaccine safety and side effects are available from three sources: prelicensure new drug investigational data, passive surveillance data associated with postlicensure use and several published studies (13,14). Prelicensure data of nearly 7,000 vaccine recipients who received over 16,000 initial doses and boosters resulted in severe local reactions (edema or induration greater than 12 cm) after 1% of the vaccinations. Moderate local reactions (edema or induration of 3–12 cm) occurred following 3% of vaccinations, and mild local reactions (erythema, edema and induration <3 cm) occurred after 20% of the vaccinations (13,14). Systemic reactions, such as fever, chills, body aches, or nausea occurred in four of the 7,000 recipients, a rate of less than 0.06% (13).

After vaccine licensure, the vaccine adverse event reporting system (VAERS) began to collect data on adverse vaccine events. Between January 1, 1990 and August 31, 2000, when nearly 2 million doses of vaccine were distributed in the United States, VAERS received 1,544 reports of adverse events. Seventy-six of these reports (approximately 5%) reflected serious events, defined by death, hospitalization, permanent disability, or life threatening illness. The most frequent adverse events were injection-site hypersensitivity, injection-site edema, injection-site pain, headache, arthralgia, asthenia, and pruritus. VAERS received two reports of anaphylaxis. Infrequently reported serious events included cellulitis, pneumonia, Guillain–Barré syndrome, seizures, cardiomyopathy, systemic lupus erythematosus, multiple sclerosis, collagen vascular disease, sepsis, angioedema, and transverse myelitis (13,14). However, analysis of these data failed to reveal a pattern of illness specifically associated with or caused by the vaccine, except for the injection-site reactions.

The third source of data on adverse anthrax vaccine events comes from published studies following the initiation of routine anthrax vaccination by the military. The large amount of anthrax vaccine given to military personnel has provided opportunities to study the safety of the vaccine. In December of 1997, the US Department of Defense began a program of vaccinating all US military personnel, the anthrax vaccine immunization program (AVIP). By April 2000, over 400,000 military personnel had received over 1.6 million doses of the vaccine. Three surveys conducted on the recipients revealed that local reactions occurred more often in women than men. Survey results failed to find any patterns of unexpected local or systemic adverse events (15). Unfortunately, the military studies have several methodological limitations that preclude drawing definitive conclusions. These limitations include relatively small sample sizes, limited power to detect rare events, attrition, observational bias, exemption of vaccine recipients with previous adverse events (selection bias), and the lack of unvaccinated control groups (14,15).

Currently, no data are available regarding the association between anthrax vaccine and chronic disease, such as infertility or cancer. In addition, no data are available regarding the safety of anthrax vaccine for children under 18 or people over 65 years, nor are there studies regarding the safety of anthrax vaccine during pregnancy. A recent study of the association between anthrax vaccine and congenital anomalies was inconclusive due to the limitations in computerized records used in the study (16).

Current supplies of anthrax vaccine are limited and the production capacity is modest. Given the costs and logistics of a large-scale vaccination program, the low likelihood of an attack in any given community, and the effectiveness of prophylactic antibiotics for those exposed, the CDC, the American college on immunization practices (ACIP) and the Civilian Biodefense Working Group do not recommend vaccination of the entire population. The ACIP recommends preexposure vaccine only for people at occupational risk, including laboratory personnel and workers in settings where repeated exposure to anthrax spores might occur. In addition, the military provides preexposure vaccination to its personnel through the AVIP. More information on AVIP, including an updated report on adverse vaccine events, is available at their Web site: http://www.anthrax.mil.

Postexposure Antibiotics

To protect the public, the highest priority is to identify people at risk of exposure and respond appropriately to protect them. The circumstances of any potential exposure rather than laboratory test results should be the main factor in decisions regarding antibiotic prophylaxis. After taking a history, clinicians should offer antibiotic prophylaxis to patients with an exposure or contact with an item or environment known or suspected to be contaminated with *B. anthracis*, regardless of laboratory tests (11). Although nasal swabs for anthrax culture can detect anthrax spores, negative cultures DO NOT rule out exposure. Therefore, nasal cultures are useful for epidemiologic purposes, but not for determining whether individual patients should receive antibiotic prophylaxis.

The latest recommendations from the CDC and the Working Group (17) recommend initiating antimicrobial prophylaxis pending additional information when:

– A patient is exposed to an air space where a suspicious material may have been aerosolized (e.g., near a suspicious powder containing letter during opening)
– A patient has shared the air space likely to be the source of an inhalational anthrax case

After initial prophylaxis, clinicians should continue antimicrobial prophylaxis for 60 days for:

– Patients exposed to an air space known to be contaminated with aerosolized *B. anthracis*
– Patients exposed to an air space known to be the source of an inhalational anthrax case
– Patients along the transit path of an envelope or other vehicle containing *B. anthracis* that may have been aerosolized (e.g., a postal sorting facility in which an envelope containing *B. anthracis* was processed)
– Unvaccinated laboratory workers exposed to confirmed *B. anthracis* cultures

Clinicians should not provide antimicrobial prophylaxis:

– For prevention of cutaneous anthrax
– For autopsy personnel examining bodies infected with anthrax when appropriate isolation precautions and procedures are followed
– For hospital personnel caring for patients with anthrax
– For persons who routinely open or handle mail in the absence of a suspicious letter or credible threat

Table 2.8 summarizes the CDC and Working Group recommendations for initial and continued postexposure prophylaxis. The Food and Drug Administration (FDA) has not approved any postexposure regimens. The recommended regimen for adults, including immunocompromised adults, is Ciprofloxacin 500 mg po BID or Doxycycline 100 mg po BID for 60 days. The antibiotic of choice for preventing inhalational anthrax in exposed pregnant women is Ciprofloxacin 500 mg twice a day for 60 days. Physicians may consider prophylactic therapy with amoxicillin, 500 mg three times daily for 60 days for instances in which the specific *B. anthracis* strain has been proven penicillin sensitive (18). However, most experts do not recommend amoxicillin as a first line drug for anthrax prophylaxis because of inadequate data about its efficacy and inadequate data regarding its ability to reach therapeutic levels at standard doses. In addition, the FDA has not approved amoxicillin for this purpose (19).

Public health experts base the 60-day recommendation on animal studies of anthrax deaths and spore clearance from the lungs following exposure. For example, one study found traces of spores in monkey lungs 100 days after exposure. Although the exact time of exposure is unknown, one anthrax case in the Sverdlovsk outbreak occurred 43 days after spore release (19).

Physicians and other health care providers must be careful in prescribing prophylactic antibiotics because they have been associated with adverse health effects among patients taking them for short-term treatment of bacterial infections. However, before the 2001 anthrax attacks, few data existed regarding the use of these antimicrobials for longer periods, such as the 60 days recommended for anthrax prophylaxis. Until then, because of the large number of patients predicted that could receive anthrax prophylaxis, the CDC recommended enhanced surveillance programs to detect and monitor adverse events associated with the medications. In addition, the CDC hoped to gain information on how to design programs to promote completion of the recommended prophylactic regimens.

The anthrax attack in the fall of 2001, which exposed large numbers of people to anthrax spores at six sites in Florida, New Jersey, Washington DC, New York City, and Connecticut, provided a real-life opportunity for studying the incidence of adverse effects associated with anthrax prophylaxis. At the time, public health authorities recommended 60-day antimicrobial prophylaxis for thousands of people at the six sites. Pending sensitivity results, authorities dispensed ciprofloxacin as the initial treatment, with the exception that pregnant women, breast feeding mothers and children received amoxicillin. Following sensitivity results, at first (10 day) and second (30 day) refill visits at four of the sites, public health officials encouraged prophylaxis recipients without contraindications to switch to doxycycline. At the Washington DC site, all patients received a 60-day supply of ciprofloxacin, while patients at the Florida site received doxycycline at their 30-day refill visit (20).

The CDC conducted a study of side effects and adherence at all six sites, including surveys administered at 10-day and 30-day refill clinics and through a phone interview at 60-days. The study defined serious adverse events based on the Code of Federal Regulations (21 CFR 314.80) and included death, a life-threatening event, inpatient hospitalization or prolongation of an existing hospitalization, persistent or substantial disability/incapacity, congenital anomalies/birth defects or an important medical event requiring medical or surgical intervention to avoid one of these outcomes.

Although more than half of the patients experienced side effects, most were mild. Serious adverse side effects were rare. Over 5,000 people reported taking at least one dose of prophylactic medication, yet prophylaxis caused no deaths and very few hospitalizations. Common types of mild side effects included gastrointestinal symptoms, such as nausea, vomiting, diarrhea, abdominal pain, heartburn, or dysphagia in nearly half of the complaints and neurologic symptoms, including headache, dizziness, lightheadedness, fainting, and seizures in about one third of the complaints. At 10 days of follow-up, the incidence of adverse events was similar for patients receiving ciprofloxacin and doxycycline; at 30 days, the rate was slightly, but significantly higher for ciprofloxacin.

After 10 days of follow-up, 7% of the nearly 3,000 participating in the survey reported seeking medical attention for side effects, while at 30 days, approximately 13% of the over 3,000 respondents reported seeking medical attention. At the 60-day phone survey, conducted on over 5,000 exposed people who took at least one dose of prophylactic antibiotics, 16% reported having sought medical care for side effects and 9% reported that their health care providers told them to discontinue prophylaxis. At the 30-day survey, seven of the people responding to the survey (0.3%) reported a serious adverse effect, including three people hospitalized. Investigators classified the association between prophylaxis and serious side effects in four of these seven patients as definite or probable, while the evidence for an association in the other three was nonexistent or not assessable. Of the four likely cases, two were associated with systemic symptoms, including a diffuse rash, while the other two were associated with swelling of the face and neck.

While most side effects were mild, the frequency of side effects from cipro-floxacin in this population was more than double that reported in the ciprofloxacin literature. Some of this difference may be due to the study design. The descriptive study following mass anthrax prophylaxis cannot substitute for a randomized clinical trial in assessing the association between a medication and symptoms. Besides study design problems, patients receiving prophylaxis for anthrax may have suffered from greater anxiety than patients receiving antibiotics for other reasons. Fear of anthrax could have caused enhanced symptom awareness in these patients, resulting in more reported symptoms. In addition, the anxiety associated with anthrax exposure itself could have caused some of the reported symptoms (20) attributed to medication side effects.

Although serious side effects were rare, adherence to the recommended regimen was low. Fewer than half of the more than 5,000 patients responding to the 60-day survey (44%) reported completing the full 60-day regimen, ranging from 21% for those exposed at a New York city postal facility to 54% exposed at a Washington DC postal facility. In addition, only 72% of respondents reported taking their medication daily, while only 19% reported taking medication "almost every day." While many patients (43%) discontinued antibiotics because of side effects, many (25%) discontinued the regimen because of a perception that they were at low risk for developing clinical anthrax. Although poor adherence was associated with the incidence of side effects, both mild and serious, perceived risk of disease had a stronger and more consistent association with adherence across the six sites (20). Of the 172 exposed people who never took prophylactic treatment, more than half reported perception of low risk as a reason for not obtaining the medication.

Given the relatively high incidence of side effects and the low rate of adherence, physicians and other health care providers prescribing antibiotic prophylaxis for anthrax exposure should monitor their patients appropriately. The association between patient perception of low risk and low prophylaxis adherence requires that clinicians understand how to predict their patients' health behaviors, which in turn requires an understanding of how their patients perceive risk (20). Clinicians must be adept at educating patients about recognizing and managing potential side effects and the consequences of their health behavior. Treating side effects can increase the likelihood that patients remain on the lengthy therapy. To enhance adherence, patient reminders such as signs and buddy systems can also be very helpful (20). Regardless of the cause of the symptoms, whether due to antibiotics themselves or anxiety, clinicians must be able to ensure that their patients receive the appropriate treatment based on the risk of exposure.

Alternative Postexposure Prophylaxis Regimens with Antibiotics with and without Vaccine

Because of the uncertainty about spore survival, the lack of effectiveness of antibiotics against the spore form, and recent studies in nonhuman primates demonstrating the effectiveness of postexposure antibiotic prophylaxis in combination with vaccine, physicians may consider two other options for postexposure prophylactic therapy. The first option is a longer period of 100 days of antimicrobial prophylaxis alone. The second alternative option is a combination of antimicrobial prophylaxis plus three doses of anthrax vaccine administered over 4 weeks.

Given the low level of adherence to the recommended 60 day regimen of antimicrobial prophylaxis following the 2001 anthrax attacks, physicians may want to consider the combined regimen for postexposure prophylaxis. On the other hand, even with low levels of adherence, no cases of anthrax occurred in people recommended to take the 60-day regimen after exposure in 2001. Although the FDA has not approved anthrax vaccine for this purpose, physicians can use the vaccine in the combined regimen as an investigational drug. (http://www.hhs.gov/news/press/2001pres/20011218.html) Like other investigational drugs, physicians should obtain informed consent from their patients, and patients may participate in an evaluation of vaccine effectiveness. Unfortunately, data are not available regarding the duration of antimicrobial prophylactic treatment in the combined regimen. Currently, the ACIP endorses a prophylactic regimen of three doses of vaccine at 0, 2, and 4 weeks combined with daily antibiotics continuing for 7–14 days after the last vaccination (21).

Regimens containing anthrax vaccine alone or in combination are not an option for pregnant women. Although there is no evidence associating anthrax vaccine with adverse pregnancy outcomes, no studies involving pregnant animals or humans have been conducted. Consequently, the FDA has not recommended or licensed the vaccine for pregnant women. In addition, the military avoids giving the vaccine during pregnancy. Physicians and other health care providers should not administer the prophylaxis option that includes anthrax vaccine to women who are pregnant or who intend to become pregnant (16).

Some exposed people may have already received a partial or complete anthrax vaccination regimen before exposure. Based on the only human clinical trial of the vaccine, in which anthrax cases occurred in those who had received less than four doses, the ACIP recommends that exposed people who have been partially or fully vaccinated receive at least 30 days of antibiotic prophylaxis while completing the vaccination regimen. However, vaccinated individuals who are working with anthrax in Biosafety Level 3 laboratories under recommended conditions or vaccinated individuals wearing appropriate personal protective equipment (PPE) while working in environments contaminated with anthrax spores do not require postexposure prophylaxis unless their respiratory protection is disrupted.

Summary of Recommendations for Postexposure Prophylaxis

Given the limited supply of vaccine, and the lack of reported cases in people given antibiotic prophylaxis following the 2001 attacks, Working Group on Civilian Biodefense continues to recommend that 60 days of antibiotics is sufficient protection postexposure.

In responding to any large biological event, public health officials will conduct an epidemiologic investigation to identify people who were likely exposed (19), and they will be establish points of dispensing centers (PODs) for mass prophylaxis (see Chap. 6). With additional CDC funding, many local public health agencies, especially those in densely populated urban areas, have already developed plans for designating and staffing these centers. Physicians and other health care providers should consider referring exposed patients to these centers, where public health authorities can monitor adherence and side effects closely. Chapter 6 describes how family physicians can participate in working with public health officials to plan, staff and refer exposed patients to PODs in their communities. Chapter 5 explains how physicians and other health care providers can work with their patients and families to reduce stress and anxiety associated with exposure to anthrax and other biological agents.

Plague

Microbiology and Epidemiology

Yersinia pestis, the organism responsible for plague, is a nonmotile, gram-negative bacillus, sometimes a coccobacillus. On staining with Wright, Giemsa, or Wayson stain, plague shows biopolar staining, giving it a characteristic "safety pin" appearance (Fig. 2.4; see color plate 2.4).

Plague exists naturally in cycles involving wild rodents such as ground squirrels and prairie dogs and their fleas in specific regions of Asia, Africa, North and South America and the extreme southeastern Europe near the Caspian Sea (22). In North America, the organism persists in rodents and other small mammals from the Pacific Coast to the Great Plains, and from southwestern Canada to Mexico (http://www.cdc.gov/ncidod/dvbid/plague/index.htm). Cycles of infection between fleas and rodents occur without human awareness, until a sporadic human case occurs following a bite from an infected flea. Occasionally, an epidemic occurs when the disease spreads

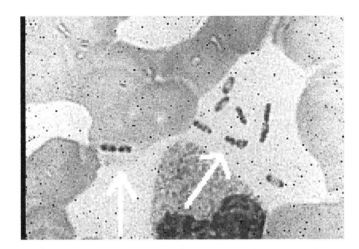

Fig. 2.4 (See color plate) Plague bacteria in blood (*arrows*). From Plague bacteria in blood. CDC Division of Vector-Borne Infectious Diseases (DVBID). http://www.cdc.gov/ncidod/dvbid/plague/p1.htm

from wild rodents to populations of rats (genus *Rattus*) living close to large human populations. Historically, large rat die-offs have preceded human epidemics as the lack of rats forced infected fleas to move to the human population.

Although the most common form of transmission of the disease to humans is through the bite of an infected flea, human infection occasionally results from the handling of body fluids or tissues of an infected animal. Rarely, inhalation of airborne infectious materials, such as laboratory-generated aerosols, has caused human disease (22). Naturally occurring plague occurs primarily in two forms, bubonic, the most common form, and primary septicemic, affecting a small minority of plague victims. Neither bubonic nor septicemic plague is transmissible person to person. Occasionally, through hematogenous transport of the organism to the lungs, patients with bubonic or primary septicemic plague develop a third form, secondary pneumonic plague. Unlike the other forms of plague, pneumonic plague is readily transmissible person to person through respiratory droplets.

From 1980 top 1994, 20 countries reported 18,739 cases to the World Health Organization (WHO), averaging 1,087 cases per year. This number probably underestimates the true incidence of plague. Many countries fail to identify and report the disease, a consequence of inadequate laboratory and surveillance infrastructure (22).

Although plague epidemics are rare, they are most likely to occur in areas with large populations of rats and poor sanitary conditions (22). Three large outbreaks of pneumonic plague occurred early in the twentieth century, two in Manchuria 10 years apart (23). The first Manchurian outbreak, from 1910 to 1911, resulted in 600,000 cases. The outbreak in Northern India caused 1,400 deaths. Studies of the Manchurian outbreaks suggested that indoor exposure, cold temperature, increased humidity and crowding were risk factors for transmission (23). More recently, in 1997 one patient in Madagascar with pneumonic plague transmitted the infection to 18 others, resulting in eight deaths (23).

Plague remains a rare but reportable disease in the United States, with 390 cases reported from 1947 to 1996. Of these cases, 84% were bubonic, 13% septicemic, and 2% were pneumonic (23). Most human cases in the United States occur in two regions: northern New Mexico, northern Arizona, and southern Colorado; and California, southern Oregon, and far western Nevada (http://www.cdc.gov/ncidod/dvbid/plague/epi.htm). Modes of transmission are known for 284 of 341 cases reported between 1970 and 1995: Flea bites were responsible for 222 (78%) cases, direct contact with an infected animal was responsible for 56 (20%) cases and inhalation of airborne materials such as respiratory droplets from infected animals was responsible for 7 (2%) cases. Los Angeles was the site of the last person-to-person transmission in the United States in 1924 (23).

In the United States, most plague cases naturally occur in the summer, when exposure to infected fleas is most likely. Most cases, especially in the Southwest, occur at or near the case's residence, and are associated with conditions that provide food and shelter for potentially infected rodents. Participation in recreational activities, especially in California, has also resulted in plague cases, although less frequently (22).

Plague as a Biologic Weapon

Like anthrax, plague has been developed and used as a biological weapon. During World War II, the Japanese army dropped infected fleas over China, causing several plague outbreaks (23). The United States and the Soviet Union both developed methods for aerosolizing plague, creating a much more efficient way of infecting large numbers of people compared to infected fleas. In 1970, the World Health Association (WHO) estimated that a dispersion of 50 kg of aerosolized plague over a city of 5 million could cause pneumonic plague in 150,000 people with 36,000 deaths (23).

In contrast to naturally occurring plague, the most likely form of terrorist-caused plague would be the more serious pneumonic form due to inhalation of a dispersed aerosol containing the organism. The quantity or organisms dispersed, the virulence of the specific strain used, and meteorological and other environmental conditions at the time of release would contribute to the size of the resulting outbreak (23). Unlike anthrax, pneumonic plague is transmissible person to person. Symptomatic people leaving the site of the release could spread the disease to others in other cities. Cases of pneumonic plague occurring in areas without enzootic infection, cases in people without other known risk factors, an atypical seasonal pattern (cases in fall, winter, or spring, rather than summer) and the absence of a rat die-off are all clues that the outbreak was manmade (23).

Clinical Presentation and Diagnosis

Bubonic Plague

Because bubonic plague results from the bite of an infected flea, it is the least likely form to be associated with a terrorist event. An infected flea can transmit thousands of plague bacilli through the skin. Once inoculated, the bacilli migrate through lymphatics to regional lymph nodes, where they resist destruction by phagocytosis. Instead, they proliferate, destroying the node architecture and causing bacteremia, septicemia and endotoxemia, leading to shock, disseminated intravascular coagulation (DIC) and coma (22,23).

Bubonic plague symptoms develop 2–8 days after the fleabite. Patients experience a sudden onset of fever, chills, and weakness. Up to 1 day after the onset of symptoms, acute regional lymphadenopathy, the bubo, develops. Buboes involve lymph nodes that drain the site where the bite occurred, and they most commonly involve the inguinal, axillary, or cervical regions (22,23). Incredibly painful, Buboes frequently prevent patients from moving the affected area. Figure 2.5 (see color plate 2.5) shows a typical bubo, which ranges in size from 1 to 10 cm. The overlying skin is erythematous (23).

Besides the incredible tenderness, buboes are warm and nonfluctuant, frequently associated with surrounding edema, but rarely lymphangitis. Occasionally, buboes

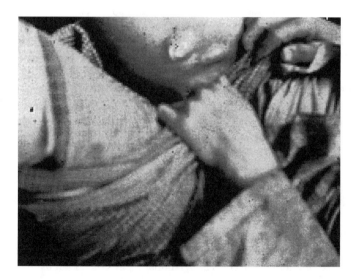

Fig. 2.5 (See color plate) Inguinal bubo on upper thigh of person with bubonic plague. From Inguinal bubo on upper thigh of person with bubonic plague. CDC Division of Vector-Borne Infectious Diseases (DVBID). http://www.cdc.gov/ncidod/dvbid/plague/p5.htm)

can become fluctuant and suppurative. Pustules and skin ulcerations sometimes occur at the site of the original fleabite (23). The case fatality rate for patients who are not treated ranges from 50 to 60% (22).

Septicemic Plague

Septicemic plague, the form of infection that results when the organism invades and multiplies within the bloodstream, can develop secondary to bubonic plague or it can develop without any lymphadenopathy (primary septicemic plague) (22). Whether primary or as a result of bubonic plague, in the United States the historic case fatality rate of septicemic plague was 50%. Patients with septicemic plague can develop septic shock, DIC, necrosis of small vessels and purpuric skin lesions (22,23). Plague meningitis occasionally results from hematogenous spread (23).

Pneumonic Plague

Pneumonic plague can occur in two ways: as a complication of septicemic plague (secondary pneumonic plague) or by direct inhalation of plague bacilli, usually from an animal or other human with plague pneumonia (primary pneumonic plague). Secondary pneumonic plague occurs when the organism spreads hematogenously to the lungs (22,23). Although primary pneumonic plague rarely occurs in the United States, it is the most likely form to be associated with a terrorist attack, because an aerosolized form of plague is the most efficient way to cause mass casualties.

Once people develop pneumonic plague, they can transmit the disease to others through respiratory droplets. A pneumonic plague outbreak would result in large numbers of patients experiencing symptoms initially resembling those of other serious respiratory illnesses (23). Table 2.10 summarizes the clinical presentation and diagnosis of pneumonic plague. After an incubation period of 1–6 days, patients would present with an acute and often fulminant course of malaise, fever, headache, myalgia, and cough with mucopurulent sputum, hemoptysis, chest pain, and clinical sepsis. Some patients with pneumonic plague may display gastrointestinal symptoms, including nausea, vomiting, abdominal pain, and diarrhea (23). Respiratory symptoms would rapidly progress to dyspnea, stridor, and cyanosis. Patients would soon develop respiratory failure, shock and a bleeding diathesis (24). Those patients not treated adequately within 18 h of onset of respiratory symptoms would be unlikely to survive (22). Without appropriate therapy, the mortality rate would be 100%.

As with anthrax, early diagnosis of plague is critical and requires a high index of suspicion. In the United States, if only a small number of cases occur, physicians may overlook pneumonic plague for a couple of reasons. First, plague pneumonia

Table 2.10 Clinical presentation and diagnosis of pneumonic plague

Epidemiology	Incubation period	Clinical signs	Diagnostic studies	Pathology
Sudden appearance of many persons with fever, cough, dyspnea, hemoptysis, and chest pain	1–7 days, usually 2–4 days	Acute onset of cough with hemoptysis Tachypnea, dyspnea and cyanosis	Pulmonary infiltrates or consolidation on chest radiograph	Lobular exudation, bacillary aggregation and areas of necrosis in pulmonary parenchyma
Gastrointestinal symptoms are common (nausea, vomiting, abdominal pain, and diarrhea)		Sepsis, shock, and organ failure Infrequent presence of a cervical bubo purpuric skin lesions and necrotic digits only in advanced disease	Sputum, blood, or lymph node aspirate for culture and gram stain Gram negative bacilli with bipolar (safety pin) staining on Wright, Giemsa, or Wayson stain	
Patients have fulminant course with high mortality			Rapid diagnostic tests available only at some health departments, the CDC and military labs	

Source: Reprinted with permission from Inglesby et al. (4) Plague as a biological weapon: medical and public health management. JAMA May 2000; 283(17):2281–2290. Copyright© 2000 American Medical Association. All rights reserved.

has similarities with other more common bacterial or viral pneumonias. Second, few US physicians have ever seen a case of pneumonic plague (23).

The sudden appearance of previously healthy patients with fever, cough, chest pain, and a fulminant course should suggest the possibility of inhalational anthrax or pneumonic plague. Hemoptysis in this setting particularly points to plague (23). Unlike naturally occurring pneumonic plague resulting from hematogenous spread of bubonic or septicemic plague, a terrorist induced primary pneumonic plague outbreak would not be associated with buboes. However, there is one exception: plague pharyngitis can occasionally follow inhalation and can be associated with cervical buboes. Pathological findings typical of primary plague, such as pulmonary disease with areas of profound lobular exudation and bacillary aggregation can also help distinguish secondary from primary pneumonic plague (23).

There are no commercially readily available rapid diagnostic tests for plague. Chest X-ray findings can vary, but bilateral infiltrates or consolidation are common (23).

Tests such as antigen detection, IgM enzyme immunoassay, immunostaining, and PCR, that might rapidly help confirm a suspected case, are available only through some state and local public health laboratories, the CDC and some military laboratories (23). Hemagglutination antibody detection assays, although routinely used, are not helpful, because it takes several days to weeks after disease onset for antibodies to develop (23). However, physicians can order sputum gram stains, which may reveal gram-negative bacilli or coccobacilli. A Wright, Giemsa, or Wayson stain may show bipolar staining (see Fig. 2.4). Direct fluorescent antibody (DFA) testing, if available, may be positive (23). Cultures of sputum, blood, or lymph node aspirates should demonstrate growth within 24–48 h after inoculation (23). Physicians should obtain these specimens before initiating antibiotic therapy and they should alert the laboratory that they are considering plague.

If cervical buboes are present, aspiration performed with a 20-gauge needle and a 10-mL syringe containing 1–2 mL of sterile saline for infusing the node can provide a specimen suitable for culture and staining (23).

If the clinical evaluation of a previous healthy patient reveals signs and symptoms suspicious of plague, the patient's physician must immediately report the case to the local health department. Chapter 6 discusses how to work with local health departments, including how to report suspected cases.

Treatment

The Working Group on Civilian Biodefense based its recommendations for treatment of pneumonic plague on reports in the literature of human disease, reports of studies in animal models, reports on in vitro susceptibility testing, and data on antibiotic safety (23). Aminoglycosides are the most efficacious treatment for pneumonic plague. In a limited, contained outbreak, either parenteral streptomycin or gentamicin is the drug of choice (23). In addition, patients with pneumonic plague will require supportive care to treat complications of gram-negative sepsis, including adult respiratory distress syndrome, DIC, shock, and multiorgan failure (23). Because the potential benefits outweigh the risks, in limited or contained situations, streptomycin, or gentamicin is the drug of choice for children (23). Due to its association with irreversible deafness in children following fetal exposure, physicians should avoid using streptomycin in pregnant women and instead give gentamicin (23). If gentamicin is not available, doxycycline is the drug of choice for pregnant women, because the benefits outweigh the risk of fetal toxicity (23).

During a pneumonic plague epidemic, all persons developing a fever of 38.5°C or above or a new cough should begin parenteral antibiotics (23). Infants with tachypnea should also receive treatment (23). In a mass outbreak, in which parenteral therapy may not be available, the Working Group recommends oral therapy for adults with doxycycline (or tetracycline or ciprofloxacin); children should receive doxycycline (see Table 2.11).

Table 2.11 Plague treatment in contained and mass casualty situation, and postexposure prophylaxis[a]

Patient category	Recommended therapy
Contained casualty setting	
Adults	*Preferred choices*
	Streptomycin, 1 g IM twice daily
	Gentamicin, 5 mg kg^{-1} IM or IV once daily or 2 mg kg^{-1} loading close followed by 1.7 mg kg^{-1} IM or IV three times daily[b]
	Alternative choices
	Doxycycline, 100 mg IV twice daily or 200 mg IV once daily
	Ciprofloxacin, 400 mg IV twice daily[c]
	Chloramphenicol, 25 mg kg^{-1} IV four times daily[d]
Children	*Preferred choices*
	Streptomycin, 15 mg kg^{-1} IM twice daily (maximum daily dose, 2 g)
	Gentamicin, 2.5 mg kg^{-1} IM or IV three times daily[b]
	Alternative choices
	Doxycycline
	If ≥45 kg, give adult dosage
	If <45 kg, give 2.2 mg kg^{-1} twice daily (maximum, 200 mg d^{-1})
	Ciprofloxacin, 15 mg kg^{-1} IV twice daily[c]
	Chloramphenicol, 25 mg kg^{-1} IV four times daily[d]
Pregnant women	*Preferred choice*
	Gentamicin, 5 mg kg^{-1} IM or IV once daily or 2 mg kg^{-1} loading dose followed by 1.7 mg kg^{-1} IM or IV three times daily
	Alternative choices
	Doxycycline, 100 mg IV twice daily or 200 mg IV once daily
	Ciprofloxacin, 400 mg IV twice daily[c]
Mass casually setting and postexposure prophylaxis[e]	
Adults	*Preferred choices*
	Doxycycline, 100 mg orally twice daily[f]
	Ciprofloxacin, 500 mg orally twice daily[c]
	Alternative choice
	Chloramphenicol, 25 mg kg^{-1} orally four times daily[d,g]
Children[h]	*Preferred choice*
	Doxycycline[f]
	If ≥ to 45 kg, give adult dosage
	If <45 kg, then give 2.2 mg kg^{-1} orally twice daily
	Ciprofloxacin, 20 mg kg^{-1} orally twice daily
	Alternative choice
	Chloramphenicol, 25 mg kg^{-1} orally four times daily[d,g]
Pregnant women[i]	*Preferred choices*
	Doxycycline, 100 mg orally twice daily[f]
	Ciprofloxacin, 500 mg orally twice daily
	Alternative choice
	Chloramphenicol, 25 mg kg^{-1} orally four times daily[d,g]

(continued)

Table 2.11 (continued)

Source: Reprinted with permission from Inglesby et al. (4) Plague as a biological weapon: medical and public health management. JAMA May 2000; 283(17):2281–2290. Copyright© 2000 American Medical Association. All rights reserved.

[a]These are consensus recommendations of the Working Group on Civilian Biodefense and not necessarily approved by the FDA. One antimicrobial agent should be selected. Therapy should be continued for 10 days. Oral therapy should be substituted when patient's condition improves

[b]Aminoglycosides must be adjusted according to renal function. Evidence suggests that gentamicin, 5 mg kg^{-1} IM or IV once daily, would be efficacious in children, although this is not yet widely accepted in clinical practice. Neonates up to 1 week of age and premature infants should receive gentamicin, 2.5 mg kg^{-1} IV twice daily

[c]Other fluoroquinolones can be substituted at doses appropriate for age. Ciprofloxacin dosage should not exceed 1 g d^{-1} in children

[d]Concentration should be maintained between 5 and 20 µg mL^{-1}. Concentrations greater than 25 µg mL^{-1} can cause reversible bone marrow suppression

[e]Duration of treatment of plague in mass casualty settings is 10 days. Duration of postexposure prophylaxis to prevent plague infection is 7 days

[f]Tetracycline could be substituted for doxycycline

[g]Children younger than 2 years should not receive chloramphenicol. Oral formulation available only outside the United States

[h]Refer to source for details. In children, ciprofloxacin dose should not exceed 1 g d^{-1}, chloramphenicol should not exceed 4 g d^{-1}. Children younger than 2 years should not receive chloramphenicol

[i]Refer to source for details and for discussion of breastfeeding women. In neonates, gentamicin loading does of 4 mg kg^{-1} should be given initially

Prevention

Vaccine and Postexposure Prophylaxis

Although the plague vaccine was effective in preventing or ameliorating bubonic disease, it was not effective in preventing pneumonic plague or reducing its morbidity. Production of the vaccine ceased in 1999. Table 2.11 summarizes the recommendations for postexposure prophylaxis and therapy for patients with pneumonic plague. Asymptomatic persons having household, hospital, or other close contact (within 2 m) with untreated patients should receive prophylactic therapy for 7 days (23). Physicians should watch case contacts closely, and begin treating for disease at the first sign of a fever or cough within 7 days of exposure. Contacts refusing antibiotic prophylaxis do not require isolation but should also receive treatment at the first sign of infection (23). Doxycycline is the drug of choice for postexposure prophylaxis (23). Table 2.11 lists the alternatives. Doxycycline is also the drug of choice as prophylaxis for exposed children and pregnant women (23). Pregnant women unable to take doxycycline should receive ciprofloxacin or another fluoroquinolone (23).

Infection Control

Because we have limited experience with pneumonic plague, there are few data helpful in making recommendations about appropriate infection control measures. Existing evidence suggests that person-to-person transmission occurs through respiratory droplets, but not through droplet nuclei (23). Wearing masks was effective in preventing person-to-person transmission of pneumonic plague in outbreaks early in the twentieth century. Therefore, current guidelines recommend the use of surgical masks to prevent transmission in future outbreaks (23).

Close contacts of confirmed cases that have received less than 48 h of antibiotic therapy should wear masks and follow droplet precautions (gowns, gloves, and eye protection) (23). In addition, people should avoid unnecessary close contact until cases receive at least 48 h of antibiotic therapy and exhibit some clinical improvement (23).

Patients suspected of having plague should be isolated until receiving 48 h of antibiotic therapy and until they begin improving clinically (23). In the event of large outbreaks, public health officials will work with private physicians to cohort cases while they receive antibiotic therapy. Hospital staff should use standard precautions for cleaning hospital rooms previously inhabited by pneumonic plague patients; body fluid contaminated clothing and bedding should receive disinfection treatment according to hospital protocols (23). Laboratory personnel should know in advance that they will be processing specimens of suspected plague patients, so they can use the appropriate biosafety precautions (23).

Bodies of plague victims can present exposure hazards, so routine strict precautions are indicated during transport and handling. Only trained personnel should handle the bodies, and precautions are the same as those for living plague patients. Personnel performing postmortem exams should avoid procedures that could generate aerosols such as bone sawing. If such procedures are necessary, personnel performing them must use high-efficiency particulate air filtered masks and negative pressure rooms (23).

Unlike anthrax spores, plague bacilli are susceptible to environmental conditions, especially sunlight and heating. Although some studies suggest that the plague bacillus can survive in soil, there is no evidence suggesting that this poses a risk to humans, and there is no need to decontaminate an area exposed to a plague aerosol. Even in a worst-case scenario, a World Health Organization analysis estimates plague organisms dispersed in an aerosol could remain viable for an hour. Clearly, by the time the first victim presented with symptoms, no organisms would remain in the environment (23).

Smallpox (Variola)

Microbiology and Epidemiology

Variola, the virus that causes smallpox, is a DNA virus. Like several similar viruses, monkeypox, vaccinia and cowpox, variola is a member of the genus Orthopoxvirus. Although all of these viruses can cause infections and cutaneous lesions in humans, only smallpox spreads easily from person to person. In the laboratory, 90% of aerosolized variola virus becomes inactive within 24 h. Low temperatures and humidities support longer virus survival. Ultraviolet light and chemical disinfectants rapidly inactivate all of the orthopoxviruses.

The variola virus received its name based on the Latin words for "spotted," *varius* or "pimple," *varus*. In the fifteenth century, Europeans began using the term "smallpox" to distinguish the infection from the "great pox," syphilis. Before the development of the smallpox vaccine, smallpox occurred worldwide, with most people getting the infection at some time in their life. Naturally occurring smallpox infection presented in two clinical forms, caused by different strains of the virus, Variola major and Variola minor. Compared to Variola minor, the more common Variola major was more severe, with a more extensive rash, higher fever and greater prostration (25). Variola major had a case fatality rate of 30% compared to the variola minor fatality rate of less than 1%.

Smallpox spread person to person through a couple of routes, respiratory and direct contact. Infected people transmitted the organism through droplet nuclei or aerosols generated from their oropharynx. Most airborne transmission occurred within 6 ft of face-to-face contact (25). Alternatively, smallpox victims with skin lesions were capable of transmitting the disease by contaminating clothing or bedding that susceptible people later wear or contact. Patients were most infectious from rash onset through the first 7–10 days of rash.

Smallpox spread slower than other viral rash illnesses like chickenpox and measles. When smallpox still occurred naturally, most people who became infected were close contacts of an index case, such as household members, close friends and health care workers. Household secondary attack rates were typically 50–60% (25). Larger outbreaks in schools were uncommon. Two reasons for this are that that transmission did not occur before rash onset and that the disease caused severe incapacitation. By the time of rash onset, victims were so ill that they did not attend school or go to other community events where they might have exposed others. Secondary cases typically occurred in hospital and household contacts.

In temperate climates, naturally occurring smallpox had a seasonal incidence similar to that of chickenpox and measles, with more cases occurring in the late winter and spring. Most likely, the association of increased survival of the virus at lower temperature and humidity contributed to the seasonal pattern. In tropical areas, there was less seasonal variation and the illness occurred year-round (25).

The age distribution of naturally occurring smallpox reflected the degree of susceptibility in different communities. In urban areas where adults had a history of natural infection or vaccination, most of the cases occurred in children. In rural areas, cases reflected the population distribution.

During the global eradication program, public health workers were able to interrupt disease transmission by isolating smallpox patients so their contact was limited to people who had already had the disease or were previously vaccinated (25). In addition, public health workers identified contacts, immediately vaccinated them, and monitored them closely, isolating them if they became ill to prevent additional transmission. This particular strategy was effective in all communities, including those with low vaccination levels (25).

The global eradication program was effective, eliminating natural smallpox infections from the world. The last case occurred in the United States in 1949. The United States discontinued routine smallpox vaccinations in 1972. Five years later, in 1977, international efforts eradicated smallpox from the world. The last case of Variola Major was in Bangladesh in 1975; the last Variola Minor case occurred in Somalia in 1977. There are no animal reservoirs or vectors for smallpox.

The susceptibility of people who received the vaccine 29 or more years ago is uncertain, because clinical studies have never measured the duration of immunity following vaccination. Given the likely susceptibility of the current US population, with most people not vaccinated or vaccinated remotely, a smallpox attack would likely affect adults as well as children (26). Because of the high case fatality rate, physicians suspecting a single case must treat it as an international health emergency and immediately contact local and state public health authorities.

Smallpox as a Biological Weapon

British soldiers were possibly the first to use smallpox as a weapon during the French and Indian Wars (1754–1767) in North America. Intending to cause disease and mortality, the soldiers took blankets used by smallpox patients and gave them to American Indians. The resulting epidemics killed more than 50% of many of the tribes. Nine years later, Jenner discovered that inoculation of cowpox protected recipients from getting smallpox. The resulting worldwide dissemination of vaccination with cowpox diminished the potential of smallpox as a bioweapon (26).

Three years after smallpox eradication, in 1980, the World Health Organization (WHO) recommended that all countries cease smallpox vaccination. In addition, WHO recommended that all laboratories destroy stocks of the virus or transfer them to either of two WHO reference laboratories, the Institute of Virus Preparations in Moscow, Russia, or the Centers for Disease Control and Prevention (CDC) in the United States. However, there may have been stocks of virus elsewhere (26,27). Although the WHO Advisory Committee on Variola Virus research recommend eradication of all smallpox stocks by June 30, 2002, the WHO Health Assembly has delayed this each year because of concerns that stocks of virus are needed for continued study (28).

Recently, a former deputy director of the Soviet Union's civilian bioweapons program alleged that the Soviet Union began developing large quantities of smallpox as a bioweapon in the early 1980s and that Russia has continued research in developing increasingly virulent strains of smallpox (26). The diminishing financial support for laboratories in Russia has led to concerns that human expertise and equipment associated with smallpox development could relocate. The possibility of existence of variola stocks, the stability of aerosolized variola, the low level of vaccination and the lethality of smallpox, increase its likelihood for use as a biological weapon.

Clinical Presentation

Acute smallpox symptoms resemble those of other acute viral infections such as influenza. After an incubation period of 12–14 days (range 7–17 days), smallpox begins with a 2–4 day nonspecific prodrome of fever, myalgias, headache, and backache. Severe abdominal pain, nausea, vomiting, prostration, and delirium may be present. Patients are not infectious until the end of the prodrome (25), when a maculopapular rash begins on the oral and pharyngeal mucosa, face and forearms, and spreads to the trunk and legs.

The Variola major rash presents in four distinct ways, ordinary, modified, flat, and hemorrhagic. The type of rash presentation is probably associated with the strength of the immune response. Ordinary smallpox is most frequent, whereas the mild modified form, seen primarily in previously vaccinated patients, is uncommon. The most severe presentations, flat and hemorrhagic, are usually fatal but are fortunately rare. Smallpox infection can also occur without a rash. A mild but uncommon variation of variola infection, variola sine eruptione (meaning smallpox without a rash) occurs generally in previously vaccinated people and involves a febrile illness alone. Asymptomatic infections are also possible, yet rare.

Ordinary Smallpox

Ordinary smallpox accounts for over 90% of the cases among unvaccinated patients. Towards the end of the prodrome, the temperature usually drops and the patient feels better. The rash then begins as small erythematous spots on the tongue and oral mucosa, followed by skin lesions 24 h later. The oral lesions grow and ulcerate quickly, releasing large amounts of virus into the saliva. Virus titers in saliva are highest during the first week of rash illness, and patients are most infectious at this time (25,26).

The skin rash usually begins with a few macules, "herald spots," on the face, particularly the forehead. Next, lesions appear on the proximal extremities, later spreading to the distal extremities and the trunk. Within 24 h, the rash is visible on the entire body. Within 2–3 days, the macules become raised papules, and by the third or fourth day, the papular lesions become vesicular. Fluid within the vesicles at first is opalescent, but within 24–48 h, it becomes opaque and turbid. A characteristic faint erythematous halo surrounds the skin lesions. Another distinctive feature of the distended smallpox lesions, their central depression or dimple, "umbilication," is less common in other vesicular or pustular rashes such as varicella.

By sixth or seventh day, all the lesions become pustular, reaching their maximum size and maturity between 7 and 10 days. The typical smallpox pustules are sharply raised, round, tense, and firm to the touch (Fig. 2.6a,b).

Deeply embedded in the dermis, the lesions feel like a "small bead" in the skin. On the eighth or ninth day of the rash, as fluid is slowly absorbed, the pustules form

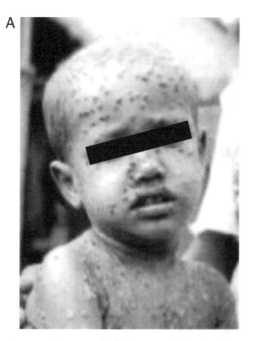

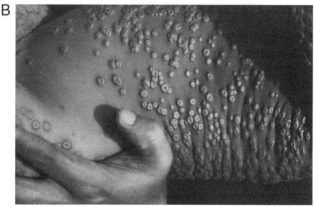

Fig. 2.6 (A and B) Patient with typical smallpox lesions. From A: CDC Public Health Image Library (PHIL). http://phil.cdc.gov/phil/quicksearch.asp, picture ID #7055. B: Hick, James. Smallpox lesions on skin of trunk. CDC: Smallpox. http://www.bt.cdc.gov/agent/smallpox/smallpox-images/smallpox2.htm)

a crust. Although the umbilication usually continues into the pustular state of the lesions, as the lesions absorb fluid, the umbilication flattens. Fever usually rises by the seventh day of illness, and the high fever continues throughout the vesicular and pustular states, until crusts have formed over all the lesions. As the patient begins to recover, the crusts separate from the lesions, leaving depigmented skin. The depigmented skin lesions develop into characteristic pitted scars.

The severity of the illness generally varies with the extent of the rash. Sometimes, the pustules on the extensor surfaces of the extremities and the face are so numerous that they become confluent. Such patients typically remain febrile and toxic even after scabs have formed over all of their lesions. Secondary bacterial infection is uncommon. Death usually results from the toxemia associated with circulating immune complexes and soluble variola antigens. The case fatality rate in the unvaccinated population is 30% (26). In one case series, patients with confluent lesions had a case fatality rate of 62% (25).

Other complications, although rare, include arthritis in up to 2% of cases, more commonly in children. Respiratory illness, viral or bacterial, and including bronchitis, pneumonia or pneumonitis, sometimes develops on the eighth day of illness. Encephalitis, indistinguishable from that seen as a complication of vaccinia, measles, and varicella, is possible. Other long-term complications include blindness, secondary to corneal lesions with subsequent scarring, and limb deformities, secondary to arthritis and osteomyelitis.

Modified Smallpox

Modified smallpox occurs typically in previously vaccinated people. The prodrome is less severe than in ordinary smallpox and patients are usually afebrile during development of the rash. Skin lesions, generally fewer in number, evolve more quickly, and are more superficial and lack uniformity compared to ordinary smallpox. Modified smallpox is rarely fatal, and is easily confused with chickenpox.

Flat (Malignant) Smallpox

"Flat-type" refers to the characteristic lesions, which are flush with the skin rather than raised vesicles. In outbreaks in India, flat-type smallpox was responsible for between 5 and 10% of cases, with most of the flat-type cases (72%) occurring in children (25). Constitutional symptoms associated with the 3–4 day prodrome are more severe than in ordinary smallpox and continue after the rash develops. Patients have a high fever and appear toxic throughout the course of the illness. Oral lesions tend to be extensive, and the skin lesions evolve slowly. By the 7 or 8 day, the flat skin lesions appear buried in the skin. In comparison to ordinary smallpox, the vesicles contain little fluid and do not develop the characteristic umbilication. Unlike ordinary smallpox, flat-type smallpox lesions are soft and velvety in texture. The lesions may contain hemorrhages. Respiratory complications are common, and the prognosis for flat-type smallpox is grave. Most cases are fatal (25).

Hemorrhagic Smallpox

Hemorrhagic smallpox, a severe but fortunately rare form of smallpox, presents with extensive bleeding into the skin, mucus membranes and the gastrointestinal tract. Studies in India revealed that hemorrhagic smallpox accounted for 2% of hospitalized patients. In comparison to flat-type smallpox, most cases of hemorrhagic smallpox occurred in adults, with the risk increased in pregnant women. The prodromal stage of hemorrhagic smallpox is severe and may be prolonged, and features fever, intense headache, backache, restlessness, a dusky flush, or occasionally pallor of the face and extreme prostration. Patients appear quite toxic. Unlike ordinary smallpox, the fever does not remit but continues throughout the course of illness.

The characteristic hemorrhages can appear early or late in the illness. In the early, fulminating form of hemorrhagic smallpox, on the second or third day of illness, patients may develop subconjunctival bleeding, bleeding from the mouth or gums, bleeding from other mucous membranes, skin petechiae, epistaxis, and hematuria. Frequently, patients die suddenly between the fifth and seventh days of illness, before any significant rash development. If patients do survive for 8–10 days, hemorrhages begin when the rash first erupts. In these patients, the rash is flat and does not progress past the vesicular stage (25).

Variola Sine Eruptione and Subclinical Smallpox

People previously vaccinated for smallpox can develop a febrile illness after exposure to a smallpox case. Typically, fever begins suddenly, reaches 39°C and is associated with headache and occasionally backache. Symptoms resolve within 48 h. Serologic studies in these patients have suggested the diagnosis of variola sine eruptione by demonstrating a significant rise in variola antibody titers following the illness (25).

Serologic studies have also shown that recently vaccinated contacts of smallpox cases can develop an actual subclinical case, without any symptoms. Persons with subclinical infection have not transmitted the infection to their contacts (25).

Diagnosis

Differentiating Smallpox from Other Rash Illness, Especially Varicella (Chickenpox)

The discovery of even one case of smallpox in the world would be an international medical and public health emergency. Therefore, the appropriate diagnosis is essential. Physicians who have never seen smallpox might confuse smallpox with varicella

Table 2.12 Distinguishing chickenpox from smallpox

	Chickenpox	Smallpox
Prodrome	None or mild	Severe, beginning 1–4 days before rash onset, with fever >101°F, other symptoms, including prostration, headache, backache, chills, abdominal pain, vomiting
Distribution of lesions	Centripetal, prominent on trunk, rarely on palms and soles	Centrifugal, most prominent on face and extremities, palms and soles involved in almost all cases
Development	Successive crops, lesions at varying stages of development	One crop, lesions at same stage of development all over the body
Lesion characteristics	Delicate, not well circumscribed, superficial, rarely become confluent, or umbilicated	Round, tense, deeply embedded, frequently become confluent and umbilicated
History	No reliable history of chickenpox disease or vaccination; 50–80% recall an exposure to chickenpox or shingles 10–21 days before onset	No history of recent exposure to chickenpox or Shingles

Source: Data from references 25 and 26

(chickenpox) but the illness and their associated rashes have distinct features. Table 2.12 summarizes the differences.

One of the most distinguishing features between smallpox and chickenpox is the presence of a prodrome, including a fever, before rash onset. Patients with smallpox characteristically have a severe febrile prodrome beginning 1–4 days before rash onset. The fever tends to be high, at least 101°F. but most frequently is between 102 and 104°F. In comparison, children with chickenpox have either no prodrome or a short, mild prodrome, and have little fever before rash onset. Chickenpox in adults may be more severe, and adults are more likely to have some fever before rash onset. However, in either adults or children, if there is no history of a febrile prodrome, smallpox is very unlikely.

Other smallpox prodromic symptoms, absent in chickenpox, include prostration, headache, backache, chills, abdominal pain, or vomiting. Unlike patients with chickenpox, patients with the smallpox prodrome are typically too sick to engage in normal activities and generally stay in bed.

Varicella and variola rashes have distinct differences in their distribution, development and appearance. The typical varicella rash has a centripetal distribution, with lesions most prominent on the trunk and rarely seen on the palms and soles. The varicella rash develops in successive groups (crops) of lesions over several days, resulting in lesions of various stages of development and resolution. Varicella lesions are superficial, the lesions appear delicate and not well circumscribed. They rarely become confluent or umbilicated.

In contrast, the vesicular/pustular variola rash has a centrifugal distribution, most prominent on the face and extremities. The palms and soles are involved in most cases. Variola lesions develop at one time (one crop), so that lesions are at the same stage of development all over the body. The variola pustules are characteristically round, tense and deeply embedded in the dermis. As variola lesions evolve, they may become confluent or umbilicated.

The patient's history is also helpful in distinguishing chickenpox from smallpox. Most patients presenting with chickenpox will have no reliable history of having the disease or the chickenpox vaccination, and most patients will recall exposure to a case of chickenpox or Shingles 10–21 days before onset of their symptoms.

Physicians may confuse several other conditions with smallpox (25). Table 2.13 lists some of these conditions:

Table 2.13 Common conditions confused with smallpox

Condition	Clues to Distinguish the Condition from Smallpox
Disseminated herpes zoster	Occurs in immunocompromised and elderly; rash looks like varicella, begins in dermatomal patterns
Impetigo	Honey-colored crusted plaques with bullae, but may begin as vesicles; regional distribution, mild or no systemic symptoms
Drug eruptions	History of medication exposure; generalized rash
Contact dermatitis	Pruritis, history of contact with allergens, location of rash suggests external contact
Erythema multiforme minor	Target, bulls eye or iris lesion, often follows recurrent herpes simplex infections, can involve palms and soles
Erythema multiforme (including Stevens–Johnson syndrome)	Mucous membranes and conjunctivae involved; may be target lesions or vesicles
Enteroviral Infection, especially hand, foot, and mouth disease	Summer and fall seasonal pattern, mild pharyngitis 1–2 days before rash onset, maculopapular lesions evolve into whitish-grey tender, flat, often oval vesicles, peripheral distribution (hands, feet, mouth, or disseminated)
Disseminated herpes simplex	Occurs in immunocompromised, lesions indistinguishable from varicella
Scabies and insect bites	Pruritis is major feature; no fever or other systemic symptoms
Molluscum contagiosum	In immunocompromised may disseminate

Adapted from Atkinson W, Hamborsky J, McIntyre L, Wolfe S. CDC: Epidemiology and Prevention of Vaccine-Preventable Diseases, 9th ed. http://www.cdc.gov/nip/publications/pink/default.htm.

In the early stages of a smallpox outbreak, perhaps before more typical cases appear, hemorrhagic smallpox can be confused with other conditions such as meningococcemia and leukemia, and flat (malignant) smallpox can be mistaken for hemorrhagic chickenpox. In some cases, the severe abdominal pain associated with the prodrome has prompted unnecessary surgical intervention (25).

To assist physicians in evaluating patients with suspicious rash illnesses, the CDC has developed three major and five minor criteria that physicians can use in determining whether patients are at high moderate or low risk for smallpox (http://www.bt.cdc.gov/agent/smallpox/diagnosis/pdf/spox-poster-1st-half.pdf. The three major criteria are:

1. Febrile prodrome (fever ≥101°F) 1–4 days before rash onset and at least one of the following systemic symptoms: prostration, headache, backache, chills, vomiting, or abdominal pain
2. Classic smallpox lesions: deep-seated, firm/hard, well circumscribed vesicles or pustules; as they evolve, the lesions may become umbilicated or confluent
3. Lesions in the same stage of development: on any one part of the body (e.g., the face or arm), all the lesions are in the same stage of development (i.e., all are vesicles or all are pustules)

The five minor criteria are:

1. Centrifugal distribution: the greatest concentration of lesions is on the face and distal extremities
2. First lesions on the oral mucosa or palate, face or forearms
3. Patient appears toxic or moribund
4. Slow evolution: lesions evolve from macules to papules to pustules over days; each stage lasts 1–2 days
5. Lesions on the palms and soles

Using an algorithm based on these criteria, the CDC has developed an interactive, case evaluation tool to help physicians and other health care providers determine whether a rash illness may be smallpox. Depending on how they respond a simple online questionnaire, the tool can help physicians and other health care providers classify the patient into a risk category and provide useful suggestions for further evaluation and treatment: http://www.bt.cdc.gov/agent/smallpox/diagnosis/riskalgorithm/index.asp. In addition, the CDC Web site includes a useful case investigation worksheet at: http://www.bt.cdc.gov/agent/smallpox/diagnosis/pdf/spox-patient-eval-wksheet.pdf.

Case Management and Reporting

Physicians and other health care providers evaluating patients who meet all three major criteria should consider them as high risk for smallpox. Physicians must isolate a suspected or confirmed case immediately while they report the case to the local and state health department. For reporting, the CDC Web site contains contact information of state health departments at: http://www.cdc.gov/other.htm#states. The National Association of County and City Health Officials (NACCHO) maintains contact information for all local health departments in the United States on its Web site at http://lhadirectory.naccho.org/phdir/. State health departments can also provide the contact information for local health departments within their states. If possible, physicians should take digital photographs of the rash, and obtain consultation with dermatology and/or infectious disease specialists. After the consultation, if public health authorities still consider the patient as high risk, they will consult with the CDC to arrange for laboratory testing for smallpox.

Infection Control

Smallpox suspect and confirmed cases require strict respiratory and contact isolation. Patients are contagious until all the crusts have separated. Before the eradication of smallpox, in-hospital transmission of smallpox was a serious problem, necessitating separate smallpox hospitals for over 200 years. Hospitalized patients can transmit smallpox through fine aerosols as well as the more common droplet spread. In Germany, one coughing smallpox patient, isolated in a single room, transmitted the disease to persons on three floors of the hospital (26). Hospital transmission by direct contact can also occur, particularly in patients with the hemorrhagic or flat-type (malignant) smallpox who frequently remain undiagnosed until near death and very contagious. Outbreaks have occurred when laundry workers handled linens and blankets used by such smallpox patients.

If faced with a high-risk case, or in a limited smallpox outbreak, physicians should take immediate action to alert infection control at the hospital and institute contact precautions and respiratory isolation. These include (25):

– Patient placement in a private, negative airflow room (airborne infection isolation) with high efficiency particulate air filtration if available; if not available, placement in a private room with the door closed at all times, except when patient or staff must enter or exit.
– Requirement that staff and visitors use appropriate PPE, including N95 or higher quality respirators (masks).
– Contact precautions should include the use of disposable gloves, gowns, and shoe covers.
– Requirements that patients wear a surgical mask when outside the negative-pressure isolation room and be gowned or wrapped in a sheet so that their rash is fully covered.
– Before contacting others, hospital personnel should remove and correctly dispose of any protective clothing.
– Personnel should place all laundry and waste in biohazard bags and autoclave the material before laundering (in hot water with bleach) or incinerating.
– Personnel handling potentially contaminated material, such as laundry workers, housekeeping staff, and laboratory personnel should also use PPE.

– If a case is confirmed, hospital personnel should receive smallpox vaccination
  before handling potentially contaminated material.

Hospitals should develop special protocols for decontaminating rooms after patients
leave (26). Standard infection control agents that hospitals use, such as hypochlorite and quaternary ammonia, should effectively clean potentially contaminated
surfaces (26).

A smallpox attack would pose difficult problems for public health officials
due to the ability of the virus to continue to spread unless stopped by isolation
of patients and vaccination/isolation of their close contacts (26). Given the
threat of aerosol transmission in hospitals, as the number of cases rises, physicians should isolate suspected patients in their homes or an alternative nonhospital facility. Such home care is reasonable, considering that supportive therapy
is the only care available to smallpox victims (26). Chapter 6 discusses alternative treatment centers that public health authorities are likely to establish during
large outbreaks.

Patients having a febrile prodrome and either one other major criterion or at least
four minor criteria are at moderate risk for smallpox. For patients at moderate risk,
physicians should alert infection control and immediately institute contact precautions and respiratory isolation. If possible, they should obtain dermatology and/or
infectious disease consultation and obtain digital photographs of the lesions. Given
a moderate risk situation, the appropriate clinical diagnosis is essential, and physicians must rule out varicella or complication of vaccinia (smallpox vaccine).
Therefore, for moderate risk patients, the history is essential, specifically the history of clinical varicella infection, history of vaccination for varicella and history
of possible exposure to vaccinia (smallpox) vaccine.

Patients without a febrile prodrome are at low risk for smallpox, as are
patients with a febrile prodrome and less than four minor criteria. Physicians
and other health care providers should manage these patients as clinically
indicated.

Smallpox Laboratory Investigation

Patients meet the smallpox clinical case definition if the algorithm classifies them
at high risk for smallpox. These cases require immediate laboratory confirmation
of smallpox. Laboratory testing to rule out other diagnoses is not a priority.
Physicians identifying a patient at high risk should immediately report the case to
their local and state health departments, who will help with the collection of the
specimen for laboratory testing. Currently, only Level D labs, at the CDC or
USAMRIID, are capable of providing initial laboratory confirmation of smallpox.

Someone either vaccinated previously or vaccinated that day should collect the
specimens while wearing a mask and gloves. They should use the blunt edge of a
scalpel to open a lesion to obtain vesicular or pustular fluid, a cotton swab to har-
vest the fluid, and forceps to pick up scabs. They should place the specimens in a

vacutainer tube, sealing the tube with adhesive tape where the stopper meets the tube. Next, they should enclose the tube in another durable, watertight container. Physicians and other health care providers evaluating high-risk patients should contact their state and local health departments for detailed directions on specimen collection and transport. The state public health laboratory will then work with the patient's physician and the CDC smallpox response team to obtain the appropriate specimen and arrange testing. Specimen collection and transport guidelines are available at http://www.bt.cdc.gov/agent/smallpox/response-plan/files/guide-d.pdf.

Electron microscopic examination of vesicular or pustular fluid or scabs can rapidly confirm the diagnosis of smallpox infection. Although the brick-shaped monkeypox and vaccinia virions appear identical to smallpox on electron microscopy, the history and clinical evaluation can rule out cowpox and vaccinia. Nucleic acid-based testing, such as PCR, can definitively distinguish between the different Orthopoxviruses. If the specimens test negative for smallpox, the patient should be evaluated for other conditions as clinically indicated. Once public health authorities confirm an outbreak of smallpox, high-risk cases would not require laboratory investigation (26).

Clinicians should not order smallpox laboratory testing for moderate or low-risk patients. Given that the global prevalence of smallpox is zero, the positive predictive value of a positive laboratory test for smallpox is extremely low, especially in patients who do not meet the case definition. Testing only high-risk patients for smallpox reduces the likelihood of false positive lab results with their attendant serious consequences.

Instead, the diagnostic priority for laboratory testing in moderate risk patients is to rule out chickenpox, the disease most commonly confused with smallpox. Therefore, moderate risk patients require rapid diagnostic testing for varicella zoster virus (VZV) (25).

Several methods are available for rapid detection of VZV in clinical specimens. Although a Tzanck smear is not diagnostic of VZV, most local hospitals with a pathology laboratory can perform the test easily and quickly. A positive Tzanck smear confirms an alphaherpes virus infection, either VZV or HSV (Herpes Simplex Virus).

Specific tests for VZV include DFA or PCR. DFA uses anti-VZV antibody conjugated to fluorescein dye to detect VZV in cells. Although the DFA is very sensitive and specific, its value is critically dependent on careful specimen collection. PCR of vesicular fluid or scabs can detect VZV DNA directly in 4–6 h. Some local health departments, all state public health laboratories and all large cities contain at least one facility, including private labs and academic health centers, capable of performing rapid diagnostic testing for VZV (25).

Treatment

Currently, the only available treatments for patients with smallpox infection are supportive therapy and antibiotics for occasional superimposed bacterial infections (26). The FDA does not approve any antiviral drug for the treatment of smallpox, although recent studies suggest that cidofovir, a nucleoside analog DNA polymerase inhibitor, might be useful. However, cidofovir requires intravenous administration and has significant renal toxicity. An infectious disease specialist would be required to administer cidofovir or any other antiviral agents under an investigational new drug protocol (25).

Prevention

Vaccine: History and Effectiveness

The term "vaccination" originated with the smallpox vaccine. In 1796, Edward Jenner developed an effective method for producing smallpox immunity by inoculating people with material from a cowpox lesion. He named the method vaccination, based on *vacca*, the Latin word for cow. During the nineteenth century, vaccinia virus, a related but genetically distinct Orthopoxvirus, replaced the cowpox virus in the vaccine (25).

By early 2004, 15 million doses of smallpox vaccine, Dryvax, were available in the United States. Dryvax, a Wyeth product, is a live virus preparation of vaccinia. The vaccine comes as a lyophilized (freeze-dried) powder in 100 dose vials containing the antibiotics polymyxin B, streptomycin, tetracycline, and neomycin. Fifty percent glycerin, containing a small amount of phenol as a preservative, serves as the diluent for reconstitution (25). Studies have shown that diluting the vaccine in a 1:5 ratio could expand the supply without reducing vaccine efficacy (25). In addition, 200 million antibiotic-free doses are in production. The CDC Web site has detailed directions on how to reconstitute and administer the vaccine at: http://www.bt.cdc.gov/agent/smallpox/vaccination/administration.asp.

Controlled studies evaluating smallpox vaccine effectiveness are not available. However, studies of exposed household case contacts demonstrated a 91–97% reduction in cases among household contacts with vaccination scars compared to contacts without scars. None of these studies investigated the association between attack rates and time since vaccination or potency of the vaccine, so they may underestimate current levels of protection in the United States (15).

Other studies have demonstrated that primary vaccination provides nearly 100% of protection for 5 years and substantial but waning immunity for 10 or more years. Subsequent booster vaccination results in antibody levels that remain high even longer, suggesting that booster vaccination can confer a longer period of immunity. Although the susceptibility of people in the United States who received the vaccine 29 or more years ago is uncertain, studies suggest such vaccinated people have less severe disease. Smallpox cases imported into Europe in the 1950s and 1960s caused fewer fatalities in vaccinated compared to unvaccinated people. The case fatality rate was 1.3% for those vaccinated less than

10 years before exposure, 7% for those vaccinated 11–20 years before exposure, and 11% among those vaccinated more than 20 years before exposure. 52% of those unvaccinated died (25).

Smallpox vaccination is also effective if given after exposure to the disease. Studies of household contacts in India and Pakistan revealed that postexposure vaccination reduced secondary cases up to 91%. The lowest secondary attack rates occurred in contacts vaccinated less than seven days after exposure. Smallpox cases that occurred were typically less severe (modified smallpox) in household contacts receiving postexposure vaccination (25).

Immediately following vaccination, the vaccinia virus begins to replicate in the skin. After 3 or 4 days, a red papule appears at the site. Two days later, the papule becomes vesicular, surrounded by erythema. After another 2 days, approximately 7 days after vaccination, the papule becomes a typical "Jennerian" pustule, a whitish, umbilicated, multilocular lesion containing turbid lymph, surrounded by erythema. The pustule may continue to expand for three additional days (26) (Fig. 2.7; see color plate 2.7).

Maximum erythema appears 8–12 days after vaccination. Some recipients develop regional lymphadenopathy and/or fever. Up to 70% of children have at least 1 day of fever greater than 39°C sometime between days 4 and 14 after vaccination. The pustule then gradually dries, with a dark crust developing 2–3 weeks after vaccination. In the third week, the crust falls off leaving a permanent scar at the vaccination site (25,26).

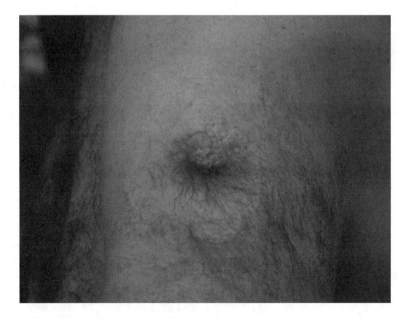

Fig. 2.7 (See color plate) Smallpox vaccination site

The response just described is a major reaction, indicating that the vaccinia virus replicated in the skin, resulting in a successful vaccination. People previously vaccinated people should develop a major reaction just like primary vaccinees, except that the lesion progresses faster. Any vaccine recipient developing a major reaction should be considered protected.

Equivocal reactions include any reaction other than the typical skin lesion, and may occur for several reasons. The recipient may be immune enough to suppress the vaccinia virus, preventing it from replicating. Alternatively, the recipient may have a hypersensitivity reaction to the vaccine. A response resulting in a peak in erythema within 48 h of vaccination represents a hypersensitivity reaction and does not indicate that viral replication occurred (26). Other possible causes of equivocal reactions include insufficiently potent vaccine or poor vaccine administration technique. After 7 days, any vaccine recipient experiencing an equivocal reaction should receive a revaccination with vaccine from a different vial (25).

Adverse Events Following Smallpox Vaccination

Local Reactions

In studies performed on previously unvaccinated adults, the average size of the pustule 2 weeks after vaccination was 12 mm, the average size of surrounding erythema was 16–24 mm and the average induration was 11–15 mm. Some vaccine recipients develop larger degrees of erythema and induration, making it difficult to differentiate a large major reaction from cellulitis. Although the large reactions will improve in 24–48 h without therapy, patients with such large reactions require an evaluation to rule out bacterial cellulitis (25).

Nearly half of the vaccinees in these studies reported mild pain at the vaccination site, with 2–3% reporting severe pain. Approximately a third of vaccine recipients developed axillary lymphadenopathy, mild in most. In 3–7% of recipients, the lymphadenopathy was moderate, causing some discomfort, but did not interfere with normal activities (25).

Mild Systemic Reactions

Fever is common following smallpox vaccination, most likely occurring 7–12 days after inoculation. In one study of Dryvax vaccine given to previously unvaccinated adults, 5–9% had a fever ≥100°F and 3% reported a temperature ≥102°F. Fever is more likely in vaccinated children. Studies have shown that about 70% of children receiving a primary vaccination develop 1 or more days with a temperature ≥100°F, with 15–20% experiencing temperatures ≥102°F (25).

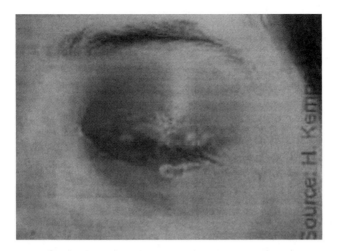

Fig. 2.8 (See color plate) Eyelid vaccinia due to inadvertent inoculation. From Kempe, H. Smallpox vaccination adverse reaction. CDC: Smallpox. http://www.bt.cdc.gov/training/smallpoxvaccine/reactions/adverse.html

Other commonly reported symptoms in vaccinated adults included headaches, myalgias, chills, nausea, and fatigue 8 or 9 days after inoculation. One or two percent reported these symptoms as severe (25).

Inadvertent Inoculation

Inadvertent inoculation, the most frequent complication of smallpox vaccination, refers to the transmission of the vaccinia virus from the inoculation site to another part of the recipient's body (autoinoculation) or to the bodies of close contacts (Fig. 2.8; see color plate 2.8). It can occur because live vaccinia virus is present at the inoculation site from about 4 days after inoculation until the crust separates from the skin. Maximum viral shedding occurs 4–14 days after inoculation. Inadvertent inoculation is responsible for approximately half of all complications for primary vaccination and revaccination. Because inadvertent inoculation frequently results from touching the vaccination site and transmitting the virus manually, the most common affected sites are the face, eyelid, nose, mouth, genitalia, and rectum. Most cases heal without any specific treatment. Inadvertent inoculation of the eye can lead to corneal scarring and subsequent vision loss. Occasionally, vaccinia immune globulin (VIG) is necessary to treat periocular lesions (26).

During the waning years of routine smallpox vaccination, in 1968, studies estimated the rate of inadvertent inoculation at 529 cases per million primary vaccinations. More recently, from January 24, 2003 to December 31, 2003, 39,213 civilian health care and public health workers received smallpox vaccination; 12 people developed inadvertent inoculation with one case involving the eye (29).

Generalized Vaccinia

Infrequently, hematogenous spread and deposition of the vaccinia virus remotely from the vaccination site causes generalized vaccinia. It occurs in people without eczema or other preexisting skin disease. Six to nine days after smallpox vaccination, vesicles and pustules appear on the skin distant from the vaccination site (Fig. 2.9; see color plate 2.9). Most generalized vaccinia rashes produce minor symptoms and minimal residual damage, and usually resolve without treatment. Occasionally patients who become toxic or are immunosuppressed require treatment with VIG. In the 1968 studies, generalized vaccinia occurred at a rate of 242 per million people receiving smallpox vaccination (25) Of the 39,213 civilians receiving vaccination in 2003, there were two cases of suspected and one case of confirmed generalized vaccinia (29).

Eczema Vaccinatum

Eczema vaccinatum, a potentially serious complication, occurs in people who have eczema, atopic dermatitis, or a history of eczema or atopic dermatitis. It can also occur in vaccine recipient contacts with these conditions. Eczema vaccinatum is

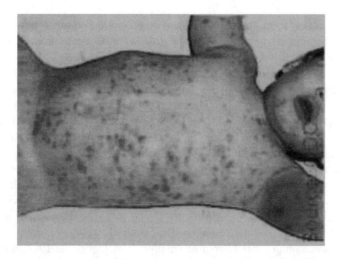

Fig. 2.9 (See color plate) Generalized vaccinia in an infant. From smallpox vaccination adverse reaction. CDC: Smallpox. http://www.bt.cdc.gov/training/smallpoxvaccine/reactions/adverse.html

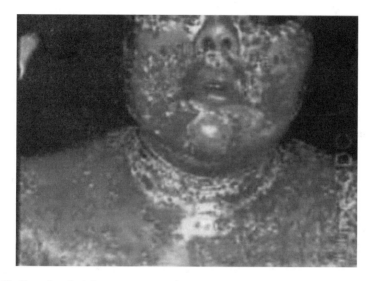

Fig. 2.10 (See color plate) Severe eczema vaccinatum in a 22 year old. From Smallpox vaccination adverse reaction. CDC: Smallpox. http://www.bt.cdc.gov/training/smallpoxvaccine/reactions/ adverse.html

due to local or systemic spread of the vaccinia virus, and can occur whether or not eczema or atopic dermatitis is active. The vaccinial lesions extend to cover most if not all of the area currently or previously affected by eczema (Fig. 2.10; see color plate 2.10) (26). Although usually mild and self-limited, eczema vaccinatum can be severe and even fatal. Severe symptoms are more likely to occur in primary vaccinees compared to those vaccinated in the past. In the 1968 studies, eczema vaccinatum occurred in at a rate of 10–39 cases per million primary vaccinations (25). Of the 39,213 civilians receiving vaccination in 2003, there were no cases of eczema vaccinatum (29).

Myopericarditis

Myocarditis symptoms following smallpox vaccination can include chest pain, fatigue, fever, palpitations, and dyspnea on exertion. Severe cases can develop severe cardiac dysfunction or dysrhythmia. Although myopericarditis occurred in vaccine recipients in the 1950s and 1960s, the strains of vaccinia used at that time were different, and the 2002 National Smallpox Vaccination program did not anticipate myopericarditis occurring among vaccine recipients (25). However, of the 39,213 civilians receiving vaccination in 2003, there were 16 suspected and five probable cases of myopericarditis (29). From March 25–31, 2003, four cases of myocarditis and/or pericarditis occurred in military vaccine recipients; added to previous cases, this resulted in a rate of 14 cases among approximately 250,000 military personnel receiving the vaccine for the first time. No cases occurred among the 115,000 military vaccine recipients vaccinated previously. Cases ranged in age from 21 to 33 and severity ranged from mild (without electrocardiogram or echocardiogram changes) to severe, specifically congestive heart failure. Onset occurred 7–19 days after vaccination. Although all military cases were hospitalized, with the most severe case requiring at least 6 days of hospitalization, none died (30).

During the military and civilian vaccination programs in 2003, several vaccine recipients experienced myocardial ischemia, including infarctions. Most of these cases had underlying risk factors for ischemic disease. In addition, the number of deaths due to cardiac disease among civilians receiving vaccination was similar to the number expected in a similar aged population in the absence of vaccination. Investigators concluded that while there is a causal relationship between smallpox vaccination and myopericarditis, there is no causal association established between smallpox vaccination and cardiac ischemia (30).

Progressive Vaccinia

Progressive vaccinia, also known as vaccinia necrosum, occurs when the vaccinial lesion fails to heal and instead progresses to involve adjacent skin with tissue necrosis (Fig. 2.11; see color plate 2.11). The lesion can spread metastatically to other parts of the skin, to bones and to viscera (26). Although progressive vaccinia occurs

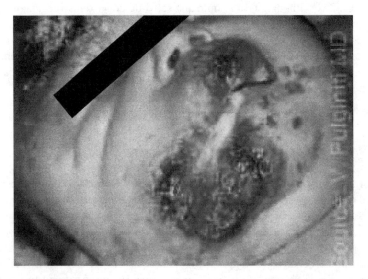

Fig. 2.11 (See color plate) Severe progressive vaccinia. From Fulginiti, V. Smallpox vaccination adverse reaction. CDC: Smallpox. http://www.bt.cdc.gov/training/smallpoxvaccine/reactions/adverse.html

primarily among primary vaccinees and revaccinees with cellular immunodeficiency, it can also occur in those with humoral immunodeficiency. Historically, progressive vaccinia was almost invariably fatal, but treatment with VIG and antiviral agents can now reduce mortality. In the 1968 studies, progressive vaccinia occurred at a rate of 1–2 cases per million vaccinees (25). While the prevalence of HIV and posttransplant immunization could lead to more cases, none of the 39,213 civilians receiving vaccination in 2003 developed progressive vaccinia, perhaps because of prescreening.

Postvaccinial Encephalitis

Historically, postvaccinial encephalitis occurred at a rate of 3–12 people per million vaccinated. It occurred exclusively in primary vaccinees. Approximately 15–25% of the cases were fatal, and approximately 25% experienced permanent neurological sequelae (25), including residual paralysis. Between 8 and 15 days after vaccination, central nervous system symptoms and signs develop, including fever, headache, vomiting, drowsiness, confusion, and sometimes spastic paralysis, meningeal signs, seizures and coma (25,26). Examination of CSF reveals a pleocytosis. Most cases are probably due to autoimmune or allergic reactions rather than central nervous system viral infection (25). There is no effective treatment for postvaccinial encephalitis. One suspect case occurred among the 39,213 civilians receiving vaccination in 2003 (29).

Fetal Vaccinia

Less than 50 cases of fetal vaccinia have occurred, usually following primary vaccination of the mother in early pregnancy. Fetal vaccinia generally causes a stillbirth or neonatal death. The vaccine is not associated with congenital anomalies. No cases occurred among the 39,213 civilians receiving vaccination in 2003 (15).

Vaccine Administration

Smallpox vaccine administration requires a bifurcated needle. Each bifurcated needle is sterile and individually wrapped. The vaccinator should first review the patient's history to ensure the patient has no contraindication to receiving the vaccine. However, during an outbreak of smallpox, case contacts should receive the vaccine regardless of the contraindications, because the vaccine is safer than the disease.

The deltoid is the recommended site for administration. Skin preparation is not necessary, unless the site is grossly contaminated. Soap and water are effective for cleaning such sites. Under no circumstances should the vaccinator prepare the skin with alcohol, because alcohol can inactivate the vaccinia virus, reducing vaccine effectiveness. The vaccinator inserts the needle into a vial of reconstituted vaccine, never inserting the same needle more than once to avoid contaminating the vial. Upon withdrawal, the vaccinator should confirm visually that a droplet of vaccine sits between the tines of the needle. The bifurcated needle design should ensure that the droplet contains an adequate vaccine dose. The vaccinator then holds the needle at right angle to the skin over the deltoid muscle, with the wrist of the vaccinator resting against the arm or other firm support (31,32).

The vaccinator then makes vigorous, rapid, perpendicular strokes into the skin within a 5 mm diameter area, with the number of strokes consistent with the package insert. People receiving a primary vaccination should receive three strokes, while secondary vaccinations require 15 strokes. The application should be vigorous enough to cause a trace of blood to appear at the site within 15–30 s. For those primary vaccinees without visible blood after three strokes, the vaccinator should perform an additional three strokes using the same bifurcated needle, without reinserting the needle into the vial. The vaccinator should dispose of the one-use needle in the appropriate biohazard container following the vaccination (31,32).

Immediately after administering the vaccine, the vaccinator should remove excess vaccine from the site by wiping the area with sterile gauze. To prevent anyone from coming in contact with vaccinia virus, the vaccinator should dispose the gauze in an appropriate biohazard receptacle. Likewise, to prevent the vaccine recipient from touching the site and transferring the vaccinia virus to another part of the body or to another individual, it is necessary to cover the site adequately (31,32). Recommended vaccine site dressings include (31,32):

– Gauze loosely held with tape.
– Vaccinated health care workers can continue to work after receiving the vaccine. However, to protect patients, they should keep the site covered with gauze or some other absorbent material, and in turn, cover this dressing with a semipermeable dressing. Several products combining an absorbent underlayer with an overlaying semipermeable layer are now available.
– In settings where close personal contact is likely, such as household contact, especially if infants and young children are present, vaccinees should cover the site with gauze or similar absorbent material, and in turn, wear clothing that covers the vaccination site.

In all cases, good hand hygiene is essential. Because semipermeable dressings are now available, people may be tempted to use them alone. However, use of semipermeable dressings alone could cause maceration with increased, prolonged irritation and itching, which in turn could encourage scratching and concomitant had contamination. Only health care workers should use semipermeable dressings, and they must place these over gauze or some similar absorbent material (31,32).

Besides proper dressing, vaccine recipient education is essential to prevent transmission of the vaccinia virus. Instructions should include (31,32):

– Avoid rubbing or scratching the site.
– Keep the site covered and change the gauze-only dressings very 1 or 2 days or sooner if wet – discard the gauze in plastic zip-lock bags.

- Change semipermeable dressings every 3–5 days.
- Keep the vaccination site dry by covering with a water-proof material while bathing.
- After showering, if the site gets wet, blot it dry with gauze, and discard the gauze appropriately. If using a towel to dry the site, do not use the towel to dry the rest of the body. Alternatively, air-dry the site before replacing the bandage.
- Do not place salves, creams or ointments on the site.
- Have a separate laundry hamper for clothing and other materials, such as bedding and towels that may contact the vaccination site – wash these items with hot water, detergent and/or bleach.
- After touching the vaccination site or materials that may have come in contact with the site, wash hands thoroughly with soap and hot water, or with alcohol-based hand rubs such as gels or foams containing at least 60% alcohol.
- When the scab falls off, discard it in a plastic zip-lock bag.
- Report any problems possibly associated with the vaccine by calling the phone number listed with patient education materials, or by calling your health care provider or visiting the emergency room.

Vaccine recipients should have the vaccination site checked for a major reaction indicating vaccination "take" 7 days after vaccination. If a major reaction is not present, the recipient should be revaccinated (32).

Hospitals vaccinating their health care workers should include a vaccination site care component in which designated staff assess dressings daily, determine if dressings need changing and change the dressing if indicated. In addition, these designated staff should assess the site for reactions and vaccine "take," provide education for vaccinees, especially regarding hand hygiene, and record and report vaccine adverse events. These designated staff should be vaccinated, but it is acceptable to have nonvaccinated staff change dressings. Of course, contact precautions are essential (32).

Contraindications to Smallpox Vaccine

For people with high-risk exposure to smallpox, there are no contraindications to the vaccine, because persons at greatest risk from vaccine complications are also at greatest risk for mortality from the disease (32). However, for preevent vaccination purposes, in the absence of circulating smallpox disease, the following groups of people should not receive smallpox vaccine (32):

- People with a history or current outbreak of eczema or atopic dermatitis; People with Darier disease (keratosis follicularis) are also at risk for eczema vaccinatum and should not receive the vaccine.
- People with other acute, chronic, or exfoliative skin conditions (such as burns, impetigo, varicella zoster, herpes, severe acne, severe diaper dermatitis with extensive areas of denuded skin, psoriasis).

- People who are immunosuppressed, such as people with HIV/AIDS, leukemia, lymphoma, generalized malignancy, solid organ transplants, or people on therapy with alkylating agents, antimetabolites, radiation or high-dose corticosteroids, (doses of ≥ 2 mg kg^{-1} body weight or 20 mg kg^{-1} of prednisone for ≥ 2 weeks). People on high doses of corticosteroids should not receive smallpox vaccine for at least 1 month after completing corticosteroid therapy, and those on other immunosuppressive medications should not receive vaccine for at least 3 months after completing treatment. Other immunosuppressed patients who should not receive smallpox vaccine include hematopoietic stem cell transplant recipients less than 24 months posttransplant and those who are more than 24 months post-transplant, but have graft versus-host disease or disease relapse (32). Patients with severe autoimmune disease, such as clinically active systemic lupus erythematosus, may also be immunocompromised and should not receive smallpox vaccine in the preevent program.
- Pregnant or breast feeding women.
- Infants under 1 year.
- People with a serious allergy to any vaccine component.
- People with household contacts who have the following conditions: a history of eczema or atopic dermatitis (regardless of disease severity or activity), other acute chronic or exfoliative skin conditions, immunosuppressive conditions, pregnancy. Household contacts include those with prolonged intimate contact, such as sexual contacts, and others who have contact with the vaccination site (32).

Preevent Smallpox Vaccine

Public health authorities have not recommended mass vaccination of the entire population for smallpox at this time for several reasons:

- Current supplies are inadequate to vaccinate the entire population, although this is improving.
- The risks of vaccine complications outweigh the likelihood of a smallpox attack. Significant populations are at greater risk of complications, including people with eczema, immune deficiency, and pregnant women.
- VIG is useful in treating some of the vaccine complications. However, like the vaccine itself, VIG is in short supply, and not enough is available to treat all the complications that could occur.

However, because of the possibility of a smallpox attack, albeit remote, in December 2002 President Bush announced his preevent vaccination plan. Instead of mass vaccination, the plan, based on recommendations from the CDC, the Advisory Committee on Immunization Practices (ACIP) and the Healthcare Infection Control Practices Advisory Committee (HICPAC) makes smallpox vaccination available for people designated by public health authorities to conduct investigation and follow-up of initial smallpox cases that might require direct patient contact (32). The continuing goal of the plan is that public health authorities ought to be able to conduct surveillance and containment if an outbreak were to occur.

Specifically, the ACIP has recommended that each state and territory establish and maintain at least one smallpox response team of vaccinated individuals. Having such smallpox response teams fits with the primary strategy to control a smallpox outbreak through surveillance and containment, which includes case isolation and vaccination of persons at risk for exposure. This strategy, which proved effective in eradicating naturally occurring smallpox, includes identification of cases through intensive surveillance, isolation of cases to prevent further transmission, vaccination of primary contacts (household contacts and other close contacts of cases) and vaccination of secondary contacts (close contacts of the primary contacts) (32).

These vaccinated smallpox response teams, at the federal, state, and local level, would be responsible for conducting diagnostic evaluation of suspected cases and initiating control measures. Teams could include medical team leaders, public health advisors, medical epidemiologists, disease investigators, diagnostic laboratorians, nurses, personnel who could administer the vaccine, security and law enforcement personnel involved in investigations, and other medical personnel assisting in evaluating suspected smallpox cases (32). Chapter 6 describes the role that family physicians could play on Disaster Medical Assistance Teams (DMATs), which could function as smallpox response teams.

In addition to the smallpox response teams, ACIP and HICPAC have recommended that every acute-care hospital identify and vaccinate a team of health care workers who might provide direct care for the first smallpox patients requiring admission or who might manage suspected case patients in emergency departments. When possible, to reduce the potential for adverse reactions to the vaccine, designated health care workers should be those who previously received smallpox vaccinations.

In the event of an outbreak, these teams would provide care 24 h d^{-1} for the first 2 days until additional health care workers receive vaccinations. Until vaccinated, other health care workers would be restricted from caring for patients with smallpox, or under emergency conditions, would be required to wear PPE (32).

The ACIP and HICPAC recommend that smallpox health care teams include:

- Emergency department staff, including physicians, and nurses
- Intensive care unit staff
- General medical unit staff, including family physicians in hospitals where they provide inpatient medical care
- Primary care house staff
- Medical subspecialists, including infectious disease specialists
- Infection control practitioners
- Respiratory therapists
- Radiology technicians
- Security personnel
- Housekeeping staff

The recommendations state that hospitals should vaccinate enough staff in each category to ensure continuity of care (32). Health care workers performing the vaccinations should first receive the vaccine to minimize the consequences of inadvertent inoculation. Laboratory workers are not included in the recommendations because the quantity of smallpox virus likely to be present in clinical specimens is low.

The original plan had three phases (27):

– Vaccination of military personnel, vaccination of State Department employees who serve oversee, and vaccination of public health and civilian health care teams (about 500,000 civilians)
– Vaccination of other medical providers and first responders (about 10 million civilians)
– Making the vaccine available to the general public
  (Adapted from Thorne CD et al., Emergency medical tools to manage smallpox 2003; 42(5): 665-681 with permission from Elsevier.)

In spite of the recommendations, less than 40,000 civilians received vaccinations in 2003, probably due to several reasons (27):

– Compared to the pre-1970 vaccination era, many more hospitalized patients are immunosuppressed, due to congenital or acquired illness, such as HIV infection, organ or bone marrow transplants, cancer, cancer therapy, eczema or other dermatological conditions, steroid or other immunosuppressive therapy, and autoimmune disease. Hospital administrators have been concerned that vaccinating large numbers of their staff might put these patients at risk of exposure and complications from the vaccinia virus.
– In addition to the patient population, many health care workers have conditions or therapy associated with immunosuppression who could be at risk for complications following exposure to staff who had received the vaccine.
– Although the CDC recommended that vaccinated hospital staff could continue to work after receiving the vaccine, and that administrative leave was not necessary, many hospital administrators were uncomfortable with this recommendation and were concerned that administrative leave for their vaccinated staff might be expensive.
– Hospital administrators felt that their liability for vaccine complications, including liability for inadvertent inoculation of patients and others in the community, was unclear.
– Hospital administrators felt that the risk and costs associated with a preevent vaccination program outweighed the risk of a smallpox attack. Even if an outbreak were to occur, given the effectiveness of the vaccine for 3 days after exposure, hospital administrators felt rapid mass vaccination efforts and quarantine of exposed individuals would probably be effective in controlling the spread of the disease.
  (Adapted from Thorne CD et al., Emergency medical tools to manage smallpox 2003; 42(5): 665-681 with permission from Elsevier.)

Some hospitals chose not to participate in the preevent smallpox vaccination program. Others have chosen to participate, but have sent fewer of their staff for vaccination compared to the number recommended by their local and state health departments. In addition to the hospital administrators, many health care workers have avoided participating because of their concerns about inadvertent inoculation of family members, concerns about compensation for lost wages if they are out of work due to side effects of the vaccine, and concern whether medical care for vaccine complications would be adequate (27).

Physician concerns about the vaccine were similar to those of other health care workers and hospital administrators. A physician survey at Yale University, conducted in the spring of 2003, revealed that fewer than 3% of physicians offered the vaccine choose to receive it. Factors associated with physician refusal included concerns that the vaccine was unnecessary; without a detailed description of the risk of a smallpox attack, physicians wanted to wait and see how safe the vaccine was. In addition, some physicians, primarily those who worked in the emergency department, had concerns about compensation for time off and liability for adverse reactions (33).

In an attempt to alleviate concerns about liability, on January 4, 2003 President Bush enacted section 304 of the Homeland Security Act. Section 304 addresses the liability of vaccine manufacturers, health care workers and public health agencies associated with federally sanctioned countermeasures against actual or potential bioterrorism. Federally recommended smallpox vaccination is a covered countermeasure. Under Section 304, if the United States Attorney General certifies that the defendant is a "covered person," and that the smallpox vaccination has caused personal injury or death, then only the federal government is liable for damages associated with the vaccination (34). Covered persons could include the vaccine manufacturer or distributor, a health care entity, such as a health department or hospital under whose auspices the vaccine was administered, a qualified person, such as a nurse or physician who administered the vaccine, or an official, agent or employee of the person or entity previously described (34). However, these protections are only available if the covered person(s) cooperate with the federal government in defense of the case. In addition, if the injury or death were due to grossly negligent, reckless, illegal, or willful misconduct, the federal government can recover the payments made to claimants from the covered person (34).

Although Section 304 satisfied some of the liability concerns, it failed to address health care worker worries about compensation for lost wages due to side effects of the vaccine (27). In addition, Section 304 did not address hospital and health care worker concerns about whether compensation would be adequate for victims of vaccine complications, including victims, such as household contacts, who were not vaccine recipients. Consequently, on April 30, 2003, the President signed a law to compensate health care workers or first responders injured by the preevent smallpox vaccination program. The law established a no-fault fund that had the following provisions (35):

– People permanently and totally disabled would receive up to $50,000 per year until retirement age, and would then transfer to a regular retirement plan
– People with less severe injuries could receive the same annual benefits with a lifetime cap of $262,000

- The surviving spouse would receive a lump sum of $262,000 for a death due to the vaccination
- A surviving spouse with children could choose the $262,000 lump sum or a payment of up to $50,000 annually until the youngest child reached 18
- Persons not satisfied with their compensation could sue under the Federal Tort Claims Act

In spite of these provisions, many hospitals and health care workers were not satisfied by the compensation provisions. By October 31, 2005, only 39,608 civilians had received the smallpox vaccine (http://www.cdc.gov/od/oc/media/pressrel/smallpox/spvaccin.htm).

Postexposure Vaccine for Prevention of Disease Transmission

The concerns about contraindications and liability associated with preevent vaccination do not apply in the event of a smallpox outbreak, because people at greatest risk from vaccine complications are also at greatest risk for mortality from the disease (32). Given the incubation period and the lag time before physicians recognized the rash as smallpox, 2 weeks or more could pass between the release of the virus and the diagnosis of the first cases. With each generation of transmission, the number of cases could expand by a factor of 10–20 (24). The best way to interrupt disease transmission is to identify, vaccinate and observe those at greatest risk of infection. Clearly, as soon as physicians make the first diagnosis, they should isolate their patients and vaccinate their household and other face-to-face contacts. Whenever possible, physicians should isolate patients in their home or other nonhospital facility to avoid further disseminating of the disease. In addition, hospitals and health care facilities treating patients with smallpox should take special precautions to ensure that all bedding and clothing of smallpox patients is autoclaved or laundered in hot water with bleach. Standard disinfectants, such as hypochlorite or quaternary ammonia, are effective for cleaning viral-contaminated surfaces.

After an aerosol release of smallpox, public health authorities will make vaccine supplies available to affected communities. Postexposure vaccination is effective in preventing infection or lowering mortality up to 4 days after exposure. Physicians should give the vaccine to suspected cases to ensure that a mistaken diagnosis does not place patients at risk for smallpox. An emergency vaccination program should also include (26):

- Health care workers at sites where smallpox patients may appear
- Other essential disaster workers including police, firefighters, transit workers, public health staff, emergency management staff
- Mortuary workers who may encounter deceased smallpox victims
- Because of the risk of dissemination, in an outbreak situation, all hospital employees and patients should receive vaccination. Immunocompromised

patients or patients with other contraindications for vaccination should receive VIG (Adapted by permission from Henderson DA, et al., (26) Copyright© 1999, American Medical Association. All Rights Reserved.)

Botulism

Microbiology and Epidemiology

The spore forming anaerobic bacillus, Clostridium botulinum, and two other Clostridia species produce a group of seven related but antigenically distinct neurotoxins (36), types A through G, responsible for human Botulism. Clostridium botulinum spores are ubiquitous, surviving in soil and aquatic habitats throughout the world. During anaerobic incubation, the spores germinate into slightly curved, gram positive, motile bacilli while producing the neurotoxins. The strains producing neurotoxins A, B, and E, are responsible for human disease, but rare cases of human botulism involving the F neurotoxin have occurred. In addition to Clostridia botulinum, Clostridia butyricum-like organisms and Clostridia baratii-like organisms have produced E and F toxins, resulting in human botulism (37).

Natural human botulism, a relatively rare disease, occurs in four epidemiologic forms: food-borne, infantile, wound, and adult botulism from intestinal colonization (38). None of these is transmissible person to person. All four forms result from absorption of the toxin into the bloodstream through the mucosa, such as the gastrointestinal tract or a wound. The toxin cannot penetrate intact skin. In the United States, fewer than 200 cases of human botulism occur each year (36).

Ingestion of food containing the preformed toxin causes food-borne botulism. Worldwide, methods of food preparation and food preservation that fail to destroy the ubiquitous spores result in sporadic cases and small outbreaks. Most cases in the United States are due to improper home canning. Since 1950, more than half of the reported food-borne outbreaks in the United States have occurred in five western states, California, Washington, Colorado, Oregon, and Alaska. Alaska has had a disproportionate share (16%) of all outbreaks, perhaps due to production and consumption of botulinum-contaminated food, such as fermented seafood, seals, whales, and other mammalian meat products (37). Commercially processed products are rarely associated with botulism, although outbreaks have resulted from cans damaged after processing (37). Before 1950, the case fatality rate for food-borne botulism was 60%; from 1950 to 1996, the case fatality rate was about 15%. In 2001, of 33 food-borne botulism cases reported in the United States, there was one fatality (39). Improved supportive care, including ventilation, and prompt administration of antitoxin have been responsible for the reduction in the case-fatality rate (38).

Infant botulism, first recognized in 1976, probably due to improved diagnostic capabilities compared to previous years, has been the most common form of reported botulism in the United States since 1980. Epidemiologically distinct from food-borne botulism, infant botulism results from endogenous production of toxin by germinating spores of *C. botulinum* in the infant's intestine rather than ingestion of the preformed toxin in food. The average annual incidence of infant botulism is 1.9 cases/100,000 births. Although the risk factors for infant botulism are not well known, foods and dust can contain spores. Some cases have been associated with ingestion of honey. Symptoms begin with constipation, followed by neuromuscular paralysis beginning with the cranial nerves and later progressing to the peripheral and respiratory musculature (38). Illness severity ranges from mild lethargy and slowed feeding to severe hypotonia and respiratory failure (38). In 2001, there were 112 reported cases of infant botulism in the United States, with one death (39).

Wound botulism, a relatively rare form of the disease, results from the production of toxin by organisms that multiply in a contaminated wound. Wounds associated with botulism may not appear obviously infected (38). Before 1980, wound botulism was most likely associated with complicated wounds, such as extensive crush injuries, compound fractures and other wounds associated with avascular areas. Since 1980, most cases have occurred in illicit drug users, including intravenous drug users with contaminated needle puncture sites or drug users with nasal and sinus wounds secondary to chronic cocaine sniffing (38). In 2001, there were 23 reported cases of wound botulism in the United States, with one death (39).

The least common form of human botulism, botulism from intestinal colonization, includes cases in patients greater than 1 year of age not associated with ingestion of contaminated food or wound infection with the only possibility being intestinal colonization (38). Stool in these patients will contain toxin and *C. botulinum*, and the suspected food may contain spores without preformed toxin. Some cases occur in patients with a history of gastrointestinal surgery or inflammatory bowel disease, conditions that could support enteric colonization of *B. botulinum* (38). In 2001, in the United States, one case of adult colonization botulism occurred in a 45 year old who survived (39).

Botulinum Toxin as a Biological Weapon

Botulinum toxin is on the "A" list of potential bioterrorist weapons because of its toxicity, its lethality, its ease of production, ease of transport, ease of use, and the need for prolonged, intensive care of affected victims (36). The colorless, odorless, and probably tasteless toxin is the most poisonous substance known (36). The most efficient route of exposure through a terrorist attack would be inhalational, causing a distribution of illness distinctly different from naturally occurring human botulism. One gram of crystalline toxin dispersed through an airborne route, could kill up to 1 million people, although technical limitations on dispersal could reduce the number of casualties (36).

Development of botulinum as a bioweapon began nearly 70 years ago, when a Japanese biological warfare group fed cultures of *C. botulinum* to prisoners during the Japanese occupation of Manchuria in the 1930s. During World War II, the United Sates biological weapons program produced botulinum toxin. Amidst concerns that Germany had developed a botulinum toxin weapon, the United States made more than 1 million doses of botulinum toxoid vaccine to protect troops for the Normandy invasion on D Day. Although President Nixon ended the US biological weapons program in 1969–1970, by then other countries had performed research on using botulinum toxin as a weapon (36).

In the 1970s, Iraq and the Soviet Union continued to produce botulinum toxin even though the international 1972 Biologic and Toxin Convention prohibited research and production of biological weapons. Following the breakup of the Soviet Union, several nations attempting to develop biological weapons recruited thousands of scientists previously working in the Soviet bioweapons program. Following the 1991 Persian Gulf War, Iraq admitted to the United Nations that it had produced a large supply of botulinum toxin, three times the amount necessary to kill the world's population through inhalation (36). Between 1990 and 1995, on at least three different occasions, the Japanese cult "Aum Shinrikyo" dispersed botulinum toxin aerosols in downtown Tokyo, other locations in Japan and at US military installations in Japan. Fortunately, none of these attacks succeeded because of faulty technique, aerosol generating equipment failure or internal sabotage (36).

In spite of potential technical difficulties, terrorists are most likely to use an aerosolized form of botulinum toxin to inflict the greatest number of casualties most efficiently. A successful point source aerosol release could incapacitate or kill 10% of people within 0.5 km downwind of the release (36). Terrorists could also use food as a vehicle for the toxin. Although food contamination would cause fewer casualties compared to an aerosol release, it would be more difficult to distinguish a food-borne attack from naturally occurring food-borne botulism. Contamination of public water supplies is unlikely for three reasons:

- Standard water treatments, such as chlorination and aeration, would rapidly inactivate the toxin (36,37)
- The slow turnover of water in larger reservoirs would effectively dilute the toxin, requiring a prohibitively large inoculum to be effective (36)
- Toxin applied to bodies of freshwater would be naturally inactivated in 3–6 days (37)

Terrorists are unlikely to use therapeutic, cosmetic botulinum toxin (FDA approved in 2002) because the commercial preparation contains only 0.3% of the injectable lethal dose and 0.005% of the lethal oral dose (37).

Clinical Presentation and Diagnosis

The clinical presentation of human botulism depends on the route of exposure and the rate and amount of toxin absorption. Food-borne botulism has an incubation period ranging from as early as 2 h or as long as 8 days after toxin ingestion (36), although most cases have an onset from 12 to 72 h. Unfortunately, we know little about the incubation period for inhalational botulism, because so few cases have occurred. In 1962, three veterinary personnel developed botulism following exposure to aerosolized botulin toxin coating the fur of laboratory animals. The time to onset of symptoms in the three cases was approximately 72 h (36), but the dose was probably small. Monkey studies revealed onset times of 12–80 h following aerosol exposures to 4–7 times the median lethal dose (36).

Once the toxin is absorbed, regardless of the route of exposure, the toxin travels by bloodstream to peripheral cholinergic synapses, essentially the neuromuscular junction, where it irreversibly binds and blocks acetylcholine release (36). As a result, all forms of human botulism, including natural and inhalational forms, result in the same neurologic symptoms. In naturally occurring food-borne botulism, bacterial metabolites besides toxin found in contaminated food may cause gastrointestinal symptoms, including abdominal cramps, nausea, vomiting, and diarrhea (36). These gastrointestinal symptoms may precede the neurologic symptoms. However, the intentional use of purified botulinum toxin may not cause gastrointestinal symptoms (36).

Neurologic symptoms develop acutely, with a symmetric, descending, flaccid paralysis beginning with the bulbar musculature (36). The presentation always includes multiple cranial nerve palsies. Severity of the disease may vary from patient to patient, with some mildly affected while others suffer from such severe paralysis that they appear comatose and require ventilatory support for months (36). The greater the amount of toxin absorbed, the more rapid the onset and severity of the paralysis. Recovery can take weeks or months, because new motor axons must reinnervate paralyzed muscle fibers (36).

Patients with botulism classically present with difficulty seeing, speaking, and swallowing (36). Clinical features of botulism include:

- Symmetrical cranial neuropathies, such as ptosis, weakened jaw clench, dysarthria, dysphonia and dysphagia, and often enlarged or sluggishly reactive pupils
- Blurred vision or diplopia
- Symmetric descending weakness in a proximal to distal pattern
- Respiratory dysfunction from respiratory muscle paralysis or upper airway obstruction
- Dry mouth and injected pharynx resulting from peripheral parasympathetic cholinergic blockade
- No sensory deficit except for rare circumoral and peripheral paresthesias secondary to hyperventilation as patients become anxious from paralysis
- No fever (botulism is an intoxication); patients can become afebrile if they develop a secondary infection, such as aspiration pneumonia
  (Adapted by permission from Arnon SS, et al. (36) Copyright© 2001, American Medical Association. All Rights Reserved.)

As the paralysis extends, patients lose head control, become hypotonic and develop generalized weakness. Dysphagia and loss of the gag reflex may necessitate intubation and usually mechanical ventilation. Deep tendon reflexes, present initially, gradually diminish, and patients may develop constipation. The case fatality rate is 60% without respiratory support. Death results from upper airway obstruction due to pharyngeal and upper airway muscle paralysis and inadequate tidal volume due to diaphragmatic and accessory respiratory muscle paralysis (36). Botulinum toxin does not penetrate the brain, so severely ill patients are not confused or obtunded. However, the associated bulbar palsies create communication difficulties and can make patients appear lethargic. Physicians can recognize botulism by its classic triad (36):

- Paralysis in symmetric, descending pattern with bulbar palsies more prominent: the "4 Ds"–diplopia, dysarthria, dysphonia, and dysphagia)
- Absence of fever
- Patient appears alert with normal mental status
  (Adapted by permission from Arnon SS, et al. (36) Copyright© 2001, American Medical Association. All Rights Reserved.)

Early recognition of an intentional airborne release of botulinum toxin requires heightened clinical suspicion. Certain features are particularly suggestive (36):

- Outbreak of a large number of cases of people with symptoms described above
- Outbreak associated with an unusual type of botulinum toxin, such as type C, D, F, or G, or type E not associated with seafood
- Although outbreak victims share geography in common (for example, airport, or work location) they lack a common dietary exposure
- Outbreaks occurring simultaneously in different locations without a common source
  (Adapted by permission from Arnon SS, et al. (36) Copyright© 2001, American Medical Association. All Rights Reserved.)

Clinicians seeing patients with findings suggestive of botulism should take a careful travel history, activity history, and a dietary history. They should ask patients if they know of anyone with similar symptoms. A single case of suspected botulism is a potential public health emergency because it reflects the possibility of contaminated food, available to others, or a release of aerosolized toxin. Therefore, clinicians must immediately report suspect cases to their hospital epidemiologist and, as required by law, to their local and state public health departments, who can coordinate shipping of antitoxin, laboratory testing and epidemiologic investigation. Given the potential public health implications of natural or terrorist-cause bioterrorism, clinicians should be prompt and persistent (36) in notifying their local and state health departments immediately when they encounter a suspect case.

Clinicians most often confuse botulism with a polyradiculoneuropathy, such as Guillain–Barré or Miller Fisher syndrome, myasthenia gravis or central nervous system disease (36) (see Table 2.14). In the United States, a cluster of cases of flaccid paralysis is more likely secondary to botulism than to Guillain–Barré syndrome or polio. In addition, compared to other causes of flaccid paralysis, unique features of botulism include (36):

- Cranial nerve palsies more severe and out of proportion to milder weakness and hypotonia from the neck down

Table 2.14 Common conditions confused with botulism

Conditions	Features that distinguish conditions from botulism
Common misdiagnoses	
Guillain–Barré syndrome[a] and its variants, especially Miller–Fisher syndrome	History of antecedent infection, paresthesias; often ascending paralysis; early areflexia; eventual CSF protein increase; EMG findings
Myasthenia gravis[a]	Recurrent paralysis; EMG findings; sustained response to anticholinesterase therapy
Stroke[a]	Paralysis often asymmetric; abnormal CNS image
Intoxication with depressants (e.g., acute ethanol intoxication), organophosphates, carbon monoxide, or nerve gas	History of exposure, excessive drug levels detected in body fluids
Lambert–Eaton syndrome	Increased strength with sustained contraction; evidence of lung carcinoma; EMG findings similar to botulism
Tick paralysis	Paresthesias; ascending paralysis; tick attached to skin
Other misdiagnoses	
Poliomyelitis	Antecedent febrile illness; asymmetric paralysis; CSF pleocytosis
CNS infections, especially of the brainstem	Mental status changes; CSF and EEG abnormalities
CNS tumor	Paralysis often asymmetric; abnormal CNS image
Streptococcal pharyngitis (pharyngeal erythema can occur in botulism)	Absence of bulbar palsies; positive rapid antigen test result or throat culture
Psychiatric illness[a]	Normal EMG in conversion paralysis
Viral syndrome	Absence of bulbar palsies and flaccid paralysis
Inflammatory myopathy[a]	Elevated creatine kinase levels
Diabetic complications[a]	Sensory neuropathy; few cranial nerve palsies
Hyperemesis gravidarum[a]	Absence of bulbar palsies and acute flaccid paralysis
Hypothyroidism[a]	Abnormal thyroid function test results
Laryngeal trauma[a]	Absence of flaccid paralysis; dysphonia without bulbar palsies
Overexertion[a]	Absence of bulbar palsies and acute flaccid paralysis

Source: Reprinted with permission from (36) Botulinum toxin as a biological weapon: medical and public health management. JAMA Feb 2001; 285(8): 1059–1070. Copyright© 2001 American Medical Association. All rights reserved. *CSF* cerebrospinal fluid, *EMG* electromyogram, *CNS* central nervous system, *EEG* electroencephalogram

[a]Misdiagnoses made in a large outbreak of botulism

- Symmetrical distribution of paralysis
- No sensory nerve involvement

   (Adapted by permission from Arnon SS, et al. (36) Copyright© 2001, American Medical Association. All Rights Reserved.)

Another condition that could be confused with botulism is nerve agent and/or atropine poisoning (28). Unlike botulinum toxin, which results in decreased secretions, nerve agent poisoning (see Chap. 3) causes patients to develop copious respiratory secretions and miotic pupils. As compared to the clear sensorium of botulism patients, atropine overdose causes nervous system excitation, including hallucinations and delirium, even though the mucous membranes are dry and patients have mydriasis (see Chap. 3).

Laboratory testing for botulism is only available at the CDC and some state public health laboratories. Physicians should not attempt to culture or identify the organism, nor should they attempt to perform a toxin analysis (37). Instead, they should work with their local and state public health officials, including the state public health laboratory, who will assist them in appropriate specimen collection and shipment. Higher-level laboratories will not accept clinical specimens without approval from the appropriate public health authorities (37).

The mouse bioassay is the standard diagnostic laboratory test for botulism (36). The procedure detects whether a type-specific antitoxin protects the mice against any botulinum toxin that may be present in the clinical specimen. The bioassay, which takes 1–2 days to complete (range 6–96 h), can detect 0.03 ng of botulinum toxin. In addition to the bioassay, anaerobic cultures of clinical specimens can isolate the organism in 7–10 days (range 5–21) days, but a mouse bioassay is necessary to confirm that the culture isolates produced the toxin (36).

Because terrorist-caused botulism would most likely be food-borne or inhalational, acceptable specimens include feces, gastric aspirate/vomitus, serum, suspected food, and environmental samples (37). Feces, gastric aspirates, or vomitus may be helpful for detecting both food-borne and inhalational botulinum toxin. A walnut-sized, 10–50 g stool sample, placed in a sterile, unbreakable, carefully labeled container, should be sufficient. Enemas are an acceptable alternative for constipated patients. To avoid diluting the toxin and confounding the mouse bioassay, a minimal amount of sterile, nonbacteriostatic water should be used. A 20 ml sample, placed in a sterile, unbreakable, carefully labeled container, should be sufficient. Similarly, 20 ml of gastric aspirate and vomitus, placed in the same type of container, is appropriate.

Clinicians caring for patients suspected of having botulism should obtain serum samples as soon as possible after the onset of symptoms. To avoid invalidating the mouse bioassay, they should obtain specimens before administering antitoxin. Serum volumes less than 3 ml will provide inconclusive results in the mouse bioassay. Therefore, at least 10 ml of serum (20 ml of whole blood), placed in a red top or serum separator tube, without anticoagulant, is an appropriate specimen. Sending whole blood is not acceptable, because it typically undergoes hemolysis during transport (37).

Several medications, including anticholinesterases such as pyridostigmine bromide, are toxic to mice, but can be dialyzed from samples before testing. To avoid interfering with the mouse bioassay, a list of the patient's medications should accompany any diagnostic samples sent. All specimens require refrigeration at 4°C (37).

In the event of a covert food-borne release of botulinum toxin, the epidemiologic analysis may reveal identify the suspect food, and public health authorities will most likely obtain the appropriate food specimens, if still available. Suspected foods require refrigeration before retrieval. Likewise, public health authorities will be responsible for obtaining the appropriate environmental swabs in the event of a food-borne or aerosol release of botulinum toxin.

Routine laboratory tests are not useful in confirming botulism. Without secondary complications, serum electrolytes, renal and liver function tests, urinalyses and electrocardiograms will be normal (38). However, several other diagnostic tests may be useful in differentiating botulism from other neurologic illnesses (see Table 2.14). Botulism has characteristic electromyographic findings, including normal nerve conduction velocity, normal sensory nerve function, a pattern of brief, small amplitude motor potentials and an incremental response (facilitation) to repetitive stimulation at 50 Hz (36). However, in the event of a large outbreak, the demand for electrophysiologic studies will overwhelm available diagnostic resources.

Cerebrospinal fluid is normal in botulism but usually abnormal with other causes of neurologic illnesses. Brain, spine, and chest imaging may reveal other causes of the neurologic symptoms, such as hemorrhage, inflammation or neoplasm (36). Myasthenia gravis patients with paralysis will obtain brief relief from a test dose of edrophonium chloride, whereas a close inspection of the skin may reveal the cause of tick paralysis (36).

These diagnostic tests may be useful in differentiating sporadic cases of botulism or limited botulism outbreaks from other causes. However, a large outbreak of flaccid paralysis is likely to overwhelm the availability of diagnostic testing. Because none of the other neurologic symptoms easily confused with botulism is likely to be associated with large numbers of cases, whether or not diagnostic tests are available, physicians should suspect a deliberate release of botulinum toxin in a large outbreak of flaccid paralysis.

An unrecognized outbreak of botulism in Canada in the 1990s, secondary to a contaminated restaurant condiment, illustrates the difficulties physicians may have in identifying a covert terrorist attack involving botulinum toxin. Over a 6-week period, before the outbreak was recognized, the restaurant continued to serve the contaminated condiment, resulting in 28 cases from two countries, all misdiagnosed. Only a retrospective analysis revealed the etiology, and that occurred only after physicians made the correct diagnosis in a mother and daughter when they returned to their home community 2000 miles away. Until then, physicians misdiagnosed four cases (14%) as suffering from psychiatric disease, including factitious symptoms.

The confusion between conversion reactions and paralysis from botulinum toxin could occur in both directions. If many casualties followed the intentional, covert release of botulinum toxin, nonexposed people could develop a hysterical paralysis as a conversion reaction secondary to anxiety. Clinicians will need to be vigilant in differentiating clinical botulism from hysterical paralysis in otherwise healthy patients.

Treatment

Although improved supportive care and prompt administration of antitoxin have reduced botulism's case-fatality rate, botulism paralysis can persist for weeks or months, requiring continued fluid and nutritional care, assisted ventilation and treatment of complications such as nosocomial infections, decubitus ulcers and deep venous thrombosis (28,36). Complete resolution of symptoms can take up to a year.

Initial treatment includes supportive care and passive immunization with equine antitoxin. The antitoxin is effective only early in the illness course, when the toxin is in the circulation, available for neutralization. Once symptoms cease progressing, the toxin is no longer present in the circulation and the antitoxin is ineffective. Patients must therefore receive the antitoxin at the first suspicion of botulism to minimize neurologic damage, and clinicians should not delay administration for microbiological testing. If the paralysis is unquestionably improving from maximal paralysis at the time of diagnosis, the antitoxin can be withheld. The antitoxin will not reverse already existing paralysis. The antitoxin may be especially helpful in food-borne cases, when the toxin continues to be absorbed through the intestine (28) and where there are no data regarding the effectiveness of using activated charcoal to reduce absorption (36).

Clinicians can obtain licensed equine antitoxin from the CDC through their state and local health departments. The CDC Web site and the Association of State and Territorial Health Officials Web site contain directories for state health departments at http://www.cdc.gov/other.htm#states and http://astho.org. The licensed vaccine is effective against the most common toxin types (A, B, and E) causing human botulism. The US Army has an investigational heptavalent (ABCDEFG) antitoxin effective against other toxin types. However, the time necessary to determine the correct toxin type makes this vaccine less useful in an outbreak (28,36).

Because the recommended dosage has changed over time, clinicians should review the package insert with public health authorities before administering the equine antitoxin. At this time, the dose of licensed antitoxin is a single 10 mL vial per patient, diluted 1:10 in 0.9% saline solution and administered through a slow intravenous infusion (36). The licensed antitoxin and the investigational heptavalent vaccine both contain amounts neutralizing antibody far greater than the highest serum toxin levels found in food-borne botulism. Therefore, patients should not require additional doses. Retesting serum for the presence of toxin can confirm the adequacy of neutralization if the clinician is concerned that the patient suffered an inordinately large exposure in an attack (36).

Because the antitoxin is a horse serum product, the most likely adverse reactions include hypersensitivity reactions, such as anaphylaxis, serum sickness, and urticaria. Unfortunately, the literature does not contain much information on botulinum antitoxin safety. From 1967 to 1977, when doses were larger than today, the frequency of hypersensitivity reactions was approximately 9%. During that time, 2% of recipients developed anaphylaxis within 10 min of receiving the antitoxin. In

1991, the investigational heptavalent antitoxin caused serum sickness in one recipient and mild hypersensitivity reactions in nine others out of 50 receiving the vaccine in an outbreak of type E food-borne botulism in Egypt (36). Since pregnant women and children have received equine antitoxin without short-term adverse effects, they should receive the standard treatment, including antitoxin (36). For fetuses, the safety of exposure to equine antitoxin is unknown. Although treatment with the investigational human-derived neutralizing antitoxin would reduce the risk of allergic reactions in pregnant women, the product is limited to suspected cases of infant botulism (36).

Because of the possibility of severe reactions, clinicians administering equine antitoxin must screen patients for hypersensitivity before administering the full dose of equine antitoxin. To screen, they should administer a small challenge dose by skin testing. Skin testing requires injecting 0.1 mL of a 1:10 dilution of the anti-toxin, using sterile physiological saline, intradermally in the forearm, using a 26 or 27 gauge needle and monitoring the site for 20 min. Any of the following reactions characterizes a positive skin test (28):

- Hyperemic areola at the injection site ≥ 0.5 cm
- Fever or chills
- Hypotension with a decrease of systolic or diastolic pressure of >20 mmHg
- Skin rash
- Respiratory difficulty
- Nausea or vomiting
- Generalized rash

Patients experiencing any of these reactions should not receive equine botulinum antitoxin. Instead, they should receive desensitization through administration of 0.01–0.1 mL of antitoxin subcutaneously, doubling the previous dose every 20 min, until they can tolerate 1.0–2.0 mL without any marked reaction (28). If available, although unlikely in an outbreak situation, an experience allergist should perform the desensitization.

Regardless of whether the patient requires desensitization, when administering the full dose intravenously, diphenhydramine and epinephrine must be available for rapid administration in case of an adverse reaction (28).

Supportive care may include hydration, enteral tube or parenteral nutrition, nasogastric suctioning for ileus, bowel and bladder care, prevention and treatment of decubitus ulcers, prevention and treatment of deep venous thromboses, intensive care, mechanical ventilation, treatment of secondary infections, and monitoring for impending respiratory failure (36,38).

Appropriate positioning may help reduce secondary complications. Although reverse Trendelenburg positioning with cervical vertebral support may be helpful for nonventilated infants, its applicability to adults with botulism is unknown (36). However, positioning the adult patient in reverse Trendelenburg makes sense because it can improve ventilation in two ways. It may reduce the amount of oral secretions entering the airway, and it may improve respiratory excursion by suspending more of the weight of the abdominal contents away from the diaphragm. Other positions, such as supine or semirecumbent positions, can have a detrimental effect on respiratory excursion and airway clearance, especially in obese patients. When using the reverse Trendelenburg position, the angle should be 20–25° (36).

Monitoring for impending respiratory failure should include continued assessment of the adequacy of gag and cough reflexes, oxygen saturation, vital capacity and inspiratory force. Control of oropharyngeal secretions is essential. Patients at risk for hypoventilation usually develop airway obstruction or aspiration. In patients with botulism, deterioration of respiratory function is an indication for controlled, anticipatory ventilation. The proportion of patients requiring mechanical ventilation has varied from 20% in a food-borne outbreak to 60% in infant botulism.

Clearly, in a large outbreak, the demand for mechanical ventilation, intensive care unit beds, and skilled personnel could overwhelm available resources. Chapter 6 will discuss the role that physicians can play in addressing the skilled workforce needs during a mass disaster.

Although antibiotics are not effective in treating botulism, patients with botulism may develop secondary infections requiring antibiotic treatment. Because aminoglycosides and clindamycin can exacerbate neuromuscular blockage, they are contraindicated for treating secondary infections (36).

Prevention

The presence of neutralizing antibody in the bloodstream, developed through either passive or active immunization could prevent botulism. Administering equine antitoxin or human hyperimmune globulin would provide passive immunity, whereas immunization with the toxoid could provide long-term active immunity. Authorities do not recommend using either approach for prophylaxis at this time for several reasons. Equine antitoxin is scarce (and expensive) and the risks of adverse reactions generally outweigh the benefits of prophylactic use. However, the decision whether or not to use the antitoxin becomes more difficult when facing a situation involving known exposure of people who are not yet ill. In a primate study, 7/7 asymptomatic monkeys given antitoxin after exposure to aerosolized botulinum toxin survived, whereas 2/4 monkeys treated after the development of neurologic signs died (36). Given the scarcity, expense and health risk of the antitoxin, the current practice in food-borne outbreaks is to closely monitor exposed, asymptomatic patients, and treat them at the first sign of illness (36). In the event of a large, terrorist-caused outbreak, the recommendation would have to be similar: exposed asymptomatic people should receive close medical observation close to critical care services (36).

Active immunization, capable of permanently eliminating the hazard posed by botulinum toxin, is available in the United State, but limited to certain populations. The CDC distributes an investigational pentavalent (ABCDE) botulinum toxoid to laboratory workers and military troops considered at risk for exposure. The heptavalent vaccine requires a primary series of injections at 0, 2, and 12 weeks, followed by a yearly booster. The vaccine has induced protective antibody levels in more than 90% or recipients after the 1-year booster (38). Although side effects tend to be mild, they increase with subsequent injections. Two to four percent of recipients report erythema, edema, or induration at the injection site, peaking in 24–48 h. After the second or third dose, 7–10% of recipients experience local reactions, and up to 20% experience local reactions after booster doses. Up to 3% of recipients develop systemic reactions, including fever, malaise, headache, and myalgia. Serious local and systemic reactions are rare.

Although more than 3,000 laboratory workers have received the pentavalent vaccine over the past 30 years, it is not administered broadly for several reasons. The toxoid is relatively scarce, expensive, requires several injections, has the side effects described previously, and the natural disease is very rare. The drawbacks of immunizing the entire population clearly outweigh the expense of preventing a very small number of cases. In addition, active immunity to botulinum toxin would preclude the use of the toxin for other medicinal purposes (36). The heptavalent vaccine would not be helpful postexposure in an outbreak scenario, because the toxoid requires several injections over several months to induce immunity. A recombinant vaccine, which may overcome these limitations, is in development (36).

Theoretically, decontamination of a site after an aerosolized or food-borne release of botulinum toxin might prevent additional exposures. Botulinum toxin is easily inactivated in the environment with bleach or heat. Unfortunately, recognition of a covert release would probably occur long after decontamination would be helpful. If epidemiologic investigation identified a possible food source, and if the food were still available in the distribution chain, public health authorities would remove the food from potential consumers and submit it for laboratory testing.

Atmospheric conditions and particle size determine the persistence of aerosolized toxin in the environment. Temperature and humidity extremes facilitate toxin degradation, and smaller particles dissipate more quickly into the atmosphere. Studies estimate that aerosolized toxin would decay between less than 1 and 4% per minute. At a 1% decay rate, insubstantial amounts of toxin would remain after 2 days (36). Although botulinum toxin can penetrate mucosal surfaces, it cannot penetrate intact skin. If a release were recognized or announced, and authorities anticipated potential airborne exposure, people could protect themselves by covering their mouths and noses with clothing, such as underwear, shirts, scarfs, or handkerchiefs. In addition, after exposure, washing with soap and water would decontaminate clothing, and a 0.1% hypochlorite bleach solution would be effective on contaminated objects and surfaces (36).

In the hospital or other health care setting, patient care requires standard precautions. Botulism patients do not require isolation, although before definitive diagnosis, those with flaccid paralysis suspected as having meningitis require droplet precautions (36).

Tularemia

Microbiology and Epidemiology

Francisella tularensis, the organism responsible for plague, is a tiny, pleomorphic, nonmotile, gram-negative, facultative intracellular coccobacillus (40,41). McCoy first recognized the zoonotic disease as a plague-like illness in Tulare County, California ground squirrels in 1911 (42). In 1922, Edward Francis described the human version of the disease now known as tularemia, hence the name of the organism (42). *Francisella tularensis* is one of the most infectious bacterial agents known, requiring inoculation with as few as ten organisms to cause human disease (43).

Tularemia, also known as "rabbit fever" and "deer fly fever," occurs throughout most of North America and Eurasia. Every state in the United States except Hawaii has reported human cases, although most cases occur in the south-central and western states, especially Missouri, Arkansas, Oklahoma, South Dakota, and Montana (Fig. 2.12; see color plate 2.12). Although the disease is endemic throughout

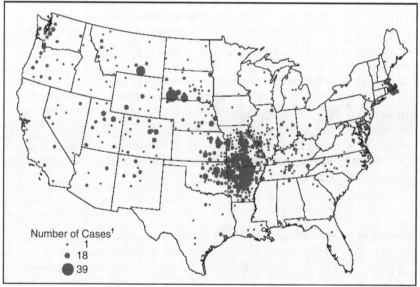

*Bases on 1,347 patients reporting country of residence in the lower continental United States. Alaska reported 10 Cases in four countries during 1990-2000.
†Circle size is proportional to the number of cases, ranging from 1-39.

Fig. 2.12 (See color plate) Reported cases of Tularemia, United States, 1990–2000. Based on 1,347 patients reporting county of residence in the lower continental United States. Alaska reported ten cases in four counties during 1990–2000. Circle size is proportional to the number of cases, ranging from 1 to 39. (From (40), public domain, Morbidity and Mortality Weekly Report 51, 9:181–185, 2002)

Eurasia, countries in northern and central Europe have reported most of the human cases (43). Given tularemia's zoonotic association with wild animals, its human distribution is almost entirely rural, although exposures with resulting cases occasionally occur in suburban and urban areas.

Within its geographic range, the organism is ubiquitous, surviving in diverse animal hosts and habitats, including contaminated water, soil, and vegetation (43). The organism can survive for weeks in water, soil, carcasses and hides, and for years in frozen rabbit meat (28). *Francisella tularensis* is resistant to extreme cold, but heat and disinfectants kill the organism readily (28). Small mammals, such as voles, mice, water rats, squirrels, rabbits, and hares serve as natural reservoirs for the organism. Vectors such as ticks, flies and mosquitoes transmit the infection through biting, but contact with a contaminated environment can also spread the disease (43). Enzootic cycles of infection generally escape human detection, but large epizootics with occasional large die-offs of animal hosts sometimes herald human tularemia outbreaks. Natural human exposure occurs through arthropod bites, handling infected animal tissues and fluids, direct contact or ingestion of contaminated water, food or soil, and inhalation of infective dusts (43). People are susceptible to infection regardless of age or gender. However, given the natural reservoirs for the disease, people, usually adult men, engaging in occupations and activities such as hunting, trapping, butchering, and farming are more likely to be exposed and develop the disease. Laboratory workers are also at risk; given the small infectious doses, activities such as examining an open culture plate can cause an infection. Fortunately, the disease is not transmissible person to person (43).

In the United States, most cases have occurred in the summer, related to insect bites, and in the winter, related to hunters' exposure to infected rabbit carcasses (40). Between 1990 and 2000, the CDC received an average of 124 case reports each year. Naturally occurring outbreaks have resulted from exposure to muskrat handling, tick bites, deerfly bites and lawn mowing or cutting brush (40). Exposures to contaminated drinking water and laboratory procedures have resulted in sporadic cases.

Tularemia as a Biological Weapon

Biological weapons manufacturers have recognized tularemia's potential as a weapon since its recognition as the cause of large waterborne disease outbreaks in Europe and the Soviet Union in the 1930s and 1940s. Francisella tularensis' reputation as a virulent laboratory hazard, with an effective dose of ten organisms, increased interest in it as a potential weapon (43).

Japanese military researchers examined tularemia as a weapon between 1932 and 1945 in Manchuria. Ken Alibeck, a former Soviet Union scientist, suggested that intentional use of tularemia caused outbreaks affecting tens of thousands of Soviet and German troops during World War II (43,44). In the 1950s and 1960s, the United States military created aerosolized Francisella tularensis as part of its offensive biowarfare program (28,43). At the same time, the United States military conducted research aimed at developing tularemia vaccines and tularemia antibiotic prophylactic and treatment regimens effective against aerosolized weapons. A component of the research program involved exposing volunteers to aerosols. By the end of the 1960s, the United States military was stockpiling Francisella tularensis as a biological weapon. Apparently, according to Ken Alibeck, the Soviet Union had a comparable program lasting into the 1990s, producing strains resistant to antibiotics and vaccines (43,44).

By 1969, the World Health Organization estimated that dispersal or an aerosol of 50 kg of Francisella tularensis over a metropolitan area of 2 million would cause 250,000 incapacitating injuries, including 19,000 deaths. Given the nature of the infection, the illness would persist for several weeks, with relapses occurring over several months. Vaccination would partially protect only a small subset of individuals. The CDC has estimated the economic cost of a tularemia attack as $5.4 billion for every 100,000 people exposed (45).

After the 1973 executive order terminated US biological weapons development, the United States destroyed its existing Francisella tularensis stocks. However, the US military has continued defensive research on Francisella tularensis and other potential bioterroist agents, including research on prevention, decontamination, surveillance, diagnosis, and treatment. The CDC removed tularemia from the list of nationally notifiable diseases in 1994, only to reinstate it in 2000, due to concerns about its potential use as a terrorist weapon (40). Given the historic epidemiology of disease and tularemia's potential as a biological weapon, an outbreak of pneumonic tularemia, especially in a low incidence area, should raise suspicion of bioterrorism (40). The risk of an attack by contaminating municipal water supplies is unlikely, because standard water treatments with chlorine would inactivate the organism (43).

Clinical Presentation and Diagnosis

Francisella tularensis can cause infection through exposure to skin or mucus membranes in the gastrointestinal tract and lungs, with the lymph nodes, lungs and pleura, spleen, liver and kidneys as the target organs (43). Once inoculated through the skin or mucus membranes, the organism multiplies in regional lymph nodes, and may disseminate throughout the body. The organism causes an initial tissue reaction characterized by focal, suppurative, necrosis. Bacteremia may be common early in the infection (43).

Aerosolized exposure, studied in monkeys, causes acute bronchiolitis within 24–48 h, depending on the size of the particles. After 72 h, inflammation develops in peribronchial tissues and the alveolar septa. Animals exposed to the smaller aerosolized particles developed bronchopneumonia characterized by tracheobronchial lymph node enlargement and 0.2–0.5 cm. inflammatory lesions throughout the lungs. In the monkey model, untreated cases develop pneumonic consolidation and organization, granuloma formation and eventually, chronic interstitial fibrosis (43). Humans exposed to aerosolized Francisella tularensis also develop hemorrhagic airway inflammation, progressing to bronchopneumonia (43).

The clinical presentation of tularemia depends on the site of inoculation, the virulence of the organism and the infecting dose. After inhalation of contaminated aerosol, the most likely type of exposure that would follow a bioterrorist attack, *F. tularensis* causes an abrupt onset of an acute, nonspecific febrile (38–40°C) illness beginning 3–5 days, with a range of 2–10 days, after exposure. Symptoms include headaches, chills and rigors, generalized body aches, most prominent in the low back, coryza and sore throat. Approximately half of all patients have a pulse-temperature disassociation. Patients frequently develop a dry or slightly productive cough and substernal chest pain or tightness with or without other symptoms or signs of pneumonia, such as dyspnea, tachypnea, pleuritic pain, purulent sputum, or hemoptysis (43). Gastrointestinal symptoms including nausea, vomiting, and diarrhea may occur. As the illness continues, diaphoresis, fever, chills, progressive weakness, malaise, anorexia, and weight loss ensue. Volunteer studies have shown that incapacitation can develop 1 or 2 days after exposure, and persist for days even after effective antibiotic treatment (43,46). Untreated patients can continue to have symptoms for weeks and even months, frequently with progressive disability. In other patients, however, tularemia pneumonia can progress rapidly to respiratory failure and death.

Complications of all forms of tularemia, usually through hematogenous spread, include secondary pleuropneumonia, sepsis and rarely meningitis (43). Tularemia sepsis is potentially dire. Following the systemic symptoms of fever, and gastrointestinal symptoms, septic patients may appear toxic, become confused or develop coma. Without prompt treatment, shock and other septic complications, including DIC and bleeding, acute respiratory distress syndrome and multiple organ failure are possible (43).

Before the antibiotic era, the case-fatality rate from the more severe type A strains was 5–15%; case-fatality rates ranged from 30 to 60% for patients with pneumonic and severe systemic tularemia. With modern treatment, the case fatality rate for type A strain infections is less than 2%. Type B infections are seldom fatal. Person-to-person transmission does not occur.

The ulceroglandular form of tularemia, the most common naturally occurring form (75–85% of cases), results from the handling of a contaminated carcass or from an infected insect bite. At the onset of systemic symptoms, a local cutaneous papule appears at the inoculation site. The papule becomes pustular, ulcerating within a few days. The resulting ulcer is tender, usually indolent, and may have a covering eschar. Typically, regional nodes enlarge and become tender within a few days after the papule appears. Despite antibiotic treatment, the affected nodes may become fluctuant and rupture (28,43).

Glandular tularemia, not quite as common (5–10% of naturally occurring cases) is similar to the ulceroglandular form but without the ulcer (28,43). Oculoglandular tularemia (1–2% of naturally occurring cases) is a special form of ulceroglandular tularemia resulting from inoculation of the eye. The ulceration develops on the conjunctiva, with associated chemosis, vasculitis, and regional lymphadenitis (27,43).

Oropharyngeal tularemia results from drinking contaminated water, ingesting contaminated food, or occasionally from inhaling infected aerosols. Patients with this form can develop stomatitis. However, more commonly, patients develop an exudative pharyngitis or tonsillitis, with our without ulceration. Patients with oropharyngeal tularemia, the ulceroglandular form of the disease confined to the throat, may develop cervical or retropharyngeal lymphadenopathy (43).

Tularemia pneumonia can result from an inhalation exposure or from hematogenous spread of the infection. An aerosol release could be expected to result in large numbers of patients experiencing systemic symptoms accompanied by signs and symptoms associated with one or more of the following conditions: pharyngitis, bronchiolitis, pleuropneumonitis and hilar lymphadenitis (43). However, many people with inhalational exposure will likely develop a clinical presentation of systemic symptoms without prominent signs or symptoms of respiratory disease.

Peribronchial infiltrates may characterize the earliest pulmonary findings. The radiographic presentation typically advances to bronchopneumonia. Pleural effusions and hilar lymphadenopathy frequently accompany the other findings (43). Nevertheless, radiographic findings may be minimal or absent, and some patients will show only one or several small, discrete infiltrates or scattered granulomatous lesions of the lung parenchyma or pleura. In previous studies, only 25–50% of patients exposed to Francisella tularensis aerosols developed radiographic evidence of pneumonia in the early stages of the disease, even though they had systemic symptoms (Fig. 2.13).

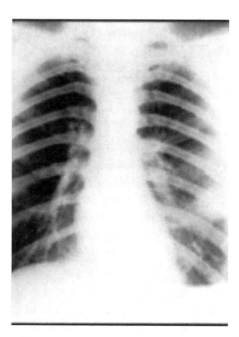

Fig. 2.13 Chest radiograph of a patient with tularemia. Note the infiltrates in left lower lung and tenting of the diaphragm, probably due to a pleural effusion, and left hilar enlargement (43). Copyright© 2001 American Medical Association. All rights reserved.)

Given its rarity, physicians and hospital laboratorians have a low index of suspicion for tularemia infection. Because of the nonspecific symptoms and absence of radiographic findings, physicians and public health authorities would have difficulty distinguishing between a terrorist attack involving tularemia and a natural outbreak of community acquired infection, especially influenza and some atypical pneumonias (43). Several epidemiologic clues that might indicate an intentional cause would include (43):

– Sudden onset of illness in a large number of people
– A large proportion of ill people will experience rapid progression of their disease from upper respiratory symptoms and bronchitis to pleuropneumonitis and sepsis
– An unusual proportion of patients with signs of atypical pneumonia, pleuritis, and hilar adenopathy
– Cases among young, previously healthy adults and children (Adapted by permission from Dennis DT, et al. (43) Copyright© 2001, American Medical Association. All Rights Reserved.)

Without specific instructions, most hospital and commercial laboratories do not routinely test for tularemia on clinical specimens. Consequently, unless clinicians suspect tularemia and order the appropriate testing, they may miss the diagnosis, or at least delay the diagnosis of *F. tularensis* infection by days or weeks. Clinicians who suspect inhalational tularemia should (43):

– Immediately obtain specimens of respiratory secretions and blood and alert the laboratory to the need for special diagnostic and safety procedures
– Immediately notify the hospital epidemiologist or infection control practitioner
– Immediately notify their state and local health departments who can then begin epidemiological and environmental investigations and arrange diagnostic specimen testing (Adapted by permission from Dennis DT, et al. (43) Copyright© 2001, American Medical Association. All Rights Reserved.)

Direct examination of secretions, exudates and biopsy specimens with direct fluorescent antibody or immunohistochemical stains can identify *Francisella tularensis*. Under light microscopy, the organism is small, stains faintly and appears pleomorphic, and is easily distinguishable from the agents causing plague and anthrax (Fig. 2.14; see color plate 2.14). Unlike Yersinia pestis, Francisella tularensis does not feature bipolar staining, and it is much smaller than the large gram-positive rods of vegetating *B. anthracis* (43).

Culture of the organism is the confirmatory test for tularemia. Pharyngeal washings, sputum specimens and fasting gastric aspirates are suitable culture specimens for patients suspected of having inhalational tularemia (43). Blood cultures seldom culture positive for patients with the disease.

Serologic tests are not helpful in suspected outbreaks of tularemia. Serum antibody levels typically reach diagnostic levels 10 or more days after illness onset, far too late for identifying or managing an outbreak. However, serologic studies may be useful for forensic or epidemiologic purposes. Most laboratory tests detect

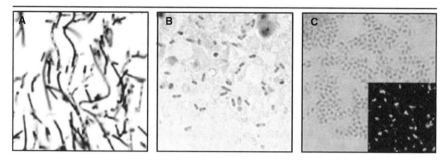

Fig. 2.14 (See color plate) Gram stain smears of the agents of anthrax (*Bacillus anthracis*) Plague (*Yersinia pestis*), and Tularemia (*Francisella tularensis*). *B anthracis* is a large (0.5–1.2 μm × 2.5–10.0 μm), chain-forming, gram-positive rod. *Y pestis* is a gram-negative, plump, non-spore-forming, bipolar-staining bacillus that is approximately 0.5–0.8 μm × 1–3 μm. *F tularensis* is a small (0.2 μm × 0.2–0.7 μm), pleomorphic, poorly staining, gram-negative coccobacillus (inset, direct immunofluorescence of smear of *F tularensis*; original magnification × 400. (From Dennis DT, et al. (43). Copyright© 2001 American Medical Association. All rights reserved.)

combined IgM and IgG antibodies. Physicians considering performing serologic studies should consult with local and state public health officials who can provide information on shipping and handling of specimens for the state public health laboratory. A fourfold increase in serum titers between acute and convalescent specimens, a single titer of at least 1:160 for tube agglutination or a 1:128 titer for microagglutination provide serologic confirmation of tularemia (43).

Notification of local and state public health officials can speed the identification of Francisella tularensis. Designated laboratories in the National Public Health Laboratory Network, including some state public health laboratories, have the capacity to preform rapid diagnostic testing using fluorescent-labeled antibodies. If alert and prepared, these laboratories can make test results available within hours of receiving the appropriate specimens.

Treatment

Contained Casualty Situation

Table 2.15 summarizes the Working Group for Civil Biodefense recommendations for antibiotic treatment in a contained casualty situation, where resources are adequate for individual case management. Streptomycin is the drug of choice, with gentamicin as an acceptable alternative in children and adults. Gentamicin is the drug of choice for pregnant women, because short courses are likely to pose only a low risk to fetuses (43). For pregnant women with a serious illness like tularemia, the benefits

Table 2.15 Tularemia treatment in a contained casualty situation[a]

Adults
 Preferred choices
   Streptomycin, 1 g IM twice daily
   Gentamicin, 5 mg kg^{-1} IM or IV once daily[b]
 Alternative choices
   Doxycycline, 100 mg IV twice daily
   Choramphenicol, 15 mg kg^{-1} IV four times daily[b]
   Ciprofloxacin, 400 mg IV twice daily[b]
Children
 Preferred choices
   Streptomycin, 15 mg kg^{-1} IM twice daily (should not exceed 2 g d^{-1})
   Gentamicin, 2.5 mg kg^{-1} IM or IV three times daily[b]
 Alternative choices
   Doxycycline, if weight ≥45 kg, 100 mg IV twice daily, if weight <45 kg, give 2.2 mg kg^{-1}
     IV twice daily
   Chloramphenicol, 15 mg kg^{-1} IV four times daily[b]
   Ciprofloxacin, 15 mg kg^{-1} twice daily[b,c]
Pregnant women
 Preferred choices
   Gentamicin, 5 mg kg^{-1} IM or IV once daily[b]
   Streptomycin, 1 g IM twice dialy
 Alternative choices
   Doxycycline, 100 mg IV twice daily
   Ciprofloxacin, 400 mg IV twice daily[b]

Source: Reprinted with permission from (40) Tularemia as a biological weapon: medical and public health management. JAMA 2001; 285(21):2763–2773. Copyright© 2001 American Medical Association. All rights reserved

[a]Treatment with streptomycin, gentamicin, or ciprofloxacin should be continued for 10 days, treatment with doxycycline or chloramphenicol should be continued for 14–21 days. Persons beginning treatment with IM or IV doxycycline, ciprofloxacin, or chloramphenicol can switch to oral antibiotic administration when clinically indicated

[b]Not a US FDA – approved use

[c]Ciprofloxacin dosage should not exceed 1 g d^{-1} in children

of gentamycin treatment clearly outweigh the low risk to the fetus. Appropriate aminoglycoside treatment should continue for 10 days for all patients.

Although tetracyclines and chloramphenicol are effective against tularemia, they are a second choice, because relapses and primary treatment failures with these bacteriostatic agents are more likely compared to the aminoglycosides. Treatment with tetracyclines or chloramphenicol should continue for at least 14 days to reduce the potential for relapse. Fluoroquinolones, already used successfully in treating tularemia in children and adults, are another promising alternative for contained casualty situations, especially in adults. Ciprofloxacin treatment should continue for 10 days. Although fluoroquinolones can cause cartilage damage in immature animals and are not FDA approved for children, short courses have not caused arthropathy in pediatric patients. Given the seriousness of tularemia infections, the benefit of treatment may outweigh the small risk in children unable to take the other preferred choices. Physicians starting patients on parenteral doxycycline, ciprofloxacin, or chloramphenicol can switch to oral antibiotic treatment when clinically indicated (43).

Neither the FDA nor the Working group approve or recommend using B-lactam or macrolide antibiotics, due to limited experience and treatment failures with these agents (43). Given the known frequency of treatment failures with bacteriostatic agents in immunocompetent patients, immunosuppressed patients should receive treatment with bacteriocidal agents, specifically aminoglycosides such as streptomycin or gentamycin (43).

Mass Casualty Situation

Table 2.16 summarizes the Working Group recommendations for tularemia treatment in a mass casualty situation. Given the lack of available resources for parenteral treatment for the volume of patients, oral agents are the preferable. Oral doxycycline or ciprofloxacin is the treatment of choice for adults and children. Children should not receive more than 1 g d^{-1} of ciprofloxacin. In a mass casualty situation, the benefits to children from short courses of doxycycline or fluoroquinolones outweigh the risks. Likewise, in mass casualty situations, oral ciprofloxacin is the best choice for pregnant women (43). If possible, due to treatment failures with bacteriostatic agents, immu-

Table 2.16 Tularemia treatment in mass casualty situations and for mass prophylaxis[a]

Adults
  Preferred choices
    Doxycycline, 100 mg orally twice daily
    Cirpofloxacin, 500 mg orally twice daily[b]
Children
  Preferred choices
    Doxycycline, if weight ≥45 kg, 100 mg orally twice daily, if weight <45 kg, give 2.2 mg kg^{-1} orally twice daily
    Ciprofloxacin, 15 mg kg^{-1} orally twice daily[b,c]
Pregnant women
  Preferred choices
    Ciprofloxacin, 500 mg orally twice daily[b]
    Doxycycline, 100 mg orally twice daily

Source: Reprinted with permission from (40) Tularemia as a biological weapon: medical and public health management. JAMA 2001; 285(21):2763–2773. Copyright© 2001 American Medical Association. All rights reserved

[a]One antibiotic, appropriate for patient age, should be chosen from among alternatives. The duration of all recommended therapies is 14 days

[b]Not a US FDA – approved use

[c]Ciprofloxacin dosage should not exceed 1 g d^{-1} in children

nosuppressed patients with tularemia should receive parenteral streptomycin or gentamycin, even in a mass casualty situation (43).

Terrorists may attempt to use drug resistant organisms in their attack. Obviously, it is imperative to obtain the appropriate specimens, perform antimicrobial susceptibility testing of isolates promptly, and alter mass treatment accordingly (43). All antibiotics useful in treating tularemia are included in the strategic national stockpile. Chapter 6 discusses how public health officials will implement mass treatment plans, and how they will involve primary care physicians.

Prevention

Tularemia Vaccine

A live attenuated vaccine, until recently an investigational drug, has been available to protect laboratory workers potentially exposed to Francisella tularensis. A retrospective study of laboratory workers revealed it was effective in reducing the incidence of acute inhalational tularemia from 5.70 cases per 1,000 person years of risk, when killed vaccine was used, to 0.27 cases per 1,000 person years of risk (43). In that study, the attenuated vaccine was less effective in preventing ulceroglandular tularemia. Although it did not appear to reduce the incidence of ulceroglandular disease, investigators felt that signs and symptoms were milder in vaccine recipients compared to controls. Volunteer studies have demonstrated that the attenuated vaccine did not protect all recipients from aerosol exposures to virulent forms of Francisella tularensis (43).

Currently, the Working Group on Civilian Biodefense does not recommend tularemia vaccination for pre- or postexposure prophylaxis of the general population for two reasons:

- The attenuated vaccine does not induce complete protection against inhalational tularemia
- It takes 2 weeks for protective immunity to develop following vaccination, far longer than the short incubation period

Consequently, the Working Group recommends continuing the program of providing the live attenuated tularemia vaccine only for laboratory personnel routinely working with the organism (43).

Postexposure Antibiotic Prophylaxis

Treatment begun with streptomycin, gentamicin, doxycycline, or ciprofloxacin during the incubation period and continuing for 14 days may prevent symptomatic infection (43). A small study in volunteers showed that oral tetracycline given within 24 h of an aerosol exposure and continued for 14 or 28 days was fully protective, whereas two out of ten volunteers treated for only 5 days developed symptomatic tularemia after stopping treatment. Once public health officials become aware that terrorists have released a *F. tularensis* aerosol, they will attempt to identify people at risk of exposure. Those exposed patients who are still asymptomatic should receive prophylactic treatment with 14 days of doxycycline or ciprofloxacin. The recommended regimen for postexposure prophylaxis for asymptomatic patients begun within the incubation period is the same regimen used for treatment of symptomatic patients in a mass casualty situation (see Table 2.16).

If health officials fail to detect the release until people start becoming ill, physicians should instruct their patients to begin a fever watch. Those who develop an unexplained fever or flu-like illness within 14 days of exposure should begin treatment as outlined in Tables 2.15 and 2.16, depending on whether the outbreak involves a contained or mass casualty scenario. Patients with tularemia do not require isolation, and close contacts of cases do not require prophylaxis because person-to-person transmission does not occur (43).

Infection Control

Given the lack of person-to-person transmission, standard hospital precautions for patient care and for disinfection of clothing and bedding are sufficient for tularemia patients. Although bodies of deceased patients require standard precautions for handling, personnel performing postmortem exams should avoid procedures that could generate aerosols, such as bone sawing (43).

Francisella tularensis can survive for long periods in a cold, moist environment. However, following an aerosol attack, it is likely the organisms would experience conditions hazardous to their survival, such as insufficient moisture and solar radiation. Therefore, it is unlikely that the organism would survive long enough for wind to create secondary dispersal with repeated exposures. Nevertheless, under certain circumstances, such as a laboratory spill or an intentional aerosol attack that may have contaminated moist surfaces, authorities recommend decontamination by spraying the area with a 10% bleach solution. After 10min, a 70% alcohol solution is effective in providing additional protection while reducing corrosion from the bleach (43). Washing with soap and water is effective in decontaminating exposed body surfaces and clothing (43).

Hemorrhagic Fever Viruses

Microbiology and Epidemiology

Several viruses, belonging to four distinct families, Arenaviridae, Bunyaviridae, Filoviridae, and Flaviviridae, cause viral hemorrhagic fever (VHF). All four VHF virus families share several characteristics (47,48):

- They are all relatively simple RNA viruses, covered or enveloped in a lipid coating.
- Their lipid envelope renders them relatively susceptible to detergents, as well as to low-pH environments and household bleach.

- They are all stable at neutral PH, especially when protein is present. Consequently, the viruses can survive in human blood for weeks after refrigeration or room temperature storage.
- They all depend on animal or insect hosts for survival. Consequently, naturally occurring human VHF has a rural distribution.
- Humans are not a natural host for any of the VHF viruses. Contact with infected animal hosts causes transmission to humans; with some of the viruses, once infected, humans can also transmit the infection person to person.
- Natural human cases and outbreaks occur sporadically irregularly and unpredictably.
- With few exceptions, there is no cure or effective drug treatment.

Arenaviruses

The arenaviruses belong to one of two subgroups, Old World and New World groups. Each arenavirus has a rodent reservoir, and a particular rodent species is responsible for transmitting each specific virus to humans. In any of the host species, the virus infects only a portion of the rodent population, frequently within a limited area of the host's geographic range. The arenaviruses do not cause clinical disease in their rodent hosts. Mother rodents can spread Old World arenaviruses to their offspring during pregnancy, resulting in maintenance of the virus in the rodent population for multiple generations (49). Adult rodents can spread New World arenaviruses to other adult rodents by fighting and biting. Rodents shed the virus into the environment through their urine or droppings. Natural outbreaks usually follow some sort of perturbation in the ecosystem that brings humans in contact with materials contaminated by rodent excretions, such as ingesting contaminated food, by catching and consuming infected rodents as a food source (50), or by contacting rodent excrement with abraded or broken skin. Inhalation of tiny particles contaminated with urine or saliva can also cause human infection.

Some of the arenaviruses, such as Lassa and Machupo, can cause secondary human person-to-person transmission, including nosocomial transmission. Humans can transmit the infection to other humans through direct contact with blood or other excretions. Airborne transmission or transmission through contact with contaminated objects, such as medical equipment, can also cause disease (49).

In West Africa, the arenavirus, Lassa Virus, causes Lassa Fever, responsible for 10–15% of adult febrile hospital admissions and up to 40% of nonsurgical deaths (48). The CDC estimates that Lassa virus infects 100,000–300,000 people annually, with approximately 5,000 deaths (50). Lassa causes pediatric disease as well as high mortality in pregnant women. Although nosocomial infections occur, most cases result from contact with the rodent species *Mastomys natalensis* (48).

In South America, the field mouse, Calomys colossus, is the host for the Junin virus, an arenavirus causing Argentine Hemorrhagic Fever. Since 1955, 300–600 cases have occurred annually in the pampas of Argentina. Other New World arenaviruses include Macupo virus, associated with Bolivian hemorrhagic fever, the Guanarito virus, recognized to cause disease in Venezuela since 1989, and the Sabia virus, first recognized in Brazil in 1990, and later associated with laboratory infections in Brazil and the United States (48).

Bunyaviruses

In Africa, insect vectors are responsible for transmitting Rift Valley Fever (RVF) infection. RVF outbreaks in humans generally follow epizootics in domestic animals such as cattle, buffalo, sheep, goats, and camels. During heavy rainfall years, Aedes mosquito eggs, naturally infected with the RVF virus, a bunyavirus, hatch, and the resulting mosquitoes transfer the infection to domestic livestock. Once livestock are infected, they can transmit the disease to other mosquito species, which can further spread the infection. Other, nonmosquito biting insects can also transmit the infection. Humans become infected following bites from mosquitoes or other blood sucking insect vectors. In addition, exposure to either the blood or body fluids of infected animals can cause infection in humans. This happens during slaughter or handling of infected animals or while touching contaminated meat during food preparation. RVF aerosols have also caused disease in laboratory workers (51).

Ticks carry Crimean–Congo hemorrhagic fever (C-CHF) virus, another bunyavirus. The C-CHF virus has caused sporadic, but severe disease in Europe, Africa, and Asia (48). The C-CHF virus is highly infective through aerosols, and hemorrhage associated with the infection has led to hospital-centered outbreaks. Arthropods are not vectors for Hantavirus, another bunyavirus subgroup. Instead, Hantavirus infections result from direct contact with infected rodents and their excretions. Human Hantavirus infection occurs in Korea, Japan and China, and a relatively new Hantavirus (Sin nombre virus) causes Hantavirus pulmonary syndrome (HPS) in the United States. From its first recognition in 1993, through June 2002, HPS was responsible for 318 reported cases in 31 states, with a case fatality rate of 37% (52).

Filoviruses

Ebola and Marburg hemorrhagic fevers are filovirus infections. In 1967, laboratory workers in Germany and Yugoslavia (including a laboratory in Marburg, Germany) acquired the first recognized Marburg hemorrhagic fever infections following exposure to blood and tissues from imported African green monkeys. The infections spread to medical personnel and family members, resulting in 31 infections and nine deaths. Since then, Marburg virus has caused sporadic, usually fatal cases among residents and travelers in Southeast Africa (48,53).

In 1976, the first recognized outbreaks of Ebola Hemorrhagic fever (Ebola HF) involving two different species of the virus occurred in northern Zaire (now the Democratic Republic of Congo) and southern Sudan. Reuse of unsterilized needles and syringes and nosocomial contact caused secondary transmission. Both viruses were highly lethal, causing a mortality rate of 92% in the Zaire outbreak (257 deaths among 277 cases) and 53% mortality in the Sudan outbreak (148 deaths among 280 cases). Since then, the Ebola virus has appeared sporadically in Africa, with small outbreaks between 1976 and 1979. Large epidemics of Ebola HF occurred in Kikwit, Zaire in 1995 and Gulu, Uganda in 2000. In 1989, an outbreak of Ebola HF occurred among cynomolgus monkeys imported to the United States from the Philippines. Although the infection caused a high mortality for hundreds of monkeys, no clinical human cases occurred. Four animal caretakers seroconverted without symptoms (48,53). Filoviruses are probably zoonotic, but the natural reservoir is still unknown. They will replicate in some bat species, suggesting that bats native to areas where a filovirus is endemic may carry the infection (53).

Flaviviruses

The flaviviruses are responsible for yellow fever, occurring throughout tropical Africa and South America, and dengue, found throughout North and South America, Asia and Africa. Mosquitoes transmit both infections. Ticks transmit the flaviviruses responsible for Kyasanur Forest Disease in India and Omsk hemorrhagic fever in the old Soviet Union.

Hemorrhagic Fever Viruses as Biological Weapons

Several factors make hemorrhagic fever viruses attractive as biological weapons. They cause human disease with horrendous morbidity and mortality, they are all highly infectious through inhalation (except for dengue) and most are quite stable as respiratory aerosols. In addition, most of the agents replicate in cell culture in concentrations sufficient to produce a weapon capable of introducing lethal doses into the air intake of an office building or airplane (2,48). Some of the agents replicate in higher concentrations, making them suitable for exposing even larger populations to lethal aerosolized doses.

The CDC has focused its efforts on four pathogens that are potential bioterrorist agents: Ebola, Marburg, Lassa, and South American VHF viruses. None of these is native to the United States, so an outbreak that epidemiologists cannot link to travel must raise suspicion of bioterrorism. Although person-to-person spread through the inhalational route in a typical outbreak situation is not common, a bioterrorist-released aerosol could cause an outbreak through inhalational exposure.

Viral Hemorrhagic Fever: Clinical Presentation and Diagnosis

The clinical presentation depends on several factors, including virulence of the specific virus, the route of exposure, the dose and the health status of the patient. All of the VHF viruses target the vascular bed. Consequently, the principal clinical features are due to microvascular damage and concomitant increases in vascular permeability (48).

After an incubation period of usually 5–10 days, with a range of 2–19 days, VHF infection causes the abrupt onset of fever, myalgias, headache, and prostration. At this stage, clinical findings may include conjunctival injection, mild hypotension, flushing, and petechiae (48). Nausea, vomiting, abdominal pain, diarrhea, cough, and sore throat are common (3). After 5 days, most patients develop a maculopapular rash, prominent on the trunk (3). As the disease evolves into full-blown VHF, patients develop shock, generalized bleeding from mucus membranes, and other symptoms secondary to neurological, hematopoietic, or pulmonary involvement (48). Bleeding manifestations include petechiae, ecchymoses, and hemorrhages (3).

Although hepatic involvement is common with VHF infection, only a small proportion of patients with RVF, C-CHF, Marburg hemorrhagic fever, Ebola hemorrhagic fever and Yellow fever develop a clinical picture dominated by jaundice and other symptoms associated with hepatic failure (48). Except for hantavirus-caused hemorrhagic fever with renal syndrome (HFRS), in which renal failure is prominent, renal failure is proportional to the degree of cardiovascular compromise. Oliguria is common in patients with VHF. The VHF mortality rate is significant, ranging from 5 to 20%, with mortality rates of 50–90% in African Ebola outbreaks (48).

Clinical features vary somewhat depending on the responsible virus. In patients suffering from the African arenavirus infection, Lassa fever, hemorrhagic manifestations are mild, and neurological complications are rare. Lassa virus infections cause mild or undetectable illness in most infected people, but about 20% of people develop severe disease. Typical Lassa fever symptoms include retrosternal pain, sore throat, back pain, cough, abdominal pain, vomiting, diarrhea, conjunctivitis, and facial swelling (50). When neurologic symptoms occur, they occur late in the course of Lassa fever and only in the most ill patients. Deafness frequently occurs in severe cases. On the other hand, for patients suffering from infection with the South American arenaviruses (Argentine and Bolivian hemorrhagic fevers), neurologic and hemorrhagic complications are prominent (48).

RVF, a bunyavirus infection, primarily affects the liver, with hemorrhagic complications occurring in a small proportion of patients. In recent Egyptian RVF outbreaks, retinitis was a frequent complication (48). On the other hand, the bunyavirus-caused C-CHF features profound hemorrhagic complications due to DIC. Affected patients may bleed profusely, with secondary transmission occurring from contact with infected blood.

Given that the natural distribution of each VHF virus is linked with the ecology of its reservoir and vectors, a high index of suspicion and a detailed travel history are essential in diagnosing naturally occurring VHF infections (48). Clinicians should suspect VHF in febrile patients with at least one of the following exposures 3 weeks before fever onset (54):

- Travel in a specific local area of a country where VHF had occurred recently
- Direct, unprotected contact with blood, other body fluids, secretions or excretions from an animal or person with VHF
- Working in a laboratory that handles hemorrhagic fever viruses

Because disease transmission is possible from contact with aerosolized excretions or contact with contaminated material in the environment, many patients may not recall either seeing or having direct contact with a rodent reservoir (48). In addition, because mosquito bites are incredibly common, patient reports of mosquito bites are not helpful in diagnosing many VHF infections. On the other hand, a history of tick bite or nosocomial exposure can be a significant clue to a suspected C-CHF (48). A history of exposure to animals in abattoirs may suggest RVF or C-CHF in a patient suspected of having a VHF infection (48).

Without one or more of the exposures listed above, the likelihood of a patient acquiring a VHF infection is remote. Even if a febrile patient has returned from an area where a VHF outbreak had occurred, the patient is much more likely to be suffering from another, more common disease, such as common respiratory viral infections, malaria or typhoid fever. Therefore, when considering VHF in such patients, clinicians should evaluate and treat patients for these more common causes while awaiting confirmatory laboratory tests for VHF (54).

Large numbers of patients presenting with VHF symptoms over a brief time in an area without endemic VHF virus should raise suspicion of a bioterrorist attack (48). Such patients would present with severe febrile illness complicated by vascular involvement, characterized by hypotension, postural hypotension, petechiae, hemorrhagic diathesis, flushing of the face and chest and nondependent edema. Other symptoms reflecting organ system involvement, such as headache, photophobia, pharyngitis, cough, nausea, vomiting, diarrhea, constipation, abdominal pain, hyperesthesia, dizziness, confusion, and tremor, are common, but they would be secondary to the vascular picture (48). If the offending agent is either the Marburg or Ebola virus, most patients may present with a macular eruption, which may be a diagnostic clue (48).

Immediate notification of a suspected case of VHF to local or state health departments and CDC is essential for rapid diagnosis, investigation, and control activities. Although laboratory findings may help, they vary based on the specific disease. For example, leukopenia may suggest VHF infection, but some patients, especially those with Lassa and Hantaan virus (a Hantavirus found in Korea, Japan and China) infections (28) may have normal or elevated white blood cell counts. While thrombocytopenia characterizes many VHF infections, it can vary. Some patients may have near normal platelet counts, and only platelet function tests might explain the bleeding diathesis. Positive tourniquet tests can help diagnose dengue hemorrhagic fever, but they are also possible in other VHF infections. Proteinuria, hematuria, or both commonly occur in VHF infections, and their absence rules out Argentine hemorrhagic fever, Bolivian hemorrhagic fever and Hanta virus infections. Although bleeding characterizes most VHF infections, hematocrits are usually normal, and even perhaps elevated if there is sufficient loss of vascular integrity associated with dehydration. Liver enzymes are frequently elevated, helping to distinguish VHF infections from simple febrile illnesses (48).

The differential diagnosis in most areas of the world has malaria at the top of the list. However, the presence of parasitemia in patients partially immune to malaria does not prove that malaria is the cause of the symptoms (48). Other confounding infections include typhoid fever, rickettsial and leptospiral diseases, nontyphoidal salmonellosis, shigellosis, relapsing fever, fulminant hepatitis, and meningococcemia. In patients with DIC, the differential diagnosis includes acute leukemia, lupus erythematosus, idiopathic or thrombotic thrombocytopenic purpura and hemolytic uremic syndrome (48).

A definitive diagnosis requires laboratory identification of the specific responsible virus. Most patients, with the exception of Hanta virus patients, will have a viremia on clinical presentation. Assays using fresh or frozen serum or plasma samples can detect and identify viruses and virus antigens. Rapid enzyme immunoassays of acute sera can detect viral antigens for Argentine hemorrhagic fever, Lassa fever, Ebola hemorrhagic fever, Marburg hemorrhagic fever, RVF, C-CHF and Yellow fever (28,55). IgM for Lassa and Hantaan infections is detectable during the acute phase of illness (28).

Enzyme-linked immunoabsorbent assays (ELISAs) for VHF infections can be performed on samples inactivated by treatment with β-propiolactone. Reverse transcriptase polymerase chain reaction (RT-PCR) tests on samples following RNA extraction using chloroform and methanol can detect most of the VHF agents rapidly. RT-PCR is particularly useful when isolation of the virus is difficult or impractical, and was effective in detecting the agent causing HPS months before it was isolated in culture (48).

In contrast to serologic tests, identification of viruses by culture takes 3–10 days for most VHF agents, and even longer for Hanta viruses. In addition, except for dengue, safe handling of the agents requires specialized microbiologic containment. Physicians should use appropriate precautions in collecting, handling, shipping, and processing specimens (28,48). Physicians identifying a patient at high risk should immediately report the case to their local and state health departments, who will help with the collection of the specimen for laboratory testing. Currently, only Level D labs, at the CDC or USAMRIID, are capable of providing initial laboratory confirmation of VHF agents other than dengue.

Isolation in cell culture and direct visualization by electron microscopy, followed by immunological identification using immunohistochemical techniques, may help if the identity of the VHF agent is unknown. In addition, immunohistochemical techniques, using formalin-fixed tissues, can retrospectively identify specific viral antigens using batteries of specific immune sera and monoclonal antibodies (48).

Treatment

Treatment for VHF infections is mostly supportive. Most patients will require close supervision, and many will require intensive care (48). Supportive care for VHF patients is similar to that provided other patients with multiple organ system failure with the additional complexity of avoiding disease transmission to other patients and staff. VHF patients require rapid, nontraumatic hospital care to prevent additional damage to the vascular bed. Transportation, especially air transportation, is usually contraindicated because drastic changes in ambient pressure can affect lung water balance. Reassurance, sedation, analgesia, and amnestic medications can help treat the restlessness, confusion, myalgias and hyperesthesia common in VHF patients. Any regimen that could increase the risk of bleeding, including aspirin and other antiplatelet or anticlotting medications, is contraindicated (48).

Patients should receive treatment for secondary infections. Unless clearly indicated, clinicians should avoid using intravenous lines, catheters and other invasive techniques that increase the risk of hemorrhage. VHF patients require attention to pulmonary toilet, specifically the usual measures necessary to avoid superinfection, and the provision of supplementary oxygen. Clinicians should avoid using steroids and other immunosuppressive agents, which have no empiric benefit, except for treatment of Hantavirus Pulmonary Syndrome (HPS) (48).

Given the diffuse vascular damage, patients will likely require multiorgan system support. Autopsies of VHF patients have revealed cardiac insufficiency. Pulmonary insufficiency is also common, and many patients with yellow fever develop hepatorenal syndrome (48). Management of bleeding should reflect that for any patient with a systemic coagulopathy, and include coagulation studies. Uncontrolled studies support vigorous administration of fresh frozen plasma, clotting factor concentrates, platelets, and the early use of heparin for preventing DIC (48). Mild bleeding manifestations do not require treatment. Severe hemorrhage requires appropriate replacement therapy as indicated. The decision to employ heparin therapy necessitates laboratory evidence of DIC and appropriate laboratory support during treatment (48).

Managing hypotension and shock is complicated in VHF patients. Dehydration results from any combination of fever, anorexia, vomiting, and diarrhea, and is more likely in hot climates. Patients lose fluid covertly through increased vascular permeability and hemorrhage. Unfortunately, VHF patients respond poorly to fluid infusions, instead developing pulmonary edema, probably secondary to myocardial impairment and increased pulmonary vascular permeability (48). Clinicians caring for these patients should consider giving asanguineous fluids, either colloid or crystalloid solutions, but should do so carefully. Dopamine might be helpful for patients with shock unresponsive to fluid replacement, but no studies are available to confirm its effectiveness. Although generally not clinically helpful, α-adrenergic vasoconstrictors are appropriate as an emergent intervention for profound hypotension. There is no evidence regarding the effectiveness of vasodilators. Likewise, corticosteroids provide another possible but untested regimen for treating shock in VHF patients (48).

Dengue and Hanta virus infections require specific considerations for treatment of shock and hemorrhage. Due to typical systemic capillary leakage, Dengue patients should receive an initial brisk crystalloid infusion, followed by albumin or other colloid if there is no response. Severe Hanta virus infections culminate in acute renal failure with oliguria during recovery. These patients require careful fluid and electrolyte management, and possibly renal dialysis (48).

Ribavirin, a nonimmunosuppressive nucleoside analogue, is effective for some of the VHF viruses. High-risk Lassa fever patients treated with ribavirin have decreased mortality, and ribavirin may reduce morbidity in all Lassa fever patients. Recommendations for Lassa fever include initial treatment with ribavirin 30 mg kg^{-1}, intravenously, followed by 15 mg kg^{-1} very 6 h for 4 days, and then 7.5 mg kg^{-1} every 8 h for an additional 6 days (48). Treatment begun within 7 days of onset is most effective. Alternative, potentially effective regimens employ either lower intravenous doses or an oral regimen, beginning with an initial ribavirin dosage of 2 g followed by 1 g d^{-1} for 10 days (48).

Significant ribavirin side effects include anemia and hyperbilirubinemia due to mild hemolysis and a reversible block of erythropoiesis. A published study in Sierra Leone and unpublished limited trials in West Africa reported that none of the patients with anemia required transfusions. Although ribavirin is contraindicated in pregnancy, pregnant women with confirmed Lassa fever should receive ribavirin because fetal death is nearly inevitable (95%) and because evacuation of uterine contents significantly increases the pregnant patient's chances of survival (48,56). Safety of ribavirin for children and infants is not well established (48).

Ribavirin, begun with similar doses within 4 days of onset, is also effective in treating Hantavirus-caused hemorrhagic fever with renal syndrome (HFRS). In addition, based studies showing its effectiveness on the Junin virus, clinicians now use ribavirin routinely as an adjunct to immune plasma in treating Argentine hemorrhagic fever (2,48). Unfortunately, because ribavirin does not penetrate the brain, it protects only the visceral and not the neurologic phase of Junin virus infection (48).

Limited studies suggest that ribavirin may be effective in treating the Arena virus causing Bolivian hemorrhagic fever and the Bunya viruses responsible for C-CHF and RVF (2,57–59). Because Bunya viruses are generally sensitive to ribavirin, it may be effective as emergency therapy for RVF, although the FDA has not yet approved it for this purpose. On the other hand, US Army Medical Research and Materiel Command (USAMRMC) studies predict that ribavirin will be ineffective against filovirus and flavivirus infections (48).

Interferon and interferon inducers significantly inhibit Bunya virus infections in animal models (60). As an adjunct to ribavirin, interferon gamma is promising for the treatment of Arena virus infections (48). There are no other antiviral agents available for treatment of VHF infections (48).

Immunotherapy, through passive immunization is helpful in treating some VHF infections. Two or more units of convalescent plasma containing adequate neutralizing antibody begun within 8 days of onset is effective treatment for Argentine hemorrhagic fever. In addition, antibody treatment is helpful in treating Bolivian hemorrhagic fever. In comparison, because of low neutralizing antibody titers and therefore the need for careful donor selection, immune plasma is less helpful in treating Lassa fever and C-CHF (48).

Someday, engineered human monoclonal antibodies may be available for targeted treatment for many of the VHF viruses. However, passive immunization therapy for HRFRS will continue to be contraindicated, because by the time the disease is recognized, most patients will have already developed an active immune response (48).

Infection Control

In Africa, reuse of contaminated needles and syringes and lack of appropriate barrier precautions to prevent exposure to blood and other body fluids (including vomitus, urine, and stool) have been responsible for transmission in healthcare settings (54). Most patients with VHF infections have significant viremia, and with the exception of dengue and classic Hanta viral infection, many have significant quantities of the virus in other secretions. Because most cases have been associated with exposures to multiple body fluids, the risk for any specific contact is not clear (54).

The risk for person-to-person transmission is highest in the late stages of illness for a couple of reasons. Viral loads are highest at this time, and exposure to body fluids is greater because of the characteristic vomiting, diarrhea, and in half of infected patients, hemorrhage (54). VHF transmission has not occurred in persons who had contact with an infected person during the incubation period, before fever onset (54).

Secondary infections among contacts and medical attendants without parental exposure have occurred. In nonhuman primate studies, mechanically generated small-particle aerosols have infected monkeys. However, epidemiologic studies involving human VHF cases reveal that the airborne route does not readily transmit VHF infection from person to person. In a nosocomial cluster of Lassa fever infections, the index patient had severe pulmonary involvement, yet investigation of the outbreak failed to determine the specific mode of transmission. At this time, we must consider airborne transmission of VHF a hypothetical possibility for procedures that generate aerosols (54). Therefore, physicians and other health care staff must use caution, but remain calm and avoid inappropriate overreaction, in evaluating and caring for patients suspected of having VHF infection. Health care providers should use appropriate infection control precautions in caring for patients with suspected VHF (54,61):

– In either a hospital or outpatient setting, place patients suspected of having VHF in a private room and initiate standard, contact, and droplet precautions. The CDC Web site has a description of these precautions at http://www.cdc. gov/ncidod/dhqp/gl_isolation.html.

- Health care staff must use barrier precautions to prevent skin or mucus membrane exposure (eyes, nose, and mouth) from patient body fluids, including blood, secretions, such as respiratory droplets, or excretions. Anyone entering the patient's room must wear PPE, including gloves and gowns, to prevent contact with potentially contaminated items or environmental surfaces. In addition, to prevent small droplet exposure, anyone coming within 3 ft of the patient should wear face shields or surgical masks and eye protection, such as goggles or eyeglasses with side shields.
- Some patients may present increased risk of transmission due to copious amounts of blood, other body fluids, vomit, or feces. In these situations, visitors should use additional protective barriers, such as plastic aprons, leg, and shoe coverings.
- Nonessential staff or visitors must not enter the room of suspected VHF patients. The facility should maintain a log of all approved visitors entering the room. Close personal contacts or medical personnel exposed to blood or body secretions from VHF patients require monitoring for fever or other symptoms during the established incubation period.
- Health care staff or other visitors leaving a suspected VHF patient's room should safely remove and dispose all protective equipment, clean and disinfect shoes soiled with body fluid. See below, under environmental control procedures, for the proper method of disposal and disinfection.
- Health care staff should use and dispose needles and other sharps according to standard precautions. The CDC has these standards available on their Web site at http://www.cdc.gov/ncidod/dhqp/gl_isolation_standard.html.
- Before performing surgical or obstetrical procedures, clinicians should consult with their local and state health departments, and the CDC, for direction regarding appropriate precautions for invasive procedures.
- Although the risk of airborne transmission is hypothetical, airborne precautions are sensible in specific situations. Hospitals should consider using airborne precautions for suspected VHF who have severe pulmonary disease or who undergo procedures that stimulate coughing and generate aerosols, such as:

  • Aerosolized or nebulized medication administration
  • Sputum induction, bronchoscopy
  • Airway suctioning
  • Intubation
  • Positive pressure ventilation via a face mask, such as biphasic intermittent positive airway pressure violation or continuous positive airway pressure ventilation

The CDC has a list of appropriate Airborne Precautions at http://www.cdc.gov/ncidod/dhqp/gl_isolation_airborne.html

Proper specimen handling is essential in preventing secondary transmission (54):

- Clinicians should alert laboratory staff about the nature of specimens before sending them to the laboratory.

- Laboratory personnel must maintain the specimens safely in the lab until they complete testing.
- Given the risks these specimens present, laboratory testing should include only the minimum number of examinations necessary for diagnostic evaluation.
- When obtaining specimens, health care staff should use appropriate infection control precautions. After placing specimens in sealed plastic bags, they should transport them in a clearly labeled, durable, leak-proof container directly to the specimen-receiving area of the laboratory. Staff should carefully avoid contaminating the external surfaces of the specimen containers.
- Laboratories should process specimens in a class II biological safety cabinet using level 3 practices. When possible, staff should pretreat serum with a combination of heat-inactivation at 56°C and polyethylene glycol *p-tert*-octylphenyl ether (Triton X-100). Although treatment with 10 uL of 10% Triton X-100 per 1 mL of serum for an hour reduces the virus titer in the serum, laboratory staff should not assume that the resulting viral titer is zero. For laboratory tests in which detergent use could alter the results, heat inactivation alone may help reduce the viral load and consequent infectivity of the sample.
- After solvent fixation, blood smears, such as those for malaria, are not infectious.
- Routine clinical laboratory testing does not include attempting to isolate or cultivate VHF viruses. Such procedures require biosafety level 4 facilities and procedures. Additional information is available on the CDC Web site at (62) http://www.cdc.gov/od/ohs/biosfty/bmbl4/bmbl4toc.htm.
- Routine cleaning and disinfection procedures are effective for decontaminating automated analyzers. Laboratory staff should disinfect analyzers after use following manufacturer recommendations or with a 5,000 parts per million solution (1:100 dilution) of sodium hypochlorite (1/4 cup of household bleach to 1 gallon of water).

Environmental infection control procedures are also essential in preventing disease transmission (54):

- Appropriately trained staff should clean and disinfect surfaces or inanimate objects contaminated with blood, other body fluids, secretions or excretions using standard procedures, as outlined in the Guidelines for Effective Environmental Infection Control in Healthcare Facilities (63) on the CDC Web site at http://www.cdc.gov/ncidod/dhqp/gl_environinfection.html.
- A US Environmental Protection Agency (EPA) registered hospital disinfectant or a 1:100 dilution of household bleach (1/4 cup per gallon of water) is effective as a disinfectant. However, for grossly soiled surfaces, such as those contaminated with vomitus or stool, staff should use a 1:10 bleach dilution.
- Staff should place soiled linens in clearly labeled leak-proof bags at the site of use, transport the bags directly to the laundry area, and launder the linens using routine healthcare laundry procedures, as outlined in the CDC guidelines to environmental infection control (63).

- Routine sewage treatment destroys the VHF viruses. Therefore, staff can dispose liquid medical waste, including feces and vomitus in the sanitary sewer. However, they should take care to avoid splashing the materials when disposing of them.
- Health care staff should carefully avoid agitating solid medical waste, such as needles, syringes and tubing, contaminated with blood or other body fluids when discarding the waste in safe containers. Staff should follow appropriate state and local public health regulations during waste treatment and disposal. If possible, on-site waste treatment using an incinerator or a gravity-displacement autoclave for decontamination can reduce handling of contaminated waste. As an alternative, off site medical waste treatment resources may be available.

The remains of patients who die from VHF infection are an additional source of contamination. Mortuary staff should minimize handling, and should not embalm the remains. Instead, they should wrap the remains in sealed leak-proof material and either cremate the remains or bury them immediately in a sealed casket. State health department and CDC should be consulted regarding precautions before considering an autopsy (54).

Anyone with a percutaneous or mucocutaneous exposure to blood, body fluids, secretions, or excretions from a suspected VHF patient should immediately wash the affected skin with soap and water. Persons with mucus membrane exposure should irrigate the area with copious amounts of water or eyewash solution. Those exposed require medical evaluation and follow-up care, especially fever monitoring twice daily for 3 weeks after exposure. Clinicians caring for exposed persons developing fever during this time should consult with an infectious disease specialist immediately (54).

Prevention

Active immunization, through an established and licensed vaccine, is currently available only for Yellow fever. A live attenuated vaccine for preventing Argentine hemorrhagic fever, effective in phase III studies in Argentina, with some cross-protection for another Junin infection, Bolivian hemorrhagic fever, is available as an investigational drug (48). Although a human live attenuated vaccine for RVF has shown promise in animal studies, more work will be necessary before the vaccine is available for humans (51). Similarly, while animal-based research efforts are progressing, no vaccine is currently available for the filovirus infections, Ebola and Marburg hemorrhagic fevers (64). Asian studies have evaluated an inactivated vaccine for Hanta virus, but the vaccine is not acceptable for US standards (48). Work is continuing on development of a Hanta virus vaccine using DNA that does not require viral culture and inactivation (65). Although research is also continuing on development of quadrivalent and recombinant vaccines for dengue fever, an effective vaccine for the public will not be available for at least 10 years (66).

Special Considerations: Intentional Contamination of Food or Water with Biologic Agents

It is difficult to predict the vulnerability of our food and water supply to a deliberate attack. Within most industrialized countries, food and water supplies are safe for consumption. However, the increased centralization of food production and water distribution in the United States gives potential saboteurs an opportunity to affect a large population (67). For large centralized food or water production and distribution systems, the potential size of an outbreak following intentional contamination increases as the contamination point gets closer to the site of production or distribution. In addition to morbidity and mortality, deliberate attacks on food and water supplies could have significant economic impact, even if the affected population is relatively small (67,68). Although the contamination was not intentional, in 1998 a US company recalled 30 million pounds of frankfurters and luncheon meat due to possible Listeria contamination, at a cost of $50–$70 million (67).

Previous examples illustrate how terrorists could contaminate food with biologic agents.

– In September 1994, members of the Rajneesh religious cult contaminated ten rural Oregon restaurant salad bars with *Salmonella* typhimurium in an attempt to influence voter turnout during an election (67). Hundreds of people became ill with salmonellosis.
– From 1964 to 1966, a Japanese microbiologist caused several outbreaks of typhoid fever and dysentery affecting over 100 people, including family members and neighbors, by contaminating food and beverages. He may have been trying to infect people so he could have access to clinical samples he needed for his doctoral thesis (67).
– In 1996, a Dallas hospital laboratory employee caused illness in 12 people by sprinkling Shigella organisms on muffins and donuts (67).

Other examples of accidental contamination demonstrate the potential size of outbreaks from contamination closer to the source of production or distribution. In 1993, an estimated 403,000 Milwaukee, Wisconsin, residents developed diarrhea due to cryptosporidia contamination of the municipal drinking water system. Four thousand people required hospitalization and authorities attributed cryptosporidiosis as the underlying or contributing cause of death for 54 Milwaukee residents (68). In 1994, cross contamination of ice cream premix transported in a truck that had carried liquid, unpasteurized eggs affected 224,000 individuals in 41 states with *Salmonella* enteritidis (67). In 2000, *E. coli* 0157:H7 contamination of the Walkerton, Ontario municipal water supply affected over 2,000 residents and caused seven deaths (68).

A few examples illustrate how the globalization of food production and distribution provides another potential source of vulnerability. United States consumers obtain more than 75% of their seasonal fresh fruit and 60% of their seafood from foreign sources (67). Contaminated Guatemalan strawberries caused an outbreak of cryptosporidiosis in 1996 and 1997, and contaminated Slovenian raspberries caused an outbreak of Norwalk virus in Canada in 1997. Frozen Mexican strawberries contaminated with Hepatitis A virus affected 151 students and school staff in Michigan in 1997 (67). In 1989, Mushrooms canned in China caused four outbreaks of staphylococcal food poisoning in the United States (67).

Drinking water is potentially vulnerable to biological (and chemical) sabotage at several locations (67,68):

– The original water source, including sites upstream from the collection point
– The water supply intake access point and the treatment facility itself
– Multiple points in the distribution system, including the pipes entering buildings and storage tanks
– Water used for food processing, bottled water, or commercial water
– Recreational waters

Federally regulated water systems serve about 90% of the population of the United States. About 53% of all drinking water in the United States comes from groundwater sources, specifically wells. The other 47% comes from surface water sources such as rivers, lakes, and reservoirs. Depending on the climate, the per capita consumption of tap water averages around 120–160 gallons each year. US consumers drink about 4 million gallons of bottled water annually; in some cities, 15–30% of residents drink bottled water due to taste concerns or fear that tap water contains chemical or infectious agents (67).

Although intentional contamination of industrialized water supplies is possible, there is no evidence anyone has been successful in carrying it out. Modern sanitation practices present several barriers preventing effective contamination of a water supply, including (67):

– Dilution
– Specific inactivation with chlorine, ozone, or other disinfectants
– Nonspecific inactivation from hydrolysis, sunlight, and microbes
– Modern filtration systems
– The small quantity of water people actually consume from their taps (approximate 1–1.5 L d^{-1})

With the exception of cryptosporidium, these factors are sufficient to inactivate most waterborne biologic agents, and they serve to protect municipal systems using surface water sources. However, contamination of wells could pose a risk, especially for the 2/3 of municipal water systems using untreated groundwater (67). Poorly operated or nonmaintained municipal water systems may pose the biggest threat to urban populations (67). In 1996–1997, disruption of chlorination due to insufficient funds resulted in nearly 9,000 cases and nearly 100 deaths from typhoid fever in Dushanbe, Tajikistan (67).

Bottled water, subject to the location and quality of its source and treatment, is not without risk. Reverse osmosis treatment, more common in the United States than in Europe, is one of the most effective protections against biological and chemical contamination (67). The 1999 Pasteurized Milk Ordinance and the national Conference on Interstate Milk Shipments have provided assurance and oversight to prevent the contamination of commercial milk supplies (67).

The keys to preventing successful biological sabotage of food and water supplies lie in tight quality control at central processing locations and effective surveillance systems that can detect disease secondary to breakdowns at more distal sites (67). Most biologic agents terrorists are likely to use to contaminate food or water cause enteric symptoms, yet less than 8% of people with gastrointestinal illness seek medical care, and fewer have stool specimens cultured (67). Public health authorities did not detect the waterborne mode of transmission or the etiologic agent of the Milwaukee cryptosporidium outbreak for 3 weeks, making it likely that smaller outbreaks could easily go undetected.

Given the importance of surveillance, primary care physicians will continue to play an important role in detecting and reporting potential food borne and waterborne illness. Clinicians seeing patients for enteric symptoms compatible with food borne or waterborne illness should attempt to identify if their patients are infected with communicable pathogens frequently associated with diarrhea and promptly report cases to their local public health officials (67).

References

1. Centers for Disease Control and Prevention. Biological and Chemical Terrorism: Strategic Plan for Preparedness and Response. Recommendations of the CDC Strategic Planning Workgroup. Morbidity and Mortality Weekly Report, 49(RR04):1–14, April 21, 2000
2. Franz, D, Jahrling, PB, Friedlander, AM, et al. Clinical Recognition and Management of Patients Exposed to Biological Warfare Agents. Journal of the American Medical Association, 278(5):399–411, 1997
3. Centers for Disease Control and Prevention. Recognition of Illness Associated with the Intentional Release of a Biologic Agent. Morbidity and Mortality Weekly Report, 50(41):893–897, 2001
4. Inglesby, TV, O'Toole, T, Henderson, DA. Anthrax as a Biological Weapon, 2002. Updated Recommendations for Management. JAMA, 287(17):2236–2252, 2002
5. Inglesby TV, Henderson DA, Bartlett JG, et al. Anthrax as a Biological Weapon. Medical and Public Health Management. JAMA, 281(18):1735–1745, 1999. Also available at http://www.bt.cdc.gov (last accessed 4/15/06)
6. Zilinskas, RA. Iraq's Biological Weapons: The Past as Future? JAMA, 278(5):418–424, 1997
7. Centers for Disease Control and Prevention. Update: Investigation of Bioterrorism-Related Anthrax and Interim Guidelines for Clinical Evaluation of Persons with Possible Anthrax. Morbidity and Mortality Weekly Report, 50(43):941–948, 2001
8. Peters, CJ, Hartley, DM. Anthrax Inhalation and Lethal Human Infection. Lancet, 359:710–711, 2002
9. Jernigan, JA, Stephens, DS, Ashford, DA, et al. Bioterrorism-Related Inhalational Anthrax: The First 10 Cases Reported in the United States. Emerging Infectious Disease, 7(6):933–944, 2001
10. Centers for Disease Control and Prevention. Notice to readers: Considerations for Distinguishing Influenza-Like Illness from Inhalational Anthrax. Morbidity and Mortality Weekly Report, 50(44):984–6, 2001
11. Centers for Disease Control and Prevention Update: Investigation of Bioterrorism-Related Anthrax and Interim Guidelines for Exposure Management and Antimicrobial Therapy, October 2001. Morbidity and Mortality Weekly Report, 50(42):909–919, 2001

12. Dixon TC, Meselson M, Guillemin J, Hanna PC. Anthrax. The New England Journal of Medicine, 341:815–26, 1999
13. Centers for Disease Control and Prevention. Use of Anthrax Vaccine in the United States. MMWR, 49(RR-15):1–20, 2000
14. Anthrax. Centers for Disease Control and Prevention, National Immunization Program. Epidemiology and Prevention of Vaccine-Preventable Illnesses. Anthrax, Chapter 20:307–322. The Pink Book. Updated Eighth Edition, 2005. http://www.cdc.gov/nip/publications/pink/anthrax.pdf (last accessed 4/07/07)
15. Centers for Disease Control and Prevention. Surveillance for Adverse Events Associated with Anthrax Vaccination – US Department of Defense, 1998–2000. MMWR, 49(16):341–345, 2000
16. Centers for Disease Control and Prevention. Notice to Readers: Status of U.S. Department of Defense Preliminary Evaluation of the Association of Anthrax Vaccination and Congenital Anomalies. MMWR, 51(6):127, 2002
17. Centers for Disease Control and Prevention. Notice to Readers: Interim Guidelines for Investigation of and Response to Bacillus Anthracis Exposures. Morbidity and Mortality Weekly Report, 50(44):987–90, 2001
18. Centers for Disease Control and Prevention. Notice to Readers: Updated Recommendations for Antimicrobial Prophylaxis Among Asymptomatic Pregnant Women After Exposure to *Bacillus Anthracis*. Morbidity and Mortality Weekly Report, 50(43):960, 2001
19. Bell, DM, Kozarsky, PE, Stephens, DS. Conference Summary. Clinical Issues in the Prophylaxis, Diagnosis and Treatment of Anthrax. Emerging Infectious Disease, 8(2):222–225, 2002
20. Shephard CW, Sorano-Gabarro, M, Zell, ER, et al. Antimicrobial Postexposure Prophylaxis for Anthrax: Adverse Events and Adherence. Emerging Infectious Disease, 8(10):1124–1137, 2002
21. Centers for Disease Control and Prevention. Notice to Readers: Use of Anthrax Vaccine in Response to Terrorism: Supplemental Recommendations of the Advisory Committee on Immunization Practices. MMWR, 51(45), 2002
22. Centers for Disease Control and Prevention. Prevention of Plague: Recommendations of the Advisory Committee on Immunization Practices. MMWR, 45(RR-14):1–15, 1996
23. Inglesby TV, Dennis DT, Henderson DA, et al. Plague as a Biological Weapon: Medical and Public Health Management. JAMA, 283(17):2281–2290, 2000. Also available at http://www.bt.cdc.gov (last accessed 4–15–06)
24. Henning KJ, Layton M. Bioterrorism. In APIC Text of Infection Control and Epidemiology. Association of Professionals in Infection Control and Epidemiology Inc. Washington, DC: Chapter 124:1–11, 2000
25. Centers for Disease Control and Prevention, National Immunization Program. Epidemiology and Prevention of Vaccine-Preventable Illnesses. Chapter 19, Smallpox: 281–306, The Pink Book. Updated Eighth Edition, 2005, http://www.cdc.gov/nip/publications/pink/smallpox.pdf
26. Henderson DA, Inglesby TV, Bartlett JG, et al. Smallpox as a Biological Weapon: Medical and Public Health Management. JAMA, 281:2127–2137, 1999. Also available at http://www.bt.cdc.gov (last accessed 4/15/06)
27. Thorne, CD, Hirshon, JM, Himes, CD, McDiarmid, MA. Emergency Medicine Tools to Manage Smallpox (Vaccinia) Vaccination Complications: Clinical Practice Guideline and Policies and Procedures. Annals of Emergency Medicine, 42(5):665–681, 2003
28. US Army Medical Research Institute of Infectious Diseases. Medical Management of Biological Casualties Handbook. Fort Detrick, Frederick, Maryland, Fifth Edition, August 2004
29. Centers for Disease Control and Prevention. Update: Adverse Events Following Civilian Smallpox Vaccination – United States 2003, MMWR, 53(5):106–107, 2004
30. Centers for Disease Control and Prevention. Update: Adverse Events Following Smallpox Vaccination – United States, 2003. MMWR, 52(13):278–282, 2003
31. Centers for Disease Control and Prevention. Smallpox Fact Sheet, Information for Clinicians, Smallpox Vaccination Method. http://www.bt.cdc.gov/agent/smallpox/vaccination/pdf/vaccination-method.pdf. (last accessed 4–08–07)

32. Wharton, M, Strikas, RA, Harpaz, F, et al. Recommendations for Using Smallpox Vaccine in a Pre-Event Vaccination Program. Supplemental Recommendations of the Advisory Committee on Immunization Practices (ACIP) and the Healthcare Infection Control Practices Advisory Committee (HICPAC). MMWR, 52(RR-7), 2003

33. Benin, AL, Dembry, L, Shapiro, ED, Holmboe, ES. Reasons Physicians Accepted or Declined Smallpox Vaccine, February Through April, 2003. Journal of General Internal Medicine, 19:85–89, 2004

34. Millock, PJ. Legal Implications of the Smallpox Vaccination Program. Journal of Public Health Management and Practice, 9(5):411–417, 2003

35. United States Department of Health and Human Services. Health Resources and Services Administration, Smallpox Vaccine Injury Compensation Program: Administrative Implement, 42 CFR Part 102, Federal Register/Vol. 68, No. 241/Tuesday, December 16, 2003/Rules and Regulations, http://publichealthlaw.law.lsu.edu/blaw/hhs/42-crf-102.pdf, also at http://www.hrsa.gov/Smallpoxinjury/frn121603.htm

36. Arnon SS, Schechter R, Inglesby TV, et al. Botulinum Toxin as a Biological Weapon: Medical and Public Health Management. JAMA, 285:1059–1070, 2001. Also available at http://www.bt.cdc.gov (last accessed 11/3/2001)

37. American Society for Microbiology. Sentinel Laboratory Guidelines for Suspected Agents Of Bioterrorism. Botulinum Toxin. http://www.asm.org/ASM/files/LEFTMARGINHEADERLIST/downloadfilename/0000000522/BotulismFinalVersion73003.pdf, last accessed 4–15–06

38. Centers for Disease Control and Prevention, National Center for Infectious Diseases, Division of Bacterial and Mycotic Diseases. Botulism in the United States 1899–1966. Handbook for Epidemiologists, Clinicians and Laboratory Workers, Atlanta, Georgia 1998

39. Centers for Disease Control and Prevention, National Center for Infectious Diseases, Division of Bacterial and Mycotic Diseases. Surveillance for Botulism. Summary of 2001 Data. http://www.cdc.gov/ncidod/dbmd/diseaseinfo/files/BotCSTE2001.pdf. Last accessed 4/15/06

40. Centers for Disease Control and Prevention. Tularemia – United States, 1990–2000. MMWR, 51(9):181–185, 2002

41. Centers for Disease Control and Prevention, American Society of Microbiology and Association of Public Health Laboratories. Basic Protocols for Level A Laboratories for Presumptive Identification of *Francisella Tularensis*. December, 2001, http://www.asm.org/ASM/files/LEFTMARGINHEADERLIST/DOWNLOADFILENAME/0000000525/tularemiaprotocol%5B1%5D.pdf, last accessed 4/15/06

42. McCoy, GW, Chapin, CW. V. *Bacterium Tularense*, The Cause of a Plague-Like Disease of Rodents. Public Health Bulletin, 53:17–23, 1912

43. Dennis, DT, Inglesby, TV, Henderson, DA, et al. Tularemia as a Biological Weapon: Medical and Public Health Management. JAMA, 285(21):2763–2773, 2001. Also available at http://www.bt.cdc.gov (last accessed 4/15/06)

44. Alibek, K. Biohazard. New Yorik, NY. Random House, 1999:29–38

45. Kauffman, AF, Meltzer, MI, and Schmid, GP. The Economic Impact of a Bioterrorist Attack: Are Prevention and Post-Attack Intervention Programs Justifiable? Emerging Infectious Disease, 2:83–94, 1997

46. Alluisi, EA, Beisel, WR, Bartonelli, PJ, Coates, GD. Behavioral Effectos of Tularemia and Sandfly Fever in Man. Journal of Infectious Disease, 128:710–717, 1973

47. Centers for Disease Control and Prevention. Viral Hemorrhagic Fevers: Fact Sheets. http://www.cdc.gov/ncidod/dvrd/spb/mnpages/dispages/vhf.htm. Last accessed 4/15/06

48. Jahrling, PB. Viral Hemorrhagic Fevers. In Sidell, FR, Takafuji, ET, Franz, DR (Eds.). Medical Aspects of Chemical and Biological Warfare. Chapter 29:591–602 Borden Institute, Walter Reed Army Medical Center. Washington DC 1997. http://www.bordeninstitute.army.mil/published_volumes/chemBio/Ch29.pdf, last accessed 4/15/06

49. Centers for Disease Control and Prevention. Arena Virus Fact Sheets. http://www.cdc.gov/ncidod/dvrd/spb/mnpages/dispages/Fact_Sheets/Arenavirus_Fact_Sheet.pdf. Last accessed 4/15/06

50. Centers for Disease Control and Prevention. Lassa Fever Fact Sheet. http://www.cdc.gov/ncidod/dvrd/spb/mnpages/dispages/Fact_Sheets/Lassa_Fever_Fact_Sheet.pdf. Last accessed 4/15/06

51. Centers for Disease Control and Prevention. Rift Valley Fever Fact Sheet. http://www.cdc.gov/ncidod/dvrd/spb/mnpages/dispages/Fact_Sheets/Rift_Valley_Fever_Fact_Sheet.pdf. Last accessed 4/15/06

52. Centers for Disease Control and Prevention. Hantavirus Pulmonary Syndrome – United States: Updated Recommendations for Risk Reduction Morbidity and Mortality Weekly Report, 51(RR-9), July 26, 2002

53. Centers for Disease Control and Prevention. http://www.cdc.gov/ncidod/dvrd/spb/mnpages/dispages/Fact_Sheets/Filovirus_Fact_Sheet.pdf. Last accessed 4/15/06

54. Centers for Disease Control and Prevention. Interim guidance for Managing Patients with Suspected Viral Hemorrhagic Fever in U.S. Hospitals. May 19, 2005. http://www.cdc.gov/ncidod/dhqp/bp_vhf_interimGuidance.html Last accessed 4/15/06

55. Bronze, MS, Huycke, MM, Machado, JL, Voskuhl, GW, Greenfield, RA. Viral Agents as Biological Weapons and Agents of Bioterrorism. American Journal of Medical Science, 323(6):316–325, 2002

56. Price, ME, Fisher-Hoch, SP, Craven, RB, McCormick, JB. A Prospective Study of Maternal and Fetal Outcome in Acute Lassa Fever Infection During Pregnancy. British Medical Journal, 297(6648):584–587, 1988

57. Whitehouse, CA. Crimean–Congo Hemorrhagic Fever. Antiviral Research, 64(3):145–160, 2004

58. Ergonul, O, Celikbas, A, Dokuzoguz, B, Eren, S, Baykam, N, Esener, H. Characteristics of Patients with Crimean–Congo Hemorrhagic Fever in a Recent Outbreak in Turkey and Impact of Oral Ribavirin Therapy. Clinical Infectious Diseases, 39(2):284–287, 2004

59. Mardani, M, Jahromi, MK, Naieni, KH, Zeinali, M. The Efficacy of Oral Ribavirin in the Treatment of Crimean–Congo Hemorrhagic Fever in Iran. Clinical Infectious Diseases, 36(12):1613–1618, 2003

60. Sidwell, RW, Smee, DF. Viruses of the Bunya- and Togaviridae Families: Potential as Bioterrorism Agents and Means of Control. Antiviral Research, 57(1–2):101–111, 2003

61. Garner, JS. Guideline for Isolation Precautions in Hospitals. Centers for Disease Control and Prevention, Division of Healthcare Quality Promotion http://www.cdc.gov/ncidod/dhqp/gl_isolation.html. Last accessed 4/15/06

62. Centers for Disease Control and Prevention and National Institutes of Health. Biosafety in Microbiological and Biomedical Laboratories. Fourth Edition, Washington DC, 1999. http://www.cdc.gov/od/ohs/biosfty/bmbl4/bmbl4toc.htm (last accessed 4/15/06)

63. Centers for Disease Control and Prevention. Guidelines for Environmental Infection Control in Healthcare Facilities. Atlanta, Ga, 2003. http://www.cdc.gov/ncidod/dhqp/gl_environinfection.html. (last accessed 4/15/06)

64. Hart, MK. Vaccine Research Efforts for Filoviruses. International Journal for Parasitology, 33(5–6):583–595, 2003

65. Custer, DM, Thompson, E, Schmaljohn, CS, Ksiazek, TG, Hooper, JW. Active and Passive Vaccination against Hantavirus Pulmonary Syndrome with Andes Virus M Genome Segment-Based DNA Vaccine. Journal of Virology, 77(18):9894–9905, 2003

66. Centers for Disease Control and Prevention. Dengue Fever home page. http://www.cdc.gov/ncidod/dvbid/dengue/index.htm. Last accessed 4/15/06

67. Khan, AS, Swerdlow, DL, Juranek, DD. Precautions Against Biological and Chemical Terrorism Directed at Food and Water Supplies. Public Health Reports, 116(1):3–14, 2001

68. Meinhardt, PL. Water and Bioterrorism: Preparing for the Potential Threat to U.S. Water Supplies and Public Health. Annual Review Public Health, 26:213–37, 2005

Chapter 3
Chemical Terrorism

Features of Chemical Terrorist Attacks

Chemical terrorism, the use of chemicals to cause human casualties or environmental destruction for political purposes, is as least as ancient as the Bible. Judges 9:45 describes the use of salt to poison soil used to grow crops (1). During the Peloponnesian War, in 429 BC, troops used smoke from lighted coals and sulfur to injure civilians barricaded in forts (2). In modern times, World War I featured the use of chemical weapons, specifically chlorine, phosgene, and mustard gas, in causing over 1 million injuries and deaths to soldiers and civilians (1). Perhaps the most horrific use of chemical weapons was the Nazi use of Zyclon B to kill over 6 million Jews and other civilian victims during the holocaust in Europe. More recently, in 1995, the cult Aum Shinrikyo used Sarin gas in attacking Tokyo subway passengers.

Chemical weapons are appealing for terrorist use for several reasons (3):

- They can cause mass casualties with minimal risk to the personnel releasing the chemicals
- Chemical weapons are relatively simple and easy to manufacture
- Resources necessary for producing chemical weapons are widely available
- They are inexpensive

Compared to biological attacks, chemical attacks are more likely to be overt, because either inhalation or skin/mucus membrane absorption of chemical agents is likely to cause immediate and obvious effects, eliciting an immediate response from law enforcement and emergency medical staff (4). Consequently, emergency medical service workers, law enforcement officers and firefighters, in addition to physicians and public health personnel, will require training in recognizing and responding to chemical agents likely used in an attack.

Not all chemical attacks may be overt, however. Covert attacks with chemicals are possible through contamination of food or water. For several reasons, authorities may fail to detect a chemical attack at the time of occurrence (5):

- Symptoms due to some chemical agents, such as ricin, may be similar to those of common illnesses, such as gastroenteritis

A. L. Melnick (ed.), *Biological, Chemical, and Radiological Terrorism.*
© Springer 2008

- Some chemical exposures, such as dimethyl mercury (neurocognitive impairment), isotretinoin (teratogenicity), or aflatoxin (cancer), may have mild or absent immediate effects, despite their long term toxicity
- Food, water, or commercial product contamination can result in illness complaints over long periods of time in multiple locations, similar to biologic attacks
- Exposure to several agents simultaneously can cause an unrecognizable, mixed clinical presentation
- Many health care providers are unfamiliar with clinical presentations due to historically rare chemical exposures

Several years ago in Belgium, terrorists contaminated chickens by adding dioxin to fat used to make animal feed. Authorities did not discover the contamination for several months, long after Europeans sold and ingested contaminated chicken meat and eggs in early 1999 (4,6). Besides pointing out the vulnerability of commercial food supplies, the experience demonstrated that our public health disease surveillance system must promptly recognize suspicious patterns of disease in animals to protect human health (4).

Several epidemiologic "clues" may be helpful in detecting the covert release of a chemical agent (5):

- An unusual increase in the number of patients presenting to physician offices and emergency departments with symptoms compatible with chemical exposure
- Unexplained deaths among young and previously healthy people
- Patients presenting with unusual, unexplained odors
- Clusters of similar illness in people with common characteristics, such as a common drinking water supply or attendance at an event
- Rapid onset of symptoms after exposure to a potentially contaminated source, such as vomiting or paresthesias within minutes after consuming a particular food
- Unexplained death of plants, fish, or animals, either domestic or wild
- A syndromic illness suggesting exposure to a known chemical, such as neurologic signs or miosis in patients with gastrointestinal symptoms or acidosis in patients with altered mental status

Depending on the route of attack and the chemical used, physicians and other health care providers may be the first to recognize illness, treat affected patients and with public health authorities, implement an appropriate emergency response to a chemical release. As with biologic attacks, physicians and other health care providers must be vigilant in recognizing an unusual temporal or geographic cluster of chemically induced illness. For example, the occurrence of similar symptoms in people who attended the same public event or gathering or patients presenting with clinical signs and symptoms suggestive of clinical syndrome related to chemical exposure should raise suspicion. Because of the public health risk, physicians must notify their local poison control center and local and state health departments if they suspect a chemical agent release. In addition, when evaluating and treating potentially exposed patients, physicians should coordinate their activities with authorities responsible for sampling and decontaminating the environment. Physicians and other health care providers able to recognize epidemiologic clues and familiar with the general characteristics of chemical agents, including the syndrome associated with exposure, could help public health and law enforcement authorities recognize and respond to intentional releases, thereby reducing morbidity and mortality (5).

General Precautions in Responding to Chemical Attacks

Depending on the chemical and the route of exposure, toxic effects will range form topical injury of the skin and respiratory mucus membranes to systemic injury due to dermal or respiratory absorption (7). Regardless of the agent used, priorities in responding to a chemical attack are the same: preserving life, stabilizing the incident and conserving the environment, including property (8). The response to chemical attacks should follow consistent principles (8):

- Containing the event
- Preventing exposure to others through secondary contamination
- Rapid decontamination
- Providing supportive care
- Administering specific antidotes as indicated

Containing the event is a law enforcement and emergency management responsibility. Containment will include isolating the area where exposure occurred, preventing anyone from entering the contaminated site and preventing people from leaving the site before decontamination. The purpose of containment is to prevent secondary contamination of other areas and people (8).

Secondary contamination, the spread of the chemical contamination to others not initially exposed, can pose a threat to responding public safety and medical personnel, including clinicians called to the site. Personnel responding to victims of chemical attacks must consider the victims contaminated until proven otherwise. Secondary contamination has caused additional casualties in hazardous chemical releases, including intentional releases such as the Tokyo subway attack. If first responders are not careful, they can exacerbate the incident by becoming victims themselves, further delaying appropriate care to others. Therefore, it is essential to protect first responders from secondary contamination. Public safety personnel, including law enforcement and fire service employees, and medical responders, including emergency medical technicians, nurses and physicians, must have appropriate training and equipment, such as personal protective equipment (PPE), to respond to hazardous events, whether accidental or intentional. Receiving health care facilities, including hospitals, must have trained staff and equipment to care for chemical casualties, some of whom might present directly without previous decontamination (8,9).

When caring for victims, rapid decontamination is an essential first step in reducing exposure. The basic purpose of decontamination is to reduce external contamination, contain the contamination present, and prevent the spread of the hazardous material. In the words of the Agency for Toxic Substances and Disease Registry (ATSDR) (9), "remove what you can and contain what you can't."

By making the victim "As Clean as Possible" (ACAP), the contamination will no longer threaten the patient or the responder (9).

Depending on the agent used in the attack, victims arriving at hospitals may still have skin and clothing contaminated with liquids and condensed vapors. These materials could cause continued exposure either through dermal absorption or through re-aerosolization and inhalation. Therefore, it is essential to remove contaminated clothing, shoes, contact lenses, and jewelry. Simply removing contaminated clothing can eliminate 80–90% of the contamination (7).

The ATSDR has developed a planning guide for managing chemically contaminated patients in emergency departments (9). All hospitals should have a plan that they have practiced in place for receiving and decontaminating these patients. Once a hospital hears that such patients are on their way, the hospital should institute a chemical emergency protocol. Hospital staff taking the call should follow a checklist to obtain appropriate information on the incoming patients, including (9):

- Type and nature of the contamination incident
- Name and phone number of the caller
- Number and ages of the patients
- Signs and symptoms
- Nature of any injuries
- Name(s) of the chemicals involved, including the correct spelling
- Extent of decontamination in the field
- Estimated time of arrival

Most states will have a designated resource center, such as a regional Poison Control Center, which can provide information for caring for specific hazardous chemical exposures, including appropriate decontamination procedures.

Special decontamination areas outside the hospital emergency department or in the field are the best locations for decontamination (7). If the decontamination area is within the hospital, its ventilation system should be separate from the rest of the hospital or turned off to prevent the spread of contamination. If it is necessary to turn the ventilation system off, the hospital should follow OSHA regulations on atmospheric monitoring, especially if health care workers are using air-purifying respirators (9,10).

Clearly, outdoors is the best place to decontaminate victims of chemical attacks, because ambient ventilation helps minimize exposure of health care workers. Through federal preparedness funding, many hospitals are beginning to purchase and practice using decontamination facilities, including outside, portable decontamination systems. If resources are limited, a warm shower nozzle, soap, a wading pool, and plastic garbage bags in a designated area outside the emergency room may suffice (9).

Essential ingredients for decontamination include (9):

- A safe area for keeping patients during the process
- A safe method for removing contaminants from the skin, hair, and mucus membranes

- A safe method for collecting and containing the waste material, including rinsate
- PPE for decontamination personnel
- Disposable or cleanable medical equipment for treatment

PPE should include (9):

- Scrub suits
- Plastic shoe covers
- Disposable chemical PPE with hoods and booties; the hood should be taped at the neck
- Polyvinyl chloride gloves, taped to the sleeves
- Appropriate respiratory protection
- Multiple layers of surgical gloves, neoprene, or disposable nitrile gloves, with the bottom glove taped. Personnel should change gloves whenever they are torn
- Eye protection

Given the layers of PPE, personnel may have difficulty recognizing and communicating with each other. To facilitate communication, personnel can wear pieces of masking tape containing their names (9).

In the ideal situation, decontamination would occur at the site of contamination. However, in a mass casualty situation, this may not be possible, and patients will arrive at the hospital still contaminated. If possible, an ED physician or nurse should meet the arriving patients and assess their condition, their degree of contamination and the body areas contaminated. Because the chemical contamination could be life threatening, health care staff should begin assessing, stabilizing, and triaging patients at the same time they begin decontamination procedures (9). Certainly, health care staff must address emergent airway, breathing, and circulatory issues at the same time they begin decontamination procedures. Once they have dealt with life threatening conditions, health care staff can attend to decontamination that is more thorough while conducting patient evaluation. Personnel must use PPE until there is no risk of exposure to contamination.

Patients with vapor exposure require clothing removal and hair washing, while those with liquid dermal exposure should receive a more thorough decontamination. Such patients present a significant risk for contaminating health care workers. Therefore, using PPE, health care workers should carefully remove the clothing, placing it in double bags. If not removed at the site of contamination, clothing removal should occur outside the ambulance or other transport vehicle, but before entry into the emergency department.

Many patients should be able to remove their own clothing, place it in the appropriate plastic bag, and do their own soap and water decontamination. If the decontamination facility is outdoors, partial tents or curtains can ensure patient privacy (9).

After removing clothing, jewelry, and contact lenses, decontamination should include gently blotting the liquid agent or brushing the dry agent from the skin, with subsequent irrigation. It is essential to remove the contaminating agent carefully, to avoid additional irritation and damage to the skin, with the concomitant risk of increased permeability.

Because intact skin is usually more resistant to hazardous substances than wounds, mucus membranes or eyes, decontamination should begin at the head, and work downward, paying close attention to contaminated eyes and open wounds (9). Wounds should receive irrigation with copious amounts of normal saline. Deep debridement and excision are necessary only if particles or pieces of contaminated material are embedded in the tissues (9). After cleaning, covering wounds with waterproof dressings can help prevent recontamination (9).

Ocular exposures require copious eye irrigation with saline or water for an extended time, while mild soap and copious amounts of tepid (never hot) water applied gently with a sponge are necessary for washing hair and skin (7–9). The decontamination process should exclude hot water, stiff brushes, and vigorous scrubbing, because these methods can cause vasodilation and abrasion, increasing the possibility for systemic absorption of the hazardous substance (9). When gently irrigating eyes, it is important to direct the stream of saline away from the medial canthus to avoid forcing contaminated material into the lacrimal duct. Likewise, gentle irrigation and frequent suctioning of contaminated nares and ear canals can prevent forcing contaminated material deeper into those cavities (9).

Contaminated children pose a special challenge, because the decontamination process is often frightening and difficult for them to understand. If possible, parents should accompany their children during the decontamination process. If a parent is not available, a nurse should accompany the child (9).

Although experts have historically recommended dilute bleach (0.5% sodium hypochlorite) for skin decontamination, with the exception of Lewisite and liquid nerve agent-exposed patients (see following discussion), this recommendation no longer stands for several reasons (7,8):

– Dilute bleach is a skin irritant, potentially increasing the permeability of the skin to the chemical agent
– Bleach can cause additional tissue damage to open wounds and eyes
– Prolonged contact time, up to 15–20 min, is necessary for inactivation of the chemical agents
– There is no evidence that dilute bleach is superior to copious soap and water washing
– There is little experience with its use for infants and young children (7)

Consequently, the use of a decontaminating solution, such as bleach or vinegar, for washing hair, is contraindicated. Instead, copious amounts of water and soap remain the optimal and nearly universal method for decontamination. Contamination from metals and strong corrosives present the only exceptions to water decontamination (8).

Health care facilities can reduce secondary contamination by removing all nonessential and nondisposable equipment from decontamination areas. Taping any surface subject to hand contact, such as doorknobs, cabinet handles, light switches, and covering floors with plastic or paper sheeting, can provide additional protection.

Taping the floor sheeting can reduce slippage, and marking the entrance to the contaminated area with a wide strip of colored tape can help warn personnel not to enter unless properly protected. In addition, contaminated personnel or equipment should not leave the area until receiving appropriate decontamination (9). An uncontaminated health care worker stationed just outside the entrance can hand in supplies and receive medical specimens for testing (9). Additional secondary contamination can be avoided by collecting runoff (rinsate) from the decontamination process for proper disposal.

The rest of this chapter will discuss diagnostic and treatment considerations for specific chemical agents. At the time that patients present to the hospital, the specific exposure may be unknown. However, it is essential to identify the chemical(s) involved as soon as possible. Information helpful for treating patients and protecting health care workers includes (9):

– The chemical name of the suspected substance
– The form of the chemical such as solid, liquid, or gas
– The duration of exposure
– Route(s) of exposure
– Potential adverse health effects
– Recommended treatment
– PPE required
– Appropriate decontamination procedures

To protect patients and health care workers, it is essential to determine the responsible hazardous chemical as early in the decontamination process as possible. Based on previous experience with hazardous exposures, the National Institute of Occupational Safety and Health (NIOSH) and the Environmental Protection Agency (EPA) recommend level B protection as a minimal precaution (see Table 3.1) before the offending substance is identified (11). However, if available evidence suggests that the substance involves the skin as a route of exposure or is dangerous by dermal absorption or corrosion, health care workers and others coming in contact with victims require the additional skin protection of Level A PPE (9).

Many of the agents and the classes of agents terrorists might use respond to specific antidotes that can reduce symptoms and hasten recovery. However, health care providers should use antidotes judiciously, because they can cause side effects and complications. For example, during the Persian Gulf War, distribution of pyridostigmine as a nerve agent prophylactic drug resulted in nine overdose cases. Autoinjectors pose a special problem, because potentially exposed people, such as troops, can use them in the field without medical consultation. During the Gulf War, over more than 200 cases of atropine toxicity necessitating medical evaluation occurred due to auto-injector administration (8,12). Some of these cases occurred because the victims mistook cooking gas for nerve gas. Clearly, health responders should use antidotes based on significant risk of exposure to specific agents (8).

Table 3.1 Personal protective equipment to prevent chemical exposures

Level	Purpose	Description
A	Greatest level of skin, respiratory and eye protection required	Positive pressure, full face-piece self-contained breathing apparatus (SCBA), or positive pressure supplied air respirator with escape SCBA, approved by the National Institute for Occupational Safety and Health (NIOSH)
		Totally encapsulating chemical-protective suit
		Chemical-resistant outer gloves, chemical-resistant inner gloves
		Chemical resistant boots with steel toes and shanks
		Disposable protective suit, gloves, and boots (depending on suit construction, may be worn over totally encapsulating suit)
		Optional: coveralls, long underwear and hard hat (under suit)
B	Highest level of respiratory protection necessary, but lesser level of skin protection needed	SCBA or positive pressure supplied air respirator with escape
		SCBA (NIOSH approved)
		Hooded, chemical-resistant clothing (overalls and long-sleeved jacket; coveralls; one of two-piece chemical-splash suit; disposable chemical-resistant overalls
		Chemical-resistant outer gloves, chemical-resistant inner gloves
		Chemical resistant outer boots with steel toes and shanks
		Optional: coveralls, chemical-resistant disposable outer boot-covers, hard hat, face shield
C	Concentration(s) and type(s) of airborne substance(s) are known and criteria for using air purifying respirators are met	Full-face or half mask, air purifying respirators (NIOSH approved)
		Hooded chemical-resistant clothing (overalls, two-piece chemical-splash suit, disposable chemical-resistant overalls
		Chemical-resistant outer gloves, chemical-resistant inner gloves
		Optional: coveralls, chemical resistant outer boots with steel toes and shanks, chemical-resistant disposable outer boot-covers, hard hat, escape mask, face shield
D	Nuisance contamination only	Coveralls
		Chemical resistant boots/shoes with steel toes and shanks
		Optional: gloves, chemical-resistant disposable outer boots, safety glasses or chemical splash goggles, hard hat, escape mask, face shield

Source: Adapted from the US Department of Labor, Occupational Safety and Health Administration (11).

Chemical Agents Terrorists Are Likely to Use

General Considerations

Chemical agents terrorists might use range from warfare agents to toxic chemicals commonly used in industry (4). Other potential chemical agents are easily obtainable, either through natural sources, such as poisonous plants, or domestic items, such as household cleaners (4). The CDC Strategic Planning Workgroup criteria for determining priority chemical agents include

- Chemical agents already known to be used as weaponry
- Availability of chemical agents to potential terrorists
- Chemical agents likely to cause major morbidity or mortality
- Potential of agents for causing public panic and social disruption
- Agents that require special action for public health preparedness (4)

Industry introduces hundreds of new chemicals internationally each month, making it impossible for physicians and other health care providers to prepare for each of them. Instead, physicians should concentrate on treating exposed persons by clinical syndrome (e.g., burns and trauma, cardiorespiratory failure, neurologic damage, and shock) rather than by specific agent (5). Potential routes of entry include inhalation, cutaneous absorption, ingestion and less likely, injection (13).

Many potential chemical agents are volatile and readily inhaled. Inhaled chemicals can cause direct injury, including asphyxia, upper airway obstruction and direct damage to pulmonary parenchyma. Other chemical agents are absorbed through the lungs, resulting in systemic symptoms. Children may be at higher risk of systemic effects due to higher metabolic and respiratory rates and increased exposure, because some of the chemical agents, such as sarin and chlorine, concentrate close to the ground (13). Direct damage from lower doses may cause airway irritation and increased secretions, which can exacerbate existing lung disease. Higher doses can cause upper airway edema, leading to airway obstruction. In addition, copious secretions, especially in infants, can cause additional obstruction. Pulmonary edema, resulting from direct alveolar exposure, can occur immediately or after delays of up to 48 h. Therefore, exposed patients will require routine airway examination to assess whether they may need emergency intubation, especially if the specific exposure is unknown (13).

The skin and eyes are the primary targets for cutaneous exposure. Cold injury results from exposure to cryogenic liquids. Different classes of agents cause skin and mucus membrane necrosis through different mechanisms: Corrosive chemicals cause an ischemic necrosis due to small vessel thrombosis and acids and alkalis cause chemical burns through coagulation necrosis and liquefaction necrosis, respectively (13). In addition, once absorbed, acids and alkalis cause systemic effects. Loss of skin integrity can lead to dehydration, especially in children. Hypothermia may occur due to cutaneous injury, the decontamination process and failure of systemic temperature regulation secondary to antidote administration (13).

Categories of chemical weapon agents terrorist might use include (4):

- *Nerve agents*: tabun (ethyl *N,N*-dimethylphosphoramidocyanidate), sarin (isopropyl methylphosphanofluoridate), soman (pinacolyl methyl phosphonofluoridate), GF (cyclohexylmethylphosphonofluoridate), VX (*o*-ethyl-[*S*]-[2-diisopropyl-aminoethyl]-methylphosphonothiolate)
- *Vesicant (blister) agents*: Lewisite (an aliphatic arsenic compound, 2-chlorovi-nyldichloroarsine), nitrogen and sulfur mustards, phosgene oxime
- *Blood agents*: hydrogen cyanide, cyanogen chloride
- *Heavy metals*: arsenic, lead, mercury
- *Volatile toxins*: benzene, chloroform, trihalomethanes
- *Pulmonary agents*: phosgene, chlorine, vinyl chloride
- *Incapacitating agents*: BZ (3-quinuclidinyl benzilate)
- *Pesticides*, persistent, and nonpersistent
- *Dioxins, furans*, and *polychlorinated biphenyls* (PCBs)
- *Explosive nitro compounds* and *oxidizers*: ammonium nitrate combined with fuel oil
- *Flammable industrial gases and liquids*: gasoline, propane
- *Poison industrial gases, liquids*, and *solids*: cyanides, nitriles
- *Corrosive industrial acids* and *bases*: nitric acid, sulfuric acid
- *Biotoxins: Ricin*

This chapter discusses several of these agents based on the Medical Management Guidelines (MMGs) for Acute Chemical Exposures (9). The Agency for Toxic Substances Disease Registry (ATSDR) developed the guidelines to help physicians and other emergency healthcare professionals manage acute chemical exposures. The guidelines, available at http://www.atsdr.cdc.gov/MHMI/mmg-n. html#bookmark02 (last accessed 5/12/06), include information on how physicians can decontaminate patients effectively, protect themselves and others from con-tamination, communicate with other involved personnel, transport patients safely and efficiently to a medical facility and provide competent medical evaluation and treatment to exposed persons. The guidelines also include patient information. Additional information on each chemical agent is also available on the CDC web site at http://www.bt.cdc.gov/agent/agentlistchem.asp.

Nerve Agents

Nerve Agents as Chemical Weapons

In the 1930s, a German scientist attempting to develop a more effective pesticide syn-thesized Tabun, the first nerve agent (13). The German army quickly developed Tabun as a chemical weapon. Following the development of Tabun came Sarin, followed by Soman in the late 1930s to early 1940s. American scientists named these German-developed chemical weapons "G" agents, resulting in the eventual designation of

Tabun as GA, Sarin as GB and Soman as GD. More stable versions of the agents, designated the V agents, arrived in the 1950s, with the British developing "Venom X" (VX) in 1952 (3,7,13). The increased stability of the less volatile and less soluble VX allows it to persist in the environment for several weeks after its release (14).

Of all known chemical warfare agents, nerve agents are the most toxic, 100–500 times more potent compared to other chemical agents (13). The nerve agents, also known as nerve gases, are clear, colorless liquids at room temperature (13,15). One of the agents, GA, reportedly has a slightly fruity odor, while GD has a slight camphor odor (16); the others are tasteless and odorless (13). The consistency and evaporation rate of the nerve agents are similar to water, making them a vapor hazard, even though they have high boiling points. Compared to the other agents, VX is less volatile, with a consistency similar to heavy lubricating oil, but it does pose a vapor hazard at temperatures exceeding 100°F (2,13). In addition, compared to the earlier G agents, VX is ten times more toxic, with a few drops on the skin sufficient to cause death (2).

Besides their toxicity, nerve agents are superior weapons because all of them easily penetrate normal clothing and all lend themselves to aerosolization (13). Significant exposure can occur through several routes, including dermal or mucus membrane absorption, inhalation, or ingestion. Nerve agents can persist in the environment for long periods, and can cause additional mortality by exposing health care workers and other responders to contaminated clothing, skin, and patient secretions (15). In addition, nerve agents are easy and inexpensive to produce and are relatively available. The Organization for the Prohibition of Chemical Weapons (OCPW) has reported to the WHO the significant amounts of nerve agents and other chemical agents stockpiled around the world (15,17) (see Table 3.2).

Mechanism of Action

Regardless of the route of exposure, nerve agents, chemically similar to organophosphate pesticides, cause symptoms by binding to acetylcholinesterase (AChE) and causing potent, irreversible inhibition of the enzyme at nicotinic and muscarinic receptors (7,13–15,18). The resulting accumulation of acetylcholine at neuromuscular junctions with concomitant overstimulation of cholinergic receptors causes a cholinergic crisis, followed rapidly by paralysis. Central nervous system symptoms and muscarinic/nicotinic effects characterize the cholinergic crisis.

Nerve Agent Exposure: Clinical Presentation and Diagnosis

The specific agent, the route of exposure and the dose absorbed determine the onset and severity of symptoms (14). Onset can range from a few minutes to 18h, depending on the extent of exposure. To best remember the clinical presentation, it helps to divide the cholinergic symptoms into three categories: central effects, muscarinic effects, and nicotinic effects.

Table 3.2 Aggregate quantities of chemical agents declared to the OPCW by its member states, as of 31 December 2002 (17)

Aggregate quantities of chemical agents declared to the OPCW by its member states, as of 31 December 2002	
Chemical agent	Total declared (tonnes)[a]
Category 1 chemical weapons[b]	
Agent Vx	15,558
Agent VX	4,032
Difluor (precursor DF)[c]	444
EDMP (precursor QL)[d]	46
Isopropanol/isopropylamine (precursor OPA)[e]	731
Lewisite	6,745
Mustard gas[f]	13,839
Mustard/lewisite mixtures	345
Runcol (agent HT)[g]	3,536
Sarin (agent GB)	15,048
Soman (agent GD)	9,175
Tabun (agent GA)	2
Unknown	5
Category 2 chemical weapons[h]	
Chloroethanol	302
Phosgene	11
Thiodiglycol	51
Chemicals declared as "riot control agents" [i]	
Adamsite, Agent CN, Agent CS, Agent CR,	
Chloropicrin, Agent OC, OC/CS mixture, MPA [sic]	
Ethyl bromoacetate, Pepperspray [sic], Pelargonic acid vanillylamide	

Source: http://www.who.int/csr/delibepidemics/chapter3.pdf, with permission from the World Health Organization.

[a] Based on figures from OPCW annual report for 2002 (*3*), rounded to the nearest tonne. Excludes chemicals declared in quantities of less than one tonne. One such chemical was the nreve-gas *O*-ethyl *S*-2-dimethylaminoethyl methylphosphonothiolate, also known as médémo or EA 1699.

[b] The CWC Verification Annex, in Part IV(A) para. 16, defines Category 1 as "chemical weapons on the basis of Schedule 1 chemicals and their parts and components".

[c] Methylphosphonyl difluoride (a binary nerve-gas component).

[d] Ethyl 2-diisopropylaminoethyl methylphosphonite (a binary nerve-gas component).

[e] A mixture of 72% isopropanol and 28% isopropylamine (a binary nerve-gas component).

[f] Including "mustard gas in oil product".

[g] A reaction product containing about 60% of mustard gas and 40% of agent T.

[h] "Chemical weapons on the basis of all other chemicals and their parts and components." The CWC goes on to define Category 3 chemical weapons as comprising "unfilled munitions and devices, and equipment specifically designed for use directly in connection with employment of chemical weapons".

[i] For chemicals declared as "riot control agents", the CWC requires disclosure of their chemical identify but not the quantities in which they are held.

Common central nervous system effects include agitation, confusion, fatigue, insomnia, memory loss, impaired judgment, slurred speech, depression, delirium, hallucinations, ataxia, seizures, loss of consciousness, coma, and central apnea. Seizures can evolve into life threatening status epilepticus (15).

The mnemonic, "SLUDGE," helps describe the prominent muscarinic symptoms:

- Salivation
- Lacrimation
- Urinary incontinence
- Diarrhea (can progress to fecal incontinence)
- Gastrointestinal distress (nausea, crampy abdominal pain)
- Emesis (14)

Other muscarinic signs and symptoms include blurred or dim vision, miosis, conjunctivitis, eye and head pain, skin flushing, diaphoresis, bradycardia, atrioventricular block, bronchospasm and genitourinary symptoms, such as frequency, urgency, and urinary incontinence (7,9).

Signs and symptoms resulting from cholinergic stimulation of nicotinic receptors in the sympathetic ganglia include tachycardia, hypertension, pallor, and metabolic abnormalities, such as hyperglycemia, hypokalemia, and metabolic acidosis, while nicotinic stimulation at the neuromuscular junction can cause muscle fasciculations, pain and weakness, including weakness of the respiratory musculature (7,14). Because muscarinic stimulation causes bradycardia, whereas nicotinic stimulation causes tachycardia, exposed patients may present with either. Although scant clinical evidence is available, two pediatric case studies of organophosphate pesticide poisoning suggest that children experience a disproportionate degree of altered sensorium and muscle weakness compared to adults (7).

The initial effects of nerve agents depend on the dose and route of exposure. A small inhalation exposure from nerve agent vapor causes a response in the eyes, nose and airway, such as miosis, conjunctival injection, eye pain, rhinorrhea, bronchoconstriction, excessive bronchial secretions, and mild to moderate dyspnea (9,13,18). Larger exposures cause central nervous system effects within seconds to minutes, including loss of consciousness, seizures, and central apnea. Death can occur within 5–10 min of a lethal dose, usually due to respiratory failure from the combined effects of respiratory muscle paralysis, loss of airway control and profuse bronchorrhea (13,14).

Mild to moderate dermal exposure causes diaphoresis and muscle fasciculations at the exposed site, as well as nausea, vomiting, diarrhea, and weakness subsequent to systemic absorption (9,18). Gastrointestinal symptoms occurring within an hour of dermal exposure are an indication of severe intoxication.

Because inhalation exposure causes respiratory effects within seconds to minutes, including rhinorrhea, chest tightness and shortness of breath, exposed patients who are asymptomatic by the time they arrive at the hospital do not require admission or treatment if inhalation was the only source of exposure. Likewise, patients with inhalation exposure exhibiting only mild symptoms, such as miosis or mild rhinorrhea, do not require admission. On the other hand, liquid exposures with concomitant dermal absorption may present with severe symptoms an hour or more after initial exposure. Therefore, patients potentially exposed to liquid agents require observation for at least 18 h (9).

Most patients who survive the acute symptoms will recover fully. However, nerve agents can cause longer term and chronic neurologic symptoms. Patients may experience an "intermediate syndrome," 1–4 days after exposure, due to altered activity at neuromuscular junction nicotinic receptors, and consisting of proximal muscle group weakness and cranial nerve palsies. Paralysis of the diaphragm and other respiratory muscles can lead to respiratory distress and even respiratory failure. With adequate ventilatory care, these patients will recover in 4–21 days. Chronic neuropsychiatric complications, which can persist for several months to years, include impairments in memory and mood, sleep abnormalities, depression, anxiety, irritability and problems with information processing (8,19). There is no evidence indicating that nerve agents are likely to have mutagenic or carcinogenic complications (8).

Laboratory tests are not helpful in diagnosing acute nerve agent exposure for a couple of reasons. Tests to detect nerve agents in urine are only available through the CDC or at five laboratory response network (LRN) laboratories across the country. While inhibition of plasma or red blood cell (more than 70%) AChE can suggest nerve agent poisoning, the normal laboratory reference ranges for AChE levels are wide and the tests are rarely available on a "stat" basis (7,20). In addition, there is no association between measured AChE activity and severity of signs and symptoms. Therefore, the final diagnosis will depend mostly on the clinical presentation, the presence of a credible threat as determined by law enforcement agencies, and the response to antidote treatment (7,20).

Treatment

Treatment of nerve agent intoxication involves four components:

- Airway and ventilatory support
- Decontamination
- Aggressive use of antidotes, especially atropine and pralidoxime
- Seizure control

Patients with respiratory compromise should receive tracheal intubation, with suctioning for excessive bronchial secretions. If the patient's condition precludes intubation, a surgical airway is necessary. Apneic patients require immediate administration of antidotes, including atropine. Some patients will exhibit resistance to ventilation because of bronchial constriction and spasm. This resistance lessons after atropine administration. In some cases, ventilation will not be possible without prior antidote administration (9).

Decontamination of patients exposed to nerve agent vapor requires removal of outer clothing and washing exposed areas, including the head and hair, with soap and water. Eye flushing is unnecessary in these patients. In contrast, decontamination of patients exposed to liquid nerve agent vapor requires removal of all clothing, washing the entire body and hair with soap and water or 0.5% hypochlorite (common bleach) followed by a water rinse, and eye irrigation with plain water or saline for 5–10 min (9). The proper procedure for flushing the eyes includes tilting the patient's head to the side, pulling the eyelids apart with fingers, and pouring water or saline slowly into the eye. Contact lenses should be removed if it is possible to do so without causing additional eye trauma. Eye bandages are contraindicated.

Because of the risk of pulmonary aspiration due to respiratory arrest, seizures, or vomiting, emergency department staff should not induce emesis. Instead, if the patient is alert and has not received charcoal previously, the patient should receive a slurry of activated charcoal. Gastric lavage, if administered within 30 min or less after ingestion, may be helpful. Staff attending to patients should consider gastric contents hazardous, and should dispose them appropriately (9).

Table 3.3 contains the CDC recommendations for treating nerve agent exposure in the field, before patients arrive at the hospital emergency department, and possibly near the site of exposure, while Table 3.4 contains the recommendations for treatment in the emergency department (http://www.atsdr.cdc.gov/MHMI/mmg166. html, last accessed 5/12/06) (18).

Table 3.3 CDC recommendations for nerve agent therapy in the field

| Patient age | Antidotes[a] | | Other treatment |
	Mild/moderate symptoms[b]	Severe symptoms[c]	
Infant (0–2 years)	Atropine: 0.05 mg kg^{-1} IM; 2-PAM Cl: 15 mg kg^{-1} IM	Atropine: 0.1 mg kg^{-1} IM; 2-PAM Cl: 25 mg kg^{-1} IM	Assisted ventilation should be started after administration of antidotes for severe exposures
Child (2–10 years)	Atropine: 1 mg IM; 2-PAM Cl: 15 mg kg^{-1} IM	Atropine: 2 mg IM; 2-PAM Cl: 25 mg kg^{-1} IM	
Adolescent (>10 years)	Atropine: 2 mg IM; 2-PAM Cl: 15 mg kg^{-1} IM	Atropine: 4 mg IM; 2-PAM Cl: 25 mg kg^{-1} IM	Repeat atropine (2 mg IM) at 5–10 min intervals until secretions have diminished and breathing is comfortable or airway resistance has returned to near normal
Adult	Atropine: 2 to 4 mg IM; 2-PAM Cl: 600 mg IM	Atropine: 6 mg IM; 2-PAM Cl: 1,800 mg IM	
Elderly, frail	Atropine: 1 mg IM; 2-PAM Cl: 10 mg kg^{-1} IM	Atropine: 2–4 mg IM; 2-PAM Cl: 25 mg kg^{-1} IM	

Source: Agency for Toxic Substances and Disease Registry. Nerve Agents (CDC public domain). http://www.atsdr.cdc.gov/MHMI/mmg166.pdf (18)

[a] 2-PAMCl solution needs to be prepared from the ampule containing 1 g of desiccated 2-PAMCl: inject 3 ml of saline, 5% distilled or sterile water into ampule and shake well. Resulting solution is 3.3 ml of 300 mg ml^{-1}

[b] Mild/moderate symptoms include localized sweating, muscle fasciculations, nausea, vomiting, weakness, dyspnea

[c] Severe symptoms include unconsciousness, convulsions, apnea, flaccid paralysis

Table 3.4 Treatment of nerve agent exposure: hospital management: CDC Recommendations for nerve agent therapy in the emergency department

| | Antidotes | | |
Patient age	Mild/moderate symptoms[a]	Severe symptoms[b]	Other treatment
Infant (0–2 years)	Atropine: 0.05 mg kg⁻¹ IM or 0.02 mg kg⁻¹ IV; 2-PAM Cl: 15 mg kg⁻¹ IV slowly	Atropine: 0.1 mg kg⁻¹ IM or 0.02 mg kg⁻¹ IV; 2-PAM Cl: 15 mg kg⁻¹ IV slowly	Assisted ventilation as needed
Child (2–10 years)	Atropine: 1 mg IM; 2-PAM Cl: 15 mg kg⁻¹ IV slowly	Atropine: 2 mg IM; 2-PAM Cl: 15 mg kg⁻¹ IV slowly	
Adolescent (>10 years)	Atropine: 2 mg IM; 2-PAM Cl: 15 mg kg⁻¹ IV slowly	Atropine: 4 mg IM; 2-PAM Cl: 15 mg kg⁻¹ IV slowly	Repeat atropine (2 mg IM or 1 mg IM for infants) at 5–10 minute intervals until secretions have diminished and breathing is comfortable or airway resistance has returned to near normal
Adult	Atropine: 2 to 4 mg IM; 2-PAM Cl: 15 mg kg⁻¹ (1 g) IV slowly	Atropine: 6 mg IM; 2-PAM Cl: 15 mg kg⁻¹ (1 g) IV slowly	Phentolamine for 2-PAM induced hypertension: (5 mg IV for adults; 1 mg IV for children)
Elderly, frail	Atropine: 1 mg IM; 2-PAM Cl: 5 to 10 mg kg⁻¹ IV slowly	Atropine: 2 mg IM; 2-PAM Cl: 5 to 10 mg kg⁻¹ IV slowly	Diazepam for convulsions: (0.2 to 0.5 mg IV for infants and children ≤5 years; 1 mg IV for children >5 years; 5 mg IV for adults)

Source: Agency for Toxic Substances and Disease Registry. Nerve Agents (CDC public domain). http://www.atsdr.cdc.gov/MHMI/mmg166.pdf (18)

[a]Mild/Moderate symptoms include localized sweating, muscle fasciculations, nausea, vomiting, weakness, dyspnea

[b]Severe symptoms include unconsciousness, convulsions, apnea, flaccid paralysis

Atropine administered repeatedly as necessary and pralidoxime (2-PAM Cl) are antidotes for nerve agent toxicity. Although atropine has no effect on nicotinic receptors, and therefore will not reverse muscle weakness or paralysis, it can reduce morbidity and mortality by reversing some of the muscarinic effects such as bronchospasm, bradycardia, salivation, diaphoresis, diarrhea, and vomiting (2). These antidotes may not be available in the field, especially in or near the site of attack. If military Mark 1 kits are available, they provide autoinjectors that automatically deliver 2 mg of atropine and 600 mg pralidoxime (9).

Once at the emergency department, patients with vapor exposure experiencing very mild symptoms, such as miosis and rhinorrhea, do not require antidote treatment with two exceptions. Those with eye or head pain or nausea and vomiting should obtain relief from topical atropine or homatropine in the eye, and they should be well enough for discharge from the hospital within an hour or so. Patients with severe rhinorrhea should experience relief from intramuscular atropine (2 mg in adults and 0.05 mg kg^{-1} in children) and should also be well enough for discharge from the hospital in an hour or so (9). Patients with miosis only should not receive topical atropine or homatropine, because both can cause visual impairment for 24 h (9).

More severely affected patients should receive atropine in doses listed in Table 3.4 (18). Severely affected adults may require a starting dose of 6 mg (9,14), with some patients requiring up to 10–20 mg in the first several hours and 100 mg cumulatively (2), although patients will rarely require more than 20 mg in the first 24 h period (8). Atropine administration should continue until respiratory secretions have resolved and ventilation has improved (2). Patients on atropine require monitoring for atropine toxicity, including delirium, hyperthermia or increased fasciculations (14). To avoid ventricular fibrillation, patients should not receive atropine while hypoxemic (19). Miosis, which may not reverse, and heart rate are not useful as clinical endpoints (2,8).

Because atropine only works on muscarinic receptors, it cannot fully reverse nerve agent-induced AChE inhibition. Pralidoxime, also known as 2-PAM Cl, can reverse the effects of AChE inhibition, such as muscle weakness and paralysis, by binding to AChE while displacing and hydrolyzing the nerve agent, thereby reactivating AChE. It is essential to give pralidoxime as soon as possible after exposure. Depending on the specific nerve agent, a process termed "aging" renders the bond between nerve agent and AChE resistant to disruption, and therefore resistant to pralidoxime therapy. The GD-AChE complex ages the fastest, with half of the Soman dose aging in 2 min, making Soman especially resistant to pralidoxime therapy. The other nerve agents, including Sarin (5 h half-time), Tabun (13 h half-time) and VX (48 h half-time), allow up to several hours or more before pralidoxime becomes ineffective (3,8).

Given that early responders may not know for certainty which nerve agent was responsible, patients suffering from nerve agent symptoms should receive pralidoxime immediately, in conjunction with atropine. The adult dose of pralidoxime (see Tables 3.3 and 3.4) is 1–2 g (15–25 mg kg^{-1}) intramuscularly (18) or 1 g (15 mg kg^{-1}) intravenously in 100 mL of saline over 15–30 min. Intravenous administration, if possible, is preferable (3). After an hour, if paralysis persists, patients should receive a second dose (21). Severely ill adult patients may benefit from an intravenous 2 g pralidoxime bolus followed by a maintenance infusion of 7.5 mg kg^{-1}h^{-1} (19). Pediatric experience with pesticide poisoning suggests that a continuous infusion may be optimal for children as well (7,22). For children, a continuous infusion of 10–20 mg kg^{-1}h^{-1} should follow a bolus of 25–50 mg kg^{-1}. More severely affected children may require a loading dose of 50 mg kg^{-1} (22).

In mass casualty situations, intravenous antidotes may not be available. In that case, the intramuscular administration is acceptable. Most Emergency Medical Systems in the United States now stock military Autoinjector units containing atropine and pralidoxime, although kits with pediatric doses may not be available. However, in critical situations, children older than 2 or 3 years of age weighing at least 13 kg might benefit from 2 mg of atropine and 600 mg pralidoxime administered intramuscularly with auto-injectors (7). Experience with the accidental atropine auto-injection in 240 Israeli children unexposed to nerve agents revealed that dire situations involving nerve gas exposure justify the risk of this practice. Although the Israeli children developed systemic anticholinergic effects, they did not develop seizures or severe dysrhythmias and none of them died (7).

Besides antidote therapy, ventilatory support, treatment of cardiac arrhythmias and management of other complications can reduce mortality significantly. Routine and early administration of benzodiazepines, such as 10 mg of Diazepam intramuscularly, can prevent seizures, including status epilepticus, as well as morphologic brain damage due to nerve agents (7,8). Patients with flaccid paralysis require electroencephalographic monitoring to detect seizures (19). A cycloplegic agent, Tropicadime 0.5%, 1–2 drops in each eye, repeated as necessary, may be useful for reversing miosis and relieving ocular pain due to blepharospasm and ciliary spasm (8,19).

Nerve Agent Intoxication: Prevention

The military has stockpiled pyridostigmine for prophylaxis of nerve agent poisoning. Although pyridostigmine inhibits AChE, unlike nerve agents, pyridostigmine induced AChE inhibition is readily reversible. Pyridostigmine works by blocking nerve agents from irreversibly inhibiting AChE. As a result, people pretreated with pyridostigmine have reservoirs of AChE that can later restore cholinergic function. The key principle for pyridostigmine effectiveness is administration before exposure to rapidly acting nerve agents. Because terrorists are unlikely to announce they are about to release a nerve agent, pyridostigmine is of little or no benefit in a civilian terrorist setting.

Vesicant Agents: Nitrogen and Sulfur Mustards, Lewisite, and Mustard-Lewisite Mixture

Vesicant Agents as Chemical Weapons

Vesicants, aptly known as blistering agents or mustard agents, are a diverse group of agents that cause significant morbidity through cutaneous burns, blisters and vesicles. All of these agents are destructive to the skin, mucus membranes, including the eyes, and respiratory tract. After development in the nineteenth century, the prototypical vesicant agent, sulfur mustard, or "mustard gas," caused over 80% of documented chemical casualties in World War I (23). More recently, in the 1980s, Iraq used vesicants in its war with Iran (14,23). Besides sulfur mustard, other common vesicant agents include nitrogen mustard and Lewisite.

Authorities consider vesicants potential terrorist weapons for several reasons (15):

– At least a dozen countries currently stockpile sulfur mustard, and it is easy and inexpensive to manufacture, making it widely available.
– Sulfur mustard is environmentally stable. After aerosolization by bomb explosion, shell blast or spraying, sulfur mustard vaporizes slowly, persisting in the environment for over a week in temperate climates (2).

- Although vesicant agents are generally not lethal (exposure is associated with a mortality rate of 2–3%), they are highly irritating, making them incredibly effective at incapacitating enemy soldiers. They cause significant, irreversible injury at three exposure sites: the eyes, the lung, and the skin (3).
- All the vesicants can cause systemic effects after cutaneous absorption.
- There is no known antidote for sulfur and nitrogen mustard.
- After exposure, sulfur and nitrogen mustards have a delayed onset of symptoms, resulting in delays of detection with concomitant increased morbidity (15).

Although Lewisite has similar effects as sulfur and nitrogen mustard, terrorists may not find it as attractive as a weapon due to its immediate effect and the existence of an effective antidote (15). When combined with mustard, Lewisite achieves a lower freezing point, making it more effective for ground dispersal and aerial spraying (24).

Mechanism of Action

After exposure to sulfur mustard, 80% of the agent evaporates, posing a hazard to the eyes, nose and respiratory tract (3). The remaining 20% is absorbed percutaneously, with 10% of the absorbed dose remaining in the skin and 90% reaching the circulation. The absorbed dose undergoes an intramolecular cyclization reaction that causes DNA alkylation, ultimately responsible for its toxicity and concomitant clinical effects, including cellular damage and blister formation (15).

DNA alkylation may not completely account for sulfur mustard's toxicity, however. Sulfur mustard may also affect intracellular enzymes and the structural components of cell membranes, causing dissolution of intracellular attachments and a cleft in the basal epidermal layer. In turn, inflammation develops, followed by edema and blisters (3). Although nitrogen mustard is less potent than sulfur, its mechanism of action is similar.

After sulfur and nitrogen mustards are absorbed and interact with body tissues, they are no longer intact molecules. Therefore, unlike nerve gas victims, the body fluids of decontaminated mustard-exposed patients pose no risk to health care providers or other responders (2). In contrast to the other vesicants, Lewisite does not require a cyclization reaction, so its effects are immediate. Through direct inhibition of thiol-containing enzymes, Lewisite disrupts energy pathways, causing ATP depletion, cell death, and clinical effects (15).

Sulfur and Nitrogen Mustard Vesicant Exposure: Clinical Presentation and Diagnosis

Table 3.5 (25,26) summarizes the clinical presentation of exposure to sulfur and nitrogen mustards. Sulfur and nitrogen mustards affect primarily the eyes, skin and respiratory tract. Most exposed patients will not have immediate symptoms, and will not

Table 3.5 The clinical presentation of exposure to sulfur and nitrogen mustards (25,26)

	Sulfur mustard	Nitrogen mustard
Dermal	Erythema and blistering. Pruritic rash develops in 4–8 h, followed by blistering in 2–18 h. Vapor exposure can cause first and second degree burns; liquid exposure leads to second and third degree burns. Burn covering more than 25% of body surface may be fatal	Erythema and blistering. Rash develops in several hours, followed by blistering in 6–12 h. Severe exposure can cause second and third degree burns
Ocular	Most sensitive tissue to sulfur. Intense conjunctival and scleral pain, swelling, lacrimation, blepharospasm, and photophobia. Effects delayed for 1 h. Miosis may occur. Severe exposure can cause corneal edema, perforation, scarring, and blindness	Intense conjunctival and scleral inflammation, pain, swelling, lacrimation, photophobia, and corneal damage; high concentration can cause burns and blindness
Respiratory	Upper and lower airway inflammation within hours of exposure and progressing over several days. Burning nasal pain, epistaxis, sinus pain, laryngitis, loss of taste and smell, cough, wheezing and dyspnea. Pseudomembrane formation and local airway obstruction	Mucosal damage within hours that may progress over days. Nasal and sinus pain or discomfort, pharyngitis, laryngitis, cough, and dyspnea. Pulmonary edema is uncommon
GI	Ingestion can cause chemical burns and cholinergic stimulation. Nausea and vomiting may occur after ingestion or inhalation. Early nausea and vomiting is usually transient and not severe. Nausea, vomiting and diarrhea occurring several days after exposure indicates GI tract damage and is a poor prognostic sign	Ingestion can cause chemical burns and hemorrhagic diarrhea. Nausea and vomiting may occur after ingestion, dermal, or inhalation exposure
CNS	High doses can cause hyperexcitability, convulsions and insomnia	High doses have caused tremors, seizures, incoordination, ataxia, and coma in laboratory animals
Hematopoietic	Bone marrow suppression and increased risk for infection, hemorrhage and anemia	Bone marrow suppression and increased risk for infection, hemorrhage and anemia
Delayed effects	Years after apparent healing of severe eye lesions, relapsing keratitis or keratopathy may develop	Potential menstrual irregularities, alopecia, hearing loss, tinnitus, jaundice, impaired spermatogenesis, generalized swelling, and hyperpigmentation
Potential sequelae	Persistent eye conditions, loss of taste and smell, and chronic respiratory illness, including asthmatic bronchitis, recurring respiratory infections, and pulmonary fibrosis	Chronic respiratory and eye conditions following large exposures

Source: From Melnick A, The family physician's role in responding to biologic, chemical, and radiological terrorism. In: Family Medicine: principles and practice (6e). Taylor R (ed). New York: Springer, 2003. Adapted by permission.

know they were exposed, making it difficult to recognize an incident. Symptoms begin after a delay of 2–24 h after exposure. The earliest symptoms suggesting exposure include eye irritation, lacrimation, cough, hoarseness and a burning sensation on the skin (14).

Skin effects generally begin 12–24 h after exposure to sulfur and nitrogen mustard, with onset dependent on concentration, climactic conditions, including temperature and humidity, and skin area exposed. The relatively moist groin and axillae are the most sensitive areas (2,15). Erythema is the first sign of skin damage, followed by development of small vesicles within the erythematous areas. The vesicles may later coalesce to form bullae. Although most blisters form within 16–24 h, in some cases, blisters can form as late as 7–12 days after exposure (15). Fluid from the blisters does not contain the mustard and does not pose a chemical contamination risk. The erythematous areas, characterized by diffuse or patchy hyperpigmentation, can go on to slough. Exposure to large doses of sulfur mustard can cause lesions with central areas of coagulation necrosis (2). Sulfur burns involving more than 25% of the body surface indicate exposure sufficient to cause systemic symptoms (3) (see Figs. 3.1 and 3.2).

Ocular effects due to sulfur or nitrogen mustard can be immediate, secondary to heavy droplet exposure, or delayed several hours secondary to vapor exposure (3). The earliest ocular symptoms are lacrimation and burning, followed by severe conjunctivitis and burns to the upper and lower eyelids. Photophobia and blepharospasm occur commonly. As the edema develops, the eyes become swollen shut. Eye recovery begins in 1–2 weeks, unless permanent damage has occurred (15). Large exposures, especially from liquid sulfur mustard in airborne droplets, can cause iritis, corneal damage, and blindness, either temporary or permanent (2,3,15). Resulting scarring and synechiae formation can restrict pupillary movement, leading to glaucoma (2). Experience from World War I revealed that 75% of ocular effects were due to mild conjunctivitis, 10% of ocular exposures were severe, and less than 1% of exposed patients developed permanent ocular damage (2).

Like chlorine, sulfur, and nitrogen mustard have high reactivity, contributing to epithelial injury of the airways. Sulfur and nitrogen mustard vapors cause dose related respiratory tract damage, beginning with the upper airways and gradually moving lower as the exposure increases (8). Symptoms begin 4–6 h after exposure. The earliest respiratory symptoms include irritation or burning of the nares, epistaxis, sinus pain, and hoarseness, pharyngeal irritation, or soreness (2,8). Tracheobronchitis typically begins several hours after exposure. Patients typically develop cough, increased secretions, wheezing, dyspnea, bronchospasm, and even laryngospasm (3). Moderate to high exposures can lead to bronchial obstruction, hemorrhagic pulmonary edema and respiratory failure (15). In addition, the irritant effects of sulfur and nitrogen mustards can produce sloughing of the mucosal lining of the large airways, resulting in pseudomembranes and damage to airway musculature (2). Bacterial pneumonia is a common complication of lower airway damage (2,15).

The earliest systemic symptoms of sulfur or nitrogen mustard exposures are nausea and vomiting, which typically begin within 2–4 h of exposure. These early gastrointestinal symptoms are self-limited and probably due to the cholinergic

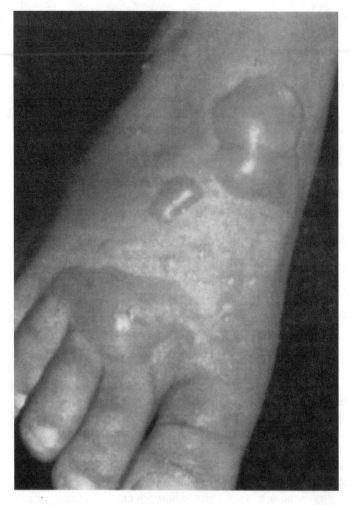

Fig. 3.1 (See color plate) Dorsum of right foot about 48 h after exposure to sulfur mustard vapor with characteristic blisters. (Courtesy of Professor Steen Christensen, Ronne, Denmark; Anitta Lild, photographer, Aarhus, Jutland.)

effects of low exposures to mustard. However, nausea and vomiting, and possibly diarrhea (seldom bloody) beginning several days after exposure have a poorer prognosis, because these symptoms are probably due to mustard-induced cytotoxic effects on the gut mucosa (2,8).

Because sulfur and nitrogen mustards are alkylating agents, large exposures can cause bone marrow suppression, similar to that seen with radiation exposure (8). A drop in the absolute lymphocyte count, particularly within the first 12–24 h after exposure, may reflect impending bone marrow suppression (3). Leukopenia develops 3–5 days after exposures, followed by thrombocytopenia and anemia (24,25).

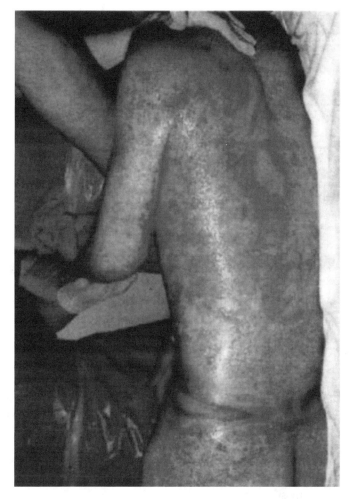

Fig. 3.2 (See color plate) Iranian soldier with mustard agent burns several weeks after exposure; injuries are beginning to heal. (Courtesy of Veijo Mehtonen, Karolinska University Hospital, Stockholm, Sweden)

Frequently, bone marrow suppression is not severe, and the bone marrow recovers 10–25 days after the exposure (3).

Available military experience indicates that less than 5% of exposed patients die from mustard exposure, although many will require a long convalescence. The most likely cause of death in severely exposed patients is massive pulmonary damage, associated with pneumonia and sepsis secondary to immunosuppression. Clues to such massive exposures include symptom onset within 4h of exposure, respiratory symptoms occurring within 6h of exposure and white blood cell counts under 200 (8).

Table 3.6 Complications of mustard exposure

Respiratory	Asthma, chronic bronchitis, bronchiectasis, airway narrowing, pulmonary fibrosis, lung, and upper airway cancer
Ocular	Chronic conjunctivitis, recurrent corneal ulcers, recurrent keratitis
Skin	Scarring, cancer
CNS	Psychological disorders
Bone Marrow	Leukemia

Source: Data from Bogucki S, et al. (8), and from the Agency for Toxic Substances and Disease Registry (25,26)

Table 3.6 lists the long-term mustard complications affecting the respiratory tract, the eyes, the skin, the central nervous system and the bone marrow (8,25,26). As alkylating agents, sulfur and nitrogen mustards are carcinogens.

Lewisite Vesicant Exposure: Clinical Presentation and Diagnosis

Unlike the other blister agents, sulfur and nitrogen mustards, Lewisite and the Mustard-Lewisite Mixture cause symptoms immediately, within minutes of exposure. Otherwise, Lewisite, a systemic poison, and Mustard-Lewisite Mixture have similar effects as sulfur and nitrogen mustard, causing irritation of the skin, eyes and airways. Table 3.7 summarizes the health effects of Lewisite and Mustard-Lewisite mixture. Immediately after dermal exposure, patients experience burning and stinging. Erythema develops within 30 min, followed by blister formation in 2–3 h (2). Compared to mustard, the skin damage from Lewisite is less severe, heals sooner, and is less likely to result in a secondary infection (8).

Ocular symptoms and signs, including burning and stinging also occur immediately after exposure, followed quickly by blepharospasm and edema, and within a few hours, iritis and corneal haziness. Blindness may result without eye decontamination within 1 min of exposure (2).

Lewisite effects on the airway are similar to sulfur and nitrogen mustard, except that Lewisite is extremely irritating to the mucus membranes. The immediate, profound irritation of the mucus membranes may drive victims away from the dispersal site, thus helping to limit exposure (8). Exposure to high concentrations of Lewisite results in pulmonary edema (8).

Large exposures to Lewisite can cause "Lewisite shock" due to increased capillary membrane permeability and subsequent protein and plasma leakage across the capillary membranes. As a result, patients suffer intravascular fluid loss, hemoconcentration, hypovolemia, and hypotension (8,24). Cutaneous exposures can produce localized edema and pulmonary edema secondary to damage at the alveolar – capillary membrane (8).

Contact with the liquid or vapor forms can cause skin erythema and blistering, corneal damage and iritis, damage to the airway mucosa, pulmonary edema, diarrhea, capillary leakage, and subsequent hypotension (21).

Table 3.7 Health effects of lewisite and mustard-lewisite mixture

Dermal	Pain and skin irritation within seconds to minutes. After exposure to the liquid form, erythema within 15–30 min and blisters within several hours, developing fully by 12–18 h. Slightly longer response times for the vapor. The blister begins as a small blister in the center of the erythematous area and expands to include the entire area
Ocular	Immediate pain and blepharospasm. Edema of conjunctiva of eyelids follows, and the eyes may be swollen shut within an hour. High doses can cause corneal damage and iritis. Lacrimation, photophobia, and inflammation of the conjunctiva and cornea may occur
Respiratory	Burning nasal pain, epistaxis, sinus pain, laryngitis, cough, and dyspnea may occur. Necrosis can lead to pseudomembrane formation and local airway obstruction. High levels of exposure can result in pulmonary edema
GI	Ingestion or inhalation of Lewisite can cause nausea and vomiting. Ingestion of the Mixture causes severe abdominal pain, vomiting and hematochezia after 15–20 min
Cardiovascular	Lewisite shock due to increased capillary permeability and subsequent intravascular volume loss, hypovolemia and organ congestion
Hepatic	Necrosis due to shock and hypoperfusion
Renal	Decreased renal function secondary to hypotension
Hematopoietic	Bone marrow suppression
Potential sequelae	Chronic respiratory and eye conditions

Source: From Melnick A. The family physician's role in responding to biological, chemical, and radiological terrorism. In: Family medicine: principles and practice (6e). Taylor R (ed). New York: Springer, 2003. Reprinted with permission.

Treatment

Management of Lewisite or Mustard-Lewisite exposure is similar to that of nitrogen and sulfur mustard exposures with two exceptions. First, patients exposed to Lewisite or the mixture will have an abrupt onset of symptoms and will likely present to emergency rooms immediately after exposure. On the other hand, because of the delayed effects, most patients with severe exposures to nitrogen or sulfur mustards will go home or elsewhere after their exposure and may only present later at emergency rooms or physicians' offices when they begin developing symptoms.

The second exception is that while an antidote is available for systemic effects of Lewisite exposure, there are no antidotes for nitrogen mustard or sulfur mustard toxicity, with one minor caveat: if given within minutes after exposure, intravenous sodium thiosulfate may prevent death due to sulfur mustard exposure (25). Otherwise, the medical management for skin, ocular, and respiratory exposure is only supportive. One guideline physicians can follow is to keep skin, eye, and airway lesions free from infection.

Regardless of the vesicant or the site where patients present, therapy begins with decontamination. Patients with vesicant-contaminated skin or clothing can contaminate rescuers and health care providers by direct contact or through off-gassing vapor. Therefore, as with other blister agents, once health care providers suspect an exposure, they should require all patients to undergo decontamination of eyes, clothing, and skin before allowing them to enter the treatment area.

Decontamination, especially within the first couple of minutes of exposure, before irreversible chemical reactions occur, can reduce tissue damage. However, even after the first 2 min, decontamination is still helpful, because it reduces continued absorption of the vesicant and because it protects health care workers (13). Because alkaline solutions will degrade Lewisite, responders treating Lewisite-exposed patients should use a dilute sodium hypochlorite (household bleach) solution in addition to the typical soap and water decontamination (2). Decontamination of patients exposed to sulfur and nitrogen mustard should only include gentle scrubbing with soap and water, not bleach, because bleach can cause deeper tissue penetration of the mustard (23). In the field, if water is not available, absorbent powders such as flour, talcum powder, or Fuller's earth can be useful for removing the chemical (24–26). Eye decontamination should consist of immediate, copious irrigation with sterile saline. Health care providers, especially first responders at risk of exposure, should wear Level A PPE until patients are fully decontaminated.

Patients exposed to sulfur or nitrogen mustard arriving at the hospital within 30–60 min of exposure will seldom have symptoms. After decontamination, patients with respiratory symptoms require placement in a critical care unit, whereas those without symptoms require observation only for at least 6 h. The sooner after exposure symptoms develop, the more likely they are to progress (25,26).

Lewisite-exposed patients arriving at the hospital within 30–60 min of exposure will likely have pain or irritation. Patients without symptoms most likely did not suffer Lewisite exposure, and they can go home, with instructions to return immediately if they develop symptoms. After decontamination, Lewisite-exposed patients with respiratory symptoms require placement in a critical care unit. Patients without symptoms, including those sent home, require observation for 18–24 h. The sooner after exposure symptoms develop, the more likely they are to progress (24).

Regardless of the specific vesicant, patients experiencing only mild conjunctivitis beginning more than 12 h after exposure are unlikely to suffer progression to serious eye injury. These patients should receive a complete eye examination, including visual acuity testing and treatment with a soothing eye solution, such as Visine or Murine. Such patients do not require admission, but should receive instructions to return home if symptoms worsen (25,26).

Conjunctivitis beginning earlier than 12 h and other ocular symptoms, such as lid swelling and signs or symptoms of inflammation, after exposure to any of the vesicants, requires inpatient treatment and observation (25,26). Staining with fluorescein is useful for assessing corneal damage that occurs in up to 10% of vesicant-exposed patients. Patients with corneal injuries should receive mydriatics, such as atropine, to relieve ciliary spasm and prevent iridolenticular adhesions (8). In addition, appropriate ocular eye treatment should include topical antibiotic drops and sterile ointment coating of lid margins to prevent the margins for sticking to each other (23– 26). Patients with ophthalmic injuries should receive a prompt evaluation by an ophthalmologist (23). Topical analgesics are acceptable for the initial eye examination, including a slit lamp test and visual acuity testing, but not after, when pain control should include systemic analgesics only (24–26). Topical steroids are controversial but may be helpful (3,13).

Small areas of erythema beginning more than 12 h after exposure to any of the vesicants are unlikely to progress to significant lesions. Burning and itching from such erythema will respond to topical calamine or other soothing lotion (2). Patients with erythema only can go home, with instructions to return if symptoms worsen (24–26). Antibiotic ointments and sterile dressings are appropriate treatments for chemical burns. Daily dressing changes and outpatient management should be sufficient for superficial burns covering a small percentage of the body surface. However, burns covering 20% or more of the body surface require inpatient treatment in a critical care unit, because this degree of injury reflects exposure to a potentially lethal dose of vesicant, even if the patient appears stable and the burns appear benign (23).

Most vesicant burns will be second degree, although liquid exposure can cause third degree burns. Although this is controversial, the ATSDR recommends unroofing blisters larger than 1 cm, while leaving smaller blisters unroofed. Blister fluid does not contain the active vesicant. Denuded areas should be irrigated two or three times daily, (using a whirlpool for very large lesions) followed by application of a topical antibiotic (24–26).

Because local inflammatory reactions may complicate some of the burn injuries, nonsteroidal antiinflammatory drugs (NSAIDs) may be helpful. Additional burn treatment may include CO_2-laser debridement, artificial skin or skin grafting (3). Large amounts of fluid loss are uncommon compared to thermal burns, but patients should still receive careful monitoring of fluids and electrolytes (2,3,23). Signs of infection and cultures revealing responsible organisms are indications for systemic antibiotics (24–26).

Regardless of the vesicant, patients with mild respiratory symptoms, such as a mild, nonproductive cough, irritation of the nose and sinuses, and/or a sore throat beginning 12 h or more after exposure, do not require hospital admission. Appropriate home-based treatment for these patients includes a cool steam vaporizer, lozenges, and cough drops, with instructions to return if symptoms worsen (24–26). On the other hand, patients with symptoms suggesting more severe exposure, such as laryngitis, shortness of breath, or a productive cough, anytime postexposure require immediate admission to the critical care unit. Immediate intubation is necessary for Lewisite exposed patients experiencing symptoms suggesting more severe exposure.

All vesicant-exposed patients, including children, with airway damage below the pharynx require oxygen and assisted ventilation as necessary with positive end expiratory pressure (PEEP). At the first sign of damage at or below the larynx, patients will require intubation and transfer to the critical care unit. Children require endotracheal tubes as large as possible to avoid tube obstruction due to epithelial debris (13). A tracheostomy may be necessary for obstructions unrelieved by bronchoscopy or direct laryngoscopy (23). Bronchodilators may be helpful for bronchoconstriction. Steroids are not of proven value, but may be worth trying for mustard-exposed patients if bronchodilators are ineffective (25,26).

Because the initial bronchitis following respiratory exposure is not infectious, patients will not benefit from administration of antibiotics. However, routine laboratory evaluation should include daily sputum cultures. Within the first several days after exposure, patients may develop a chemical pneumonitis, reflected by fever, elevated white blood cell counts and pulmonary infiltrates, but this pneumonitis is typically sterile. An infectious etiology is uncommon until the third or fourth day after exposure. Patients should receive antibiotics only after identification of a causative organism, not prophylactically (8,25,26). Patients with pulmonary edema should not receive diuretics, because vesicant-caused pulmonary edema is not cardiogenic (3).

Due to the risk of bleeding and perforation, patients who have ingested vesicants should not have emesis induced. Physicians may consider careful orogastric lavage for mustard exposed patients with large ingestion exposures within 30 min of exposure, but they should weigh the benefits of this treatment against the risk of hemorrhage and perforation. There is no evidence supporting the effectiveness of activated charcoal (25,26). Antiemetics may be helpful in relieving nausea and vomiting (24).

All vesicant-exposed patients should have a CBC performed daily. Treatment of bone marrow suppression should include infection precautions, transfusions, and aggressive treatment of infections as indicated (3). Studies indicate that granulocyte colony-stimulating factor (GCSF) may be useful for bone marrow suppression secondary to nitrogen mustard exposure (25,26). Bone marrow transplantation may be useful, but evidence is limited. Any mustard-exposed patient with a marked decrease in white blood cell count requires reverse isolation in an oncology or burn unit (25,26).

British Anti-Lewisite (BAL), also known as Dimercaprol, is a chelating agent than can reduce systemic effects from Lewisite. BAL works by binding the arsenic group in Lewisite and displacing it from tissue binding sites. If applied topically within minutes, after decontamination, BAL may prevent or reduce the severity of cutaneous and ocular toxicity (8).

However, because of toxic side effects, only patients who have signs of shock or significant pulmonary injury should receive systemic BAL (24). Only trained personnel, in consultation with a regional poison control center, should provide BAL chelation therapy. BAL comes in 3 mL ampules containing 100 mg mL^{-1} (2). The standard BAL dosage is 3–5 mg kg^{-1}, up to 400 mg, intramuscularly every 4–12 h for four doses (24). Adjustment of the regimen should depend on the severity of the exposure and the patient's symptoms. Preexisting renal disease, pregnancy (except in life-threatening circumstances) and concurrent iron therapy are contraindications to BAL therapy. Because peanut oil is the vehicle used for BAL, patients with peanut allergies should not receive BAL (2).

By stabilizing the Dimercaprol-arsenic complex, alkalinization of the urine may protect the kidneys of patients undergoing BAL treatment. If patients develop renal insufficiency, they should receive hemodialysis to remove the Dimercaprol-arsenic complex. Side effects at the lower 3 mg kg^{-1} BAL dosage are primarily pain at the injection site. At the higher 5 mg kg^{-1} dosage, potential side effects include nausea, vomiting, headache, burning sensation of the lips, mouth, throat and eyes, lacrimation, rhinorrhea, salivation, muscle aches, burning and tingling in the extremities, tooth ache, diaphoresis, chest pain, anxiety and agitation (24).

Prevention

Because terrorists are unlikely to announce they are about to release a vesicant agent, there are no effective preventive measures for vesicant exposure. Recognition of the exposure and rapid, effective decontamination of victims is essential to prevent secondary exposure and additional cases.

Blood Agents: Cyanide (Hydrogen Cyanide, Cyanogen Chloride, Sodium Cyanide, Potassium Cyanide)

Blood Agents as Chemical Weapons

Because cyanide gases are highly volatile and lighter than air, they are ineffective outdoors as military weapons (2). However, inhaled indoors, or through ingestion of the crystal form, they reach concentrations that are fast acting, with high mortality. Recognizing this potential, the Nazis used hydrocyanic acid (Zyklon B) to murder millions of civilians in gas chambers during World War II (27). In 1984, seven Chicago residents died after ingesting cyanide-laced Extra Strength Tylenol capsules (28). Cyanide was the agent responsible for the mass suicides in Guyana (13). More recently, in 1995, weeks after the Tokyo subway Sarin attack, authorities found a crude apparatus containing cyanide gas precursors, acid and a cyanide salt, in a Tokyo subway restroom (27,28). According to the presiding judge at their trial, terrorists may have attempted to use cyanide as part of the New York City World Trade Center bombing in 1993, but the blast destroyed the cyanide (29).

Besides their lethality, blood agents are attractive as chemical weapons due to their availability and affordability. Cyanide is ubiquitous. Natural sources include plants such as peach pits, apple, and pear seeds, elderberry leaves and hydrangeas (13). In industry, cyanide contributes to the manufacture of paper, textiles, plastics, and it is a component of chemicals used in developing photographs. The metallurgy industry uses cyanide salts for electroplating, metal cleaning, and removing gold from its ore, and exterminators use cyanide gas for pest control in ships and buildings (30). Mixing cyanide salts with an acid is an easy and reliable method for producing cyanide gas (31).

Mechanism of Action

Cyanide can exist as a solid (sodium or potassium salt), liquid, or vapor. Hydrogen cyanide and cyanogen chloride are clear liquids, becoming gases above 26°F (2). Cyanide gas reportedly smells like bitter almonds, but because 20–40% of the general population cannot detect the odor, its presence is an unreliable indicator of possible exposure (2,21,31). Cyanogen chloride has a pungent, biting odor (21).

Hydrogen cyanide gas is rapidly absorbed through the lungs, producing symptoms within seconds to minutes. Due to greater lung surface per body weight ratios and increased minute volumes per weight, children are at particular risk for inhalation exposure. Skin or eye absorption is also rapid, with systemic symptoms beginning immediately or after a 30–60 min delay. Due do a relatively larger surface area to body weight ratio, children are also at increased risk from dermal exposures. Ingestion of cyanide salts can also be rapidly fatal (31).

Once inhaled, absorbed through the skin, or ingested, cyanide acts at the cellular level by binding to the ferric ion in mitochondrial cytochrome oxidase, effectively blocking the enzyme responsible for oxidative phosphorylation. As a result, cells lose the ability to synthesize ATP, causing impairment of ATP-dependent processes and a shift to anaerobic metabolism, leading to cellular anoxia and lactic acidosis (7,8,31).

Clinical Presentation and Diagnosis

Progressive tissue hypoxia without cyanosis is the hallmark of cyanide exposure. The rapidity of onset and the severity of symptoms are dependent on the degree of exposure. The central nervous system is particularly sensitive to hypoxia. Immediately after large inhalation exposures, patients develop hyperventilation, hypertension and tachycardia due to effects on the chemoreceptor body (8). Failure of brain aerobic metabolism results in a loss of consciousness within 1 min, with respiratory depression and cardiac arrest following a few minutes later (21).

Either inhalation of smaller cyanide concentrations or dermal exposure to cyanide can result in a slower progression of symptoms. Early symptoms of milder exposures include hyperventilation, headaches, dyspnea and central nervous system symptoms of anxiety, personality changes and agitation. In addition, patients may experience flushing, lightheadedness, dizziness, diaphoresis, nausea, vomiting, and weakness. If exposure continues and worsens, symptoms can progress to drowsiness, tetanic spasm, lockjaw, hallucinations, seizures, loss of consciousness, coma, apnea, and cardiac arrest (7,8,13,21,31). Cyanogen chloride, acidic in a moist environment, also produces ocular, nasal and airway irritation (8,13).

Patients who survive the acute exposure may suffer brain damage from direct neurological effects, hypoxia or insufficient circulation. Personality changes, memory deficits, disturbances in voluntary muscle movements, intellectual deterioration and extrapyramidal syndromes are potential chronic sequelae (21,31). Some patients may experience delayed toxicity involving the basal ganglia, with Parkinsonian features developing earlier than dystonia. Chronic symptoms can include dysarthria, eye movement abnormalities, and ataxia, with cavitation of the putamen and globus pallidus on magnetic resonance imaging. Cortical, cerebellar, and diencephalic abnormalities are also possible. Unfortunately, and probably due to cell loss in lenticular structures, parkinsonian and dystonic symptoms do not respond to dopaminergic drug therapy (21). There is no evidence that blood agents are carcinogenic, and exposures have not caused reproductive or developmental effects in animals or humans (31).

Cyanide poisoning is a possibility in any acyanotic patient with a rapid onset of CNS symptoms and symptoms of hypoxia, including cardiorespiratory collapse (15,31). The patient's blood, skin, and fundi may appear cherry red (27). Although the diagnosis is primarily clinical, the bitter almond smell in breath or gastric washings may be helpful, with the caveat that the attending clinician and health care staff may be among the 20–40% of people unable to detect the characteristic odor. Laboratory findings include normal oxygen saturations despite respiratory distress (2), a large anion gap metabolic acidosis (due to lactic acid), and high venous blood high oxygen content due to inability of the tissues to extract and use oxygen (2,7,8). Most hospital laboratories do not have the capability to measure plasma cyanide levels, but even if they did, results would rarely be available soon enough to have an impact on patient management (2,21). Plasma thiocyanate levels may be useful, but the time it takes to confirm levels does not justify a delay in treatment (15).

Treatment

The first step in patient management is to reduce exposure by moving victims to areas with good ventilation and by providing thorough decontamination. Because blood agents are volatile and do not remain on the skin, dermal decontamination is rarely necessary for cyanide gas exposures. However, at the time of presentation, it may not be clear whether patients were exposed to cyanide in liquid form or solution. Therefore, victims should have wet clothing removed and double bagged and their skin and hair washed with plain water for 2–3 min followed by washing twice with mild soap and water rinse. Eye contamination requires 5 min of irrigation with plain water or saline as well as removal of contact lenses. Although victims exposed only to cyanide gas do not present a secondary contamination risk, responders should still use Level A or B PPE (see Table 3.1), because of the possibility of liquid or solution exposure (2). Responders should not attempt mouth-to-mouth resuscitation (13). Patients with liquid exposures pose a risk of secondary contamination through direct contact or by off-gassing vapor (31).

Patients who have ingested cyanide should not have emesis induced. Instead, activated charcoal may be helpful, but should be administered as soon as possible after exposure, due to the rapid absorption of cyanide. Patients who are alert, asymptomatic and have an alert gag reflex should receive a slurry of activated charcoal at 1 gm kg^{-1}, at an adult dose of 60–90 g and a pediatric dose of 25–50 g. Children may accept charcoal through a soda can and straw more readily. Gastric lavage may be appropriate for conscious patients identified soon after ingestion exposure. Because gastric washings and vomitus of cyanide ingestion victims are potentially hazardous, the lavage tube should be connected to an isolated wall suction unit or other closed container (31). Responders should use PPE to prevent exposure to contaminated gastrointestinal material.

Asymptomatic patients who have ingested hydrogen cyanide solutions or those with direct skin or eye contact require observation in the emergency department for at least 4–6 h. Those who remain asymptomatic should be discharged with instructions to return if symptoms develop. The ATSDR Medical Management guidelines include a useful patient information sheet (31).

Patients suffering from mild or moderate exposures may only require supportive care and observation (8,21). More severe exposures necessitate basic life support, including mechanical ventilation, 100% oxygen, circulatory support with crystalloid and vasopressor agents, sodium bicarbonate for correction of the metabolic acidosis and seizure control with benzodiazepines (7,21).

Patients with severe cyanide exposures should receive antidotal therapy in the intensive care unit (31). The specific antidote treatment may vary by country and medical practice, but the universal two-stage regimen is based on cyanide's mechanisms of action. The first stage of antidotal treatment requires the displacement of cyanide from cytochrome oxidase. Nitrites or other methemoglobinemia inducing agents can accomplish this first task (2,7,8,21). The second state of treatment involves giving sodium thiosulfate or some other sulfur donor to convert the cyanide through hepatic metabolism into a form that the body can excrete (2,7,8,21). In the United States, cyanide antidote kits (CAKs) typically include amyl nitrite perles and intravenous infusions of sodium nitrite and sodium thiosulfate (31). Physicians should check with their hospitals proactively to make sure CAKs are available.

In an emergent situation, before obtaining intravenous access, amyl nitrite can be administered by breaking the perles onto a gauze pad and holding the saturated gauze under the patient's nose and mouth, over the Ambu-valve intake or under the lip of the face mask, for 30 s every minute or by emptying an ampule into a respiratory reservoir (21,31). If there is an insufficient response to oxygen and amyl nitrite, once intravenous access is available, the patient should receive an infusion of 300 mg sodium nitrite (one ampule, 10 mL of a 3% solution) over no less than 5 but up to 20 min. Pediatric doses range from 0.12 to 0.33 mL kg^{-1} body weight up to 10 mL infused similarly (31). For recurrent or persistent symptoms, adult and pediatric patients can receive an additional half dose of sodium nitrite.

Both amyl nitrite and sodium nitrite oxidize the ferrous iron in hemoglobin, creating measurable levels of methemoglobin. Patients receiving sodium nitrite infusions require close require constant monitoring of blood pressure and close observation for cyanosis and shock, both manifestations of methemoglobinemia.

Methemoglobin levels should approximate 20% of total hemoglobin, certainly below the 35–40% levels associated with deficits in oxygen carrying capacity of the blood (8,21,31). In disaster situations, when doing the calculations, it is reasonable to assume that total hemoglobin levels are normal (13). Unfortunately, the usual methods of monitoring methemoglobin levels are not reliable in cyanide poisoning and may underestimate the level of inactive hemoglobin. Therefore, the patient's clinical condition and not the methemoglobin level should guide the decision to give doses beyond the additional half dose (31). Development of hypotension necessitates a reduction of the infusion rate. Although a 1% methylene blue infusion can treat excessive methemoglobinemia, it can also cause an intravascular release of cyanide, making it inadvisable (21).

Following the sodium nitrite infusion, patients should receive the second stage of antidotal therapy, an intravenous infusion of sodium thiosulfate. The typical adult dose is 50 mL of a 25% solution (12.5 g) given over 10–20 min; the average pediatric dose is 1.65 mL kg^{-1} of the same solution. If there is an inadequate clinical response, adult and pediatric patients may receive an additional half dose 30 min later (31). Because sodium thiosulfate treatment is effective and relatively innocuous, it is acceptable to administer it to patients with mild to moderate exposure or if the diagnosis is uncertain (7). Patients with combined carbon monoxide and cyanide exposures due to smoke inhalation should probably receive sodium thiosulfate only, because the combination of methemoglobinemia and carboxyhemoglobinemia can result in severe tissue hypoxia (13,32).

Hydroxocobalamin (vitamin B_{12a}), another antidote, is a potential alternative to sodium nitrite treatment. It works by binding with cyanide to form nontoxic cyanocobalamin (vitamin B_{12}). Although effective and relatively safe in experimental models, the concentration available in the United States requires large infusion volumes and has a short shelf life due to light instability, and reports of anaphylactoid reactions have limited its use (8,13,21). Further studies using higher concentrations available in European formulations may eventually lead to its use as an outpatient alterative to sodium nitrite treatment in the United States (7,32). Other alternatives currently used or undergoing clinical trials in Europe include cobalt salts, limited by their toxicity, aldehydes, and aminophenol derivatives. These alternative treatments are not currently available in the United States (7).

In addition to antidotal therapy, administration of 100% oxygen can help with cyanide detoxification, possibly by affecting the binding of cyanide to cytochrome oxidase (13). Hyperbaric therapy may be considered, but only after standard treatment has failed, or if the patient has concurrent carbon monoxide poisoning (13).

Pulmonary Agents

Pulmonary Agents as Chemical Weapons

Pulmonary agents, also known as choking agents or lung irritants (33), attack the upper and lower respiratory tract, including the nose, throat, and lung parenchyma, ultimately causing pulmonary edema. Chlorine and phosgene, typical pulmonary agents, saw their first use during World War I. In 1915, the German army attacked allied troops in their trenches by detonating canisters containing chlorine gas. The resulting overpowering green vapor cloud caused heavy British and French casualties. After experiencing such triumph with chlorine gas, the German army quickly developed another, similar chemical agent, phosgene, which they also used with success (3). Although chlorine and phosgene are not as deadly as nerve gases, they are readily available industrial chemicals (3,7). Other potential, easily available pulmonary agents used in industry include ammonia, sulfur dioxide, and nitrogen dioxide (15).

Mechanism of Action

Pulmonary agents exist as gases, vapors or aerosolized liquids or solids. Vapors are gases resulting from heating a liquid or solid agent or exposing a liquid or solid agent to a drop in ambient pressure. Several factors contribute to the site and degree of damage caused by pulmonary agents:

– Gases or solid particles less than 2 mm in size are capable of causing damage to the entire respiratory tract, including airways and pulmonary alveoli, whereas damage from larger particles may cause damage to airways only, due to inability of the particles to pass through the bronchioles.
– Whereas gases and vapors cause damage only during exposure, deposited particles remaining in the respiratory tract can continue to cause damage after exposure ceases.
– Agents vary in toxicity; the inherent toxicity of the specific agent, its atmospheric concentration and the duration of exposure all contribute to injury severity.
– Water solubility affects the site and severity of injury. Moderate exposure to highly water-soluble pulmonary agents, such as ammonia and sulfur dioxide, can cause immediate injury to exposed skin and mucus membranes of the eyes and upper respiratory tract. Victims experiencing such immediate injuries usually flee the area of exposure before suffering exposure sufficient to cause alveolar damage. However, in enclosed situations where victims cannot evacuate, prolonged exposure will cause alveolar damage. Phosgene, nitrogen dioxide, and other pulmonary agents with low water-solubility tend to cause minimal immediate injury to skin and mucus membranes. The resulting lack of symptoms may cause unknowingly exposed victims to remain close to the source of exposure, allowing them to experience exposures sufficient to cause injury to the lower airways and alveoli. Chlorine and other agents with intermediate water-solubility are likely to cause diffuse damage to skin, mucus membrane, upper airway and alveoli (15).

Chlorine, a choking, yellow green gas, interacts with water to generate hydrochloric and hypochlorous acids. The resulting generation of free oxygen radicals penetrate cell membranes, form chloramines and oxidize sulfur-containing amino acids, causing cell injury and death (15). Chlorine, with intermediate water-solubility, typically causes injury to the entire respiratory tract.

Phosgene, also known as carbonyl chloride, carbon oxychloride, carbonic acid dichloride, and chloroformyl chloride, has a characteristic moldy hay or green corn odor, with greater pungency at higher concentrations (34). Toxic effects can occur below the odor threshold (34). Phosgene, like chlorine, generates hydrochloric acid. However, its carbonyl group also participates in acylation reactions at the alveolar-capillary membrane, resulting in membrane dysfunction and pulmonary edema (7,15). In addition, phosgene causes lipid peroxidation and production of leukotrienes, causing further cell injury and inflammation (15). Because of its low water-solubility, phosgene causes extensive lung damage with minimal concomitant upper airway injury. Development of pulmonary parenchymal injury, manifesting as adult respiratory distress syndrome, can develop after a latent period of 24 h following phosgene exposure (15).

Ammonia, used extensively in industry and agriculture, is a highly water-soluble gas. It interacts with water to form ammonium hydroxide, causing alkaline burns of the eyes and other mucosal surfaces and upper airway. Prolonged, extensive exposure can injure the lung parenchyma and lead to respiratory failure (15).

Sulfur dioxide, a highly water-soluble, colorless gas, interacts with water on tissue surfaces to form sulfuric acid, with resulting injury to the eyes, nasopharynx, oropharynx, and upper airway. Extensive exposure can cause injury to the lung parenchyma, manifesting as acute respiratory distress syndrome (15). Late sequelae may include chronic lung disease, such as bronchiolitis obliterans and reactive airway dysfunction syndrome (RADS) (15). Nitrogen dioxide interacts with water to form nitric acid, leading to tissue injury, pulmonary edema, and potentially chronic lung diseases such as bronchiolitis obliterans (15).

Clinical Presentation and Diagnosis

Although the mechanism of action varies among the pulmonary agents, the respiratory tract injuries and concomitant clinical manifestations are similar (15). Because of the similarity, it may be difficult to determine the specific agent soon after the exposure incident. Early symptoms of exposure to pulmonary agents include generalized burning of mucus membranes of the eyes, nasopharynx, oropharynx, and upper respiratory tract. Victims may suffer from profuse lacrimation, rhinorrhea, coughing, hoarseness, dyspnea, and odynophagia (15). Chest tightness is an early symptom in patients exposed to chlorine, and is more prominent in patients with preexisting hyperreactive airways (8).

Initial physical findings in pulmonary agent exposure may include conjunctivitis, corneal injury, and nasopharyngeal and oropharyngeal injury and edema. Patients may develop stridor and respiratory distress secondary to inflammation of glottic structures, excessive secretions and/or laryngospasm (2,15).

Patients with airway injuries will develop cough, which may be croupy, wheezing, dyspnea, and sputum production. Victims of chlorine exposure commonly develop exertional dyspnea and inspiratory cough (8). Many of the pulmonary agents directly damage bronchial epithelial cells, resulting in mucus production and bronchospasm. In addition to respiratory distress, findings in affected patients may include rhonchi and wheezes on auscultation (15).

Depending on the exposure, alveolar damage can occur suddenly or after a prolonged latency phase. Exposure to high concentrations of agents such as chlorine or phosgene destroys alveolar epithelial cells and adjacent capillary endothelial cells, causing acute respiratory distress syndrome and death (15). Phosgene, in high doses, passes through the lungs into the pulmonary circulation, where it causes hemolysis. The resulting erythrocyte fragments obstruct pulmonary blood flow, causing sludging. Cor pulmonale can develop within minutes, causing death before other typical phosgene exposure symptoms evolve (34).

Exposure to chlorine or phosgene commonly results in a delayed onset of acute lung injury. Although moderate exposure to chlorine results in immediate upper airway symptoms, development of pulmonary edema occurs over 2–4 h. Severe chlorine exposures can cause pulmonary edema within 30–60 min, whereas massive exposures can cause sudden death secondary to laryngospasm (8). In contrast, phosgene exposure presents with more peripheral airway symptoms and a longer delay to symptom onset.

Massive exposure to phosgene can cause pulmonary edema within 2–6 h. However, in most victims, after a prolonged asymptomatic latency phase of up to 15 h, possibly 24–72 h (8), with phosgene exposure, patients can progress to acute respiratory distress syndrome/noncardiogenic pulmonary edema. Phosgene-induced injury to alveolar epithelial cells, with concomitant injury to pulmonary capillary endothelial cells sharing the same basement membrane, results in leakage of protein rich fluid into the interstitium between alveoli and into the alveolar spaces (15). Halfway through the latency phase, 2–8 h after exposure, the chest X-ray may reveal early signs of pulmonary edema, such as blurred enlargement of the hila and poorly defined patches or strip shadows, predominantly in the central portions of the lung (34). X-ray findings may have some prognostic significance: well-defined, small nodular opacifications indicate a better prognosis compared to large, patchy opacifications (34). Eventually, towards the end of the latency phase, patients develop profound dyspnea. Chest auscultation reveals diffuse crepitations, and patients suffer from significant respiratory distress (15,34). At this point, pulmonary function tests may demonstrate decreased pulmonary compliance and flow rate, with decreased vital capacity and decline in 1-s forced expiratory volume, and a disruption in gas exchange, with a decrease in carbon monoxide diffusion capacity (15,34). Airway obstruction may not respond to sympathomimetics and other bronchodilators (34).

As the symptoms progress, patients may develop frank pulmonary edema, manifested by progressive dyspnea, diffuse crackles on chest auscultation and cyanosis (34). In phosgene-exposed patients, chest X-rays may indicate pulmonary edema before development of these symptoms and physical findings (34). Pulmonary arterial pressure remains normal. However, as arterial oxygen tensions decrease, patients may develop ischemic changes on EKG. Some patients may develop a fever up to 40°C (104°F). Frequently, patients will develop copious amounts of frothy, protein-rich sputum and tracheal secretions. 24–30 h after phosgene exposure, patients may die due to asphyxiation and cardiac failure secondary to pulmonary edema (34).

Clearly, the clinical response to pulmonary agent exposures, especially those with low water solubility, such as phosgene, can vary, depending on the exposure. Patients with moderate exposures to phosgene may be asymptomatic, yet the prognosis may be poor. Clinicians treating phosgene-exposed patients should be aware of several caveats and one prognostic aid (34):

– Although phosgene reportedly has a characteristic odor, the smell has no value as a warning, because toxic effects can occur below the odor recognition threshold, and because other smells can mask the odor.

- Immediate irritation of mucus membranes, including the eyes, has no prognostic significance, because prolonged exposure to doses insufficient to cause such symptoms is capable of causing significant lung damage.
- Development of pulmonary edema can occur hours after exposure without any prodromal clinical symptoms.
- The length of the latency period is helpful as a prognostic indicator, because the shorter the latency period, the worse the prognosis.

Exertional dyspnea and reduced exercise tolerance can persist for several months or years in patients following phosgene exposure (8). Long-term sequelae of pulmonary agent exposure include chronic bronchitis, bronchiectasis, interstitial pulmonary fibrosis, airway hyperreactivity and large airway obstruction. Bronchiolitis obliterans and bronchiolitis obliterans organizing pneumonia are two distinct late sequelae from injury to small, distal airways. Some patients will develop Reactive Airway Dysfunction Syndrome (RADS), manifested by episodic cough, dyspnea, and chronic airway hyperreactivity, with wheezing after inhaling cold air or nonspecific pulmonary irritants (15,34). Chronic problems are more common in smokers and patients with preexisting lung disease (34). Human phosgene exposure has not been associated with increased incidence of cancer or adverse pregnancy outcomes (34).

Treatment

Management of pulmonary agent exposure begins with removal of the victim from the exposure site to fresh air and decontamination. Personnel caring for victims should use Level A or Level B PPE (Table 3.1) until completing decontamination (2). The first step in decontamination is to remove clothing that appears contaminated and jewelry. Patients with eye symptoms should receive a saline lavage to the eyes, and removal of contact lenses if present. After irrigation, use of a mydriatic may help prevent future synechiae formation (2). Patients should receive a thorough ophthalmological evaluation, if available, including visual acuity testing, fluorescein staining and slit lamp examination. In addition to mydriatics/cycloplegics such as homatropine, patients with corneal defects require antibiotic ointment and a pressure patch, followed by ophthalmologic referral (34). Patients with cutaneous or oropharyngeal symptoms should receive saline lavage to the affected areas (15).

After completing decontamination, the only effective management consists of close observation for the development of respiratory distress and supportive care. There are no known antidotes for pulmonary agent exposure. Patients exposed to phosgene or diphosgene require monitoring for a minimum of 12h because of the possibility of delayed symptoms (2). Strict bed rest is essential for patients with mild and moderate exposures, because any exertion, even minimal exertion, can shorten the clinical latent period and increase the severity of respiratory symptoms (8). In symptomatic patients, physical activity can cause clinical deterioration and even death (8). Supportive care consists of managing secretions, bronchospasm, hypoxia, and pulmonary edema.

The development of upper airway irritation, coughing, and stridor may indicate impending upper airway compromise. After exposure to chlorine, some adults and children have obtained symptomatic relief from administration of nebulized 3.75% sodium bicarbonate (7). Because patients can develop progressive upper airway injury and accumulate copious secretions, clinicians caring for these patients with upper airway symptoms should consider early intubation. Unfortunately, extensive glottic inflammation may preclude translaryngeal intubation, and some patients may require surgical establishment of an airway (15). Patients with any respiratory dysfunction should receive supplemental, humidified oxygen (2,15).

Nebulized bronchodilators, such as albuterol, may be helpful for patients with mild and moderate bronchospasm, with systemic steroids added for severe wheezing (2). All patients require monitoring for the development of acute lung injury and acute respiratory distress syndrome, which may occur up to 12–24 h after phosgene exposure. Some patients will develop severe pulmonary damage without upper airway or pharyngeal symptoms (15). Clinicians should consider ordering serial chest X-rays beginning 2 h after exposure (34). Patients developing manifest ARDS/pulmonary edema will require intubation with positive pressure ventilation, PEEP and high concentrations of oxygen (15,34). Superimposed bacterial infections require antibiotic therapy (2).

Other supportive therapies recommended for treatment of pulmonary edema include steroids and diuretics. In animal studies, earlier administration of steroids reduced pulmonary edema and lowered mortality rates, but there is no evidence systemic steroid treatment would be effective in humans. The recommended treatment for patients with pulmonary edema is parenteral prednisone, 1 g iv repeatedly, and aerosolized dexamethasone (34). There is scant evidence supporting the use of diuretics in treating pulmonary agent-caused pulmonary edema in patients without cardiac failure who are not fluid overloaded. Most animal studies reveal negative effects from diuretics, and some authorities view them as contraindicated. Certainly, clinicians treating pulmonary agent exposed patients should strive to maintain fluid balance and avoid fluid overload (34). If diuretics are necessary, patients require close monitoring of pulmonary wedge pressure to avoid excessive diuresis, which could predispose the patient to developing hypotension given the presence of air trapping and positive pressure ventilation (8).

Other, nontested, proposed regimens of dubious value include prostaglandin E_1, surfactant, antihistamines, asparaginase, calcium, atropine, anticoagulants, e-amino caproic acid, urease, hypothermia, and extra-corporeal oxygenation (34).

Postexposure Prophylaxis

Animal studies and human case reports have led to several proposed postexposure prophylactic regimens for asymptomatic patients exposed to pulmonary agents, specifically phosgene, to prevent development of complications. Unfortunately, all of these treatments lack evidence in systemic studies, and asymptomatic patients may find at least one of the treatments unacceptable:

- *Theophylline:* aminophylline and other β_2 agonists, such as nebulized isoproterenol, by increasing intracellular cyclic AMP, may be protective. In most, but not all animal studies, giving aminophylline 10 min after exposure, and repeated intraperitoneally after 2 and 4 h, reduced development of pulmonary edema. In another animal study, while aminophylline was effective, a related methyl xanthine, pentoxifylline, was not effective in preventing pulmonary edema. Unfortunately, there is no evidence recommending for or against using theophylline to prevent development of pulmonary edema in humans exposed to phosgene or other pulmonary agents (15,34).
- *N-acetyl cysteine (NAC):* in animal studies, NAC administered intratracheally 45–60 min after high-dose phosgene exposure significantly reduced development of pulmonary edema (15,34). The appropriate dose for humans would be 20 mL of a 20% NAC solution administered via nebulizer. However, there is no evidence for using this regimen in humans, and the FDA has not approved its use for prophylactic treatment of phosgene exposure (34).
- *Ibuprofen:* studies in rats, mice, and rabbits revealed that parenteral or intraperitoneal administration of ibuprofen during the asymptomatic phase following phosgene exposure was effective in preventing pulmonary edema. However, there is no evidence of its effectiveness in human victims and the FDA has not approved its use for this purpose. In addition, a dose comparable to those used in the animal studies, would require giving patients at least 25–50 mg kg^{-1} orally (34).
- *Steroids:* results from animal studies suggest that intravenous steroids, at doses ranging from 450 mg to 1 g of prednisolone, administered after exposure, may be effective in preventing pulmonary edema (15,34). Some experts have also recommended using an inhaled steroid, such as aerosolized dexamethasone or beclomethasone as a prophylactic agent (34). It is unclear whether any of these regimens would be useful in preventing pulmonary edema secondary to exposure to phosgene or any other pulmonary agent (15).
- *Positive airway pressure ventilation:* some experts recommend using positive pressure ventilation during the early, asymptomatic phase following phosgene exposure to prevent pulmonary edema. While positive pressure ventilation may reduce fluid accumulation, stabilize the intra-alveolar surfactant film and suppress arteriovenous shunts, many asymptomatic patients will find the treatment unacceptable (34). In addition, resources for providing prophylactic positive pressure ventilation may not be available in a mass-casualty situation.

RICIN

Ricin as a Chemical Weapon

Ricin, derived from the beans of the castor plant (Ricinus communis) is one of the most potent and easily produced toxins known. Early recognition of these characteristics led the United States to develop ricin as a chemical weapon during World

War I (35). Although the entire castor plant is poisonous, the seeds contain the highest concentration of ricin (36). For hundreds of years, countries all over the world have cultivated the plant for its oil, specifically for use as a laxative and for lubrication. Castor oil has many industrial and commercial uses, having served as a lubricant for racing engines (Castrol-R racing motor oil) and as an additive in paints and varnishes. One of its derivatives, sebacic acid, is a component in the production of nylon and alkyd resins, and contributes to the manufacture of plasticizers, lubricants, diffusion pump oils, cosmetics, and candles (35). India is currently the world leader in production, followed by China and Brazil (35).

The toxicity of the plant and its seeds has been common knowledge for centuries, particularly because of its effect on livestock. One seed, if chewed, can be fatal for a child (36). Besides its toxicity, ricin is attractive as a chemical agent because of its ease of extraction from the ubiquitous plant. The aqueous residue, or mash, following extraction of oil from the plant contains 5% ricin by weight (36). A simple procedure, using chemistry techniques familiar to undergraduate students, is sufficient to separate the toxin from the mash (36). Once produced, the toxin is relatively stable, making it suitable for dispersion as an aerosol, for injection or for contaminating food and water supplies (36). Given that the global production of castor beans exceeds 1 million tons each year, ricin is readily available.

Although far less toxic than botulinum toxin, given its availability, toxicity, stability, and ease of production, ricin has a colorful history of use as a chemical weapon. During World War II, the United States and Britain developed and tested, but never used, a bomb containing ricin, code-named "compound W" (35). In 1978, in London, using a weapon designed as an umbrella, an assassin killed Georgi Markov, a Bulgarian dissident, by injecting him in the thigh with a small metal pellet containing ricin (35,36). More recently, according to CNN news reports, Russian special forces found a recipe for ricin production while searching the body of a Chechen rebel, and plans for ricin production were found in Kabul, Afghanistan in November 2001 (35–38). Within the United States, in 1995, four US tax protesters belonging to a group called the "Minnesota Patriots Council" received convictions for possessing ricin and conspiring to use it to murder law enforcement officials by mixing it with the solvent DMSO (39). In addition, in 1995, a Kansas City oncologist fed her husband food contaminated with ricin in an unsuccessful murder attempt. In another domestic case, authorities arrested an Alaskan pipeline worker for possessing castor beans; 2 years earlier, Canadian customs agents found large quantities of ricin in his car while he was attempting a border crossing (35).

On October 15, 2003, authorities found an envelope with a threatening note accompanied by a sealed container containing ricin. Both items had undergone processing at a mail processing and distribution facility in Greenville, South Carolina (40). The note contained language threatening to poison water supplies if authorities did not meet certain demands. Fortunately, the subsequent investigation found no evidence of environmental contamination and no cases of ricin-associated illness. However, the CDC warned clinicians and public health officials to be vigilant for illnesses that could be related to ricin exposure (40).

Mechanism of Action

Ricin acts at the cellular level through an enzymatic inhibition of protein synthesis (35,36). Containing two polypeptide chains connected by a single disulfide bond (35,37,40,41), ricin is a member of the A–B family of toxins, which includes bacterial toxins such as diphtheria, pseudomonas, cholera, Shiga, and anthrax toxins (35). Within this family, the B chain facilitates bonding to cellular receptors and delivery of the toxin to the cell, whereas, once in the cell, the A chain possesses the catalytic activity that inactivates protein synthesis. Ricin's B-chain has lectin (agglutination) properties that facilitate binding to molecules on cell surfaces, triggering endocytosis of the toxin. Cellular uptake is slow, about 10% per hour at body temperature, resulting in a lag time between exposure to ricin and development of toxic effects (35). Once in the cell, cellular transport brings the A-chain through the Golgi complex to the cytoplasm where it enzymatically disrupts the 28S ribosomal unit, thereby inactivating protein synthesis (36).

Clinical Presentation and Diagnosis

Like many other biologic and chemical agents, the clinical presentation secondary to ricin exposure depends on the dose and route of exposure (41). Although terrorists might likely use ricin in aerosolized form, there are limited data on clinical symptoms following inhalation exposure due to the lack of historic inhalational cases, and animal studies are limited (35). Sublethal human aerosol exposures accidentally occurring in the 1940s caused an acute onset of several symptoms 4–8 h after exposure, including fever, chest tightness, cough, dyspnea, nausea, and arthralgias (41). Several hours later, profuse sweating heralded the termination of most of the symptoms (39). Animal models suggest that injury to the respiratory tract, including necrosis and severe alveolar flooding, would cause death from acute respiratory distress syndrome and respiratory failure following lethal human inhalation exposures (39). Human symptoms secondary to lethal inhalation doses would most likely include progressive cough and dyspnea, accompanied by cyanosis and pulmonary edema. In animal models, the time to death following inhalation exposure was dose dependent, with death occurring within 36–72 h (39,41).

In addition to symptoms and physical findings, diagnostic clues for inhalational exposure may include bilateral pulmonary infiltrates on chest X-ray, arterial hypoxemia, neutrophilic leukocytosis and a bronchial aspirate rich in protein compared to plasma, characteristic of high permeability pulmonary edema (39). Unlike many biologic agents, ricin intoxication would progress despite treatment with antibiotics.

Data on exposure through ingestion are also limited. There are no reported cases of ingestion of pure ricin toxin. Nevertheless, the signs and symptoms of exposure to the pure toxin are probably similar to those following ingestion of masticated castor beans (40). However, even this type of exposure is rare in humans, and case reports are uncommon. Depending on the dose, toxicity ranges from mild to severe symptoms, progressing to death. The incidence of mortality following castor bean ingestion may be exaggerated. One review of reported cases of castor bean ingestion from the early 1900s until 1984 revealed only three deaths, two verified by autopsy, and all occurring before 1935 (35,42) when modern treatment was unavailable.

Gastrointestinal symptoms following ricin ingestion may result from necrosis of gastrointestinal epithelium. Based on 10 nonfatal reported cases, initial symptoms begin 1–5 h following ricin ingestion. Symptoms can include nausea, vomiting, diarrhea, and abdominal cramps, and flu like symptoms, such as myalgias and arthralgias and dehydration (35,39). Fever can also occur. Larger exposures can cause persistent vomiting and massive diarrhea, perhaps bloody, potentially leading to substantial fluid loss, dehydration and hypovolemic shock (40). Severe exposures can cause hepatic, splenic, renal necrosis and failure (15,40). One case report was a 20-month-old child who developed hepatotoxicity 48–72 h after ingesting castor beans; laboratory tests revealed resolution of the hepatotoxicity 1 month later (35,43).

Parenteral ricin exposure is unlikely a result of a terrorist attack. Limited experience suggests that intramuscular injection may cause local necrosis of muscles and regional lymph nodes with moderate involvement of visceral organs (39). The only documented cases include a single human trial using low doses of intravenous ricin as a chemotherapeutic agent (40), an attempted suicide involving an intentional injection of ricin in the thigh, and the 1978 assassination of Georgi Markov (35). In the chemotherapy trial, intravenous ricin caused flu-like symptoms with fatigue and myalgias for several days. One patient developed weakness within 5 h, vomiting and fever within 24 h, followed by shock, multiorgan failure and death in three days (40). The patient who attempted suicide using an intramuscular injection presented 16 h after exposure with swelling of the injection site without necrosis. He developed a persistent temperature of 39°C for 8 days with nausea and anorexia, but recovered completely 10 days after exposure. One day after the umbrella attack, Markov was admitted to the hospital with high fever and inflammation at the puncture wound site on the back of his thigh, accompanied by a leukocyte count of 33,000 cu mm⁻¹. He had a fever and sudden drop in blood pressure and died 3 days after the incident (35,44).

Laboratory testing for ricin is limited, especially for inhalational exposures. The two common methods that can detect ricin in blood or other body fluids are the radioimmunoassay and the enzyme-linked immunosorbent assay (ELISA). Because ricin binds quickly and the body metabolizes it efficiently before excretion, the length of time necessary for these tests limits their usefulness for inhalation exposures (35). Besides testing body fluids, the CDC and member LRN state public health laboratories have a time-resolved fluorescence immunoassay that can test preparations of suspected ricin-containing substances and environmental specimens for the presence of ricin (40).

As with other biologic and chemical agents, symptoms of ricin exposure may resemble a typical respiratory or gastrointestinal illness. Physicians may suspect an intentional exposure to ricin based on epidemiologic clues suggestive of a chemical release, such as an unusual increase in the number of patients seeking care for similar symptoms, an unexpected progression of such symptoms in a group of patients or a credible threat of chemical release in the community (5). Person to person transmission does not occur.

Treatment

There are no known antidotes for ricin and treatment is primarily supportive. Depending on the route of exposure and symptoms, treatment may include intravenous fluids, vasopressors, respiratory support and cardiac monitoring (40). Dialysis will not remove ricin. Patients suffering from exposure through ricin ingestion should receive gastrointestinal decontamination based on the same principles used for other ingested toxins (40). Oral activated charcoal may reduce gastrointestinal absorption of ricin. Patients should receive activated charcoal as soon as possible, if there is no vomiting. Doses range from 25 to 100 g for adults, 25 to 50 g for children aged 1–12 years and 1 g kg^{-1} for infants. Although the efficacy of gastric lavage is controversial, physicians suspecting substantial gastrointestinal exposures should consider lavage if the patient presents to the hospital within 1 h of ingestion (40). Patients suspected or confirmed with ricin ingestion should not receive ipecac, whole bowel irrigation or cathartics.

All patients, regardless of the route of exposure, require monitoring for hypotension, hepatotoxicity and bone marrow suppression because of the risk of cardiac effects, liver damage, and multiple organ failure (35). Physicians and other health care providers suspecting ricin intoxication should immediately report the case(s) to their regional poison control center and local and state public health departments. The regional poison control center can provide guidance and information helpful in managing patients. Although ricin is not absorbed through the skin, patients with ricin containing powder on their skin should receive decontamination in a designated area outside of the main emergency department. Anyone potentially exposed to ricin-containing material should wash their hands thoroughly with soap and water and refrain from any hand-to-mouth activities (40).

Prevention

Ricin's potent immogenicity raises hope for development of an effective vaccine (36). Animal studies reveal that either active or passive immunization may be effective for intravenous or intraperitoneal exposures but only if given within a few hours after exposure (35). The vaccine is not effective against aerosolized toxin, the form terrorist would most likely use.

Special Considerations: Intentional Contamination of Food or Water with Chemical Agents

The last chapter discussed difficulties predicting the likelihood of intentional contamination of food and water with biological agents, and how the potential number of people affected increases as the contamination occurs closer to the site of production or distribution. The same is true for chemical contamination. Toxins make good weapons for contaminating food and water because they are usually odorless, colorless, and tasteless. In addition, many toxins, such as Botulinum toxin, are heat stable, allowing them to survive cooking, and are biologically active in microgram dosages (45).

Some historic examples illustrate how chemical contamination might occur. In 1946, one of the largest and most lethal terrorist attacks in the twentieth century resulted in arsenic poisoning of several thousand SS soldiers housed in US prisoner of war camp near Nuremberg, Germany in 1946. Nakam, a vengeance group, infiltrated the bakery supplying bread to the camp and spread an arsenic-based poison on the loaves (45). In 1978, a terrorist group attempting to damage Israel's economy claimed responsibility for contaminating Israeli citrus fruit with mercury (45). The contamination caused the hospitalization of a dozen children in Holland and Germany. In 1989, the United States recalled all Chilean grapes following allegations that terrorists had laced the fruit with minute quantities of cyanide (45). According to press reports, in 1992, Kurdish rebels may have tried to contaminate the water supply of a Turkish military base with potassium cyanide (45).

Potential chemical food contaminants terrorists could use include (45):

– Pesticides
– Heavy metals, such as lead or mercury
– Nonmetal ions such as fluorine, bromine, and iodine
– Food additives, such as bromate, gluatamate, nitrite, salicylate, sorbate, and sulfite
– Detergents, such as anionic detergents and quaternary amines
– Fat soluble vitamins
– Plant toxins, such as phytohemagglutinins, which can survive cooking temperatures and cause gastrointestinal symptoms
– Fungi produced heat-stable mycotoxins, such as vomitoxin, sometimes found in moldy grain
– Dioxin

Some of these substances can cause "natural" outbreaks, making detection of intentional contamination difficult. For example, from the early 1960s to the mid-1980s, consumption of food made with moldy grain caused at least 35 outbreaks affecting nearly 8,000 people in China. In 1987, nearly 100 people in India became ill after eating wheat products contaminated with mycotoxins after heavy rains (45).

Potential drinking water chemical contaminants terrorists could use include (45,46):

- Pesticides
- Inorganics, such as arsenic, barium, chromium, lead, mercury, and silver
- Radionuclides, such as radon, radium, and uranium
- Biologic toxins such as Botulinum toxin or Ricin
- Prions

Fortunately, several factors, including dilution, specific inactivation by chorine, ozone or other disinfectants, nonspecific inactivation by natural factors such as sunlight and microbes, filtration, and the small quantity of water individuals consume reduce the risk of disease from intentional contamination of water supplies (45). A few water treatment facilities add activated carbon to filter media to control taste, odor, and other chemical problems. These filters may provide additional protection against some of the organic toxins (45). The international recall of Perrier bottled water due to concerns about benzene contamination is evidence that bottled water is susceptible to contamination (45).

The keys to preventing successful chemical sabotage of food and water supplies are the same as those for biological sabotage: tight quality control at central processing locations and effective surveillance systems that can detect disease secondary to breakdowns at more distal sites (45). One clue indicating intentional contamination at a distal point of distribution would be a localized outbreak in a specific neighborhood, indicating contamination of a selected marketed food product or point in a posttreatment water distribution system (46). Primary care physicians will continue to play an important role in detecting potential food borne and water-borne chemical illness and promptly reporting cases to their local public health officials (46).

References

1. Malloy, CD. A History of Biological and Chemical Warfare and Terrorism. In Novick, LF and Marr, JS (Eds.). Public Health Issues in Disaster Preparedness. Aspen Publishers, Gaithersburg, Maryland, 85–92, 2001
2. Bozeman, WP, Dilbero, D, Schauben, JL. Biologic and Chemical Weapons of Mass Destruction. Emergency Medicine Clinics of North America, 20:975–993, 2002
3. Goozner, B, Lutwick, LI, Bourke, E. Chemical Terrorism: A Primer for 2002. Journal of the Association for Academic Minority Physicians, 13(1):14–18, 2002
4. Centers for Disease Control and Prevention. Biological and Chemical Terrorism: Strategic Plan for Preparedness and Response. Recommendations of the CDC Strategic Planning Workgroup. Morbidity and Mortality Weekly Report 49(RR04):1–14, April 21, 2000
5. Centers for Disease Control and Prevention. Recognition of Illness Associated with Exposure to Chemical Agents – United States, 2003. Morbidity and Mortality Weekly Report, 52(39):938–940, October 3, 2003

6. Ashraf, H. European dixoin-contaminated food crisis grows and grows [news]. Lancet, 353:2049, 1999
7. Henretig, FM, Cieslak, TJ, Eitzen, EM. Biological and Chemical Terrorism. Journal of Pediatrics, 141(3):311–326, 2002
8. Bogucki, S and Weir, S. Pulmonary Manifestations of Intentionally Released Chemical and Biological Agents. Clinics in Chest Medicine, 23:777–794, 2002
9. Agency for Toxic Substances and Disease Registry (ATSDR). Managing Hazardous Material Incidents (MHMI), Vols. 1–3. Atlanta, GA: US Department of Health and Human Services, Public Health Service, 2001. http://www.atsdr.cdc.gov/MHMI (last accessed 5/26/07)
10. US Department of Labor. Occupational Safety and Health Administration. Regulations (standards – 29 CFR): Hazardous Waste Operations and Emergency Response. 1910.120 Washington, DC 2002 http://www.osha.gov/pls/oshaweb/owadisp.show_document?p_table = STANDARDS&p_id = 9765. Last accessed 4/15/06
11. US Department of Labor, Occupational Safety and Health Administration. General Description and Discussion of the Levels of Protection and Protective Gear – 1910.120, Appendix B http://www.osha.gov/pls/oshaweb/owadisp.show_document?p_table = STANDARDS&p_id = 9767 Last accessed 4/15/06
12. Barach, P, Rivking, A, Israeli, AT, et al. Emergency Preparedness and Response During the Gulf War. Annals of Emergency Medicine, 32(2):224–233, 1998
13. Lynch, EL, Thomas, TL. Pediatric Considerations in Chemical Exposures. Are We Prepared? Pediatric Emergency Care, 20(3):198–205, 2004
14. Noeller, TP. Biological and Chemical Terrorism: Recognition and Management. Cleveland Clinic Journal of Medicine, 68(12):1001–1016, 2001
15. Greenfield, RA, Brown, BR, Hutchins, JB, et al. Microbiological, Biological and Chemical Weapons of Warfare and Terrorism. American Journal of the Medical Sciences, 323(6):326–340, 2002
16. Agency for Toxic Substances and Disease Registry. ToxFAQs for Nerve Agents (GA, GB, GD, VX). April 2002. http://www.atsdr.cdc.gov/tfacts166.html. Last accessed 4/15/06
17. World Health Organization. Public Health Response to Biological and Chemical Weapons: WHO Guidance. Chapter 3: Biological and Chemical Agents, 2004 http://www.who.int/csr/delibepidemics/chapter3.pdf (last accessed 4/15/06)
18. Agency for Toxic Substances and Disease Registry. Nerve Agents. http://www.atsdr.cdc.gov/MHMI/mmg166.pdf Last accessed 4/15/06
19. Belson, MG, Schier, JG, Patel, MM. Case Definitions for Chemical Poisoning. Centers for Disease Control and Prevention, MMWR 54(RR01):1–24, January 14, 2005
20. Lee, EC. Clinical Manifestations of Sarin Nerve Gas Exposure. Journal of the American Medical Association, 290(5):659662, 2003
21. Martin, CO, Adams, HP. Neurological Aspects of Biological and Chemical Terrorism. Archives of Neurology, 60(1):21–25, 2003
22. Schexnayder, S, James, LP, Kearns, GL, Farrar, HC. The Pharmacokinetics of Continuous Infusion Pralidoxime in Children with Organophosphate Poisoning. Journal of Toxicology: Clinical Toxicology, 36:549–555, 1998
23. Davis, KG, Aspera, G. Exposure to Liquid Sulfur Mustard. Annals of Emergency Medicine, 37(6):653–656, 2001
24. Agency for Toxic Substances and Disease Registry. Medical Management Guidelines. Blister Agents Lewisite (L) ($C_2H_2AsCl_3$) Mustard-Lewisite Mixture (HL) http://www.atsdr.cdc.gov/MHMI/mmg163.html. Last accessed 4/15/06
25. Agency for Toxic Substances and Disease Registry. Medical Management Guidelines. Blister Agents. Sulfur Mustard Agent H or HD ($C_4H_8Cl_2S$) CAS 505-60-2, UN 2927; and Sulfur Mustard Agent HT CAS 6392-89-8. http://www.atsdr.cdc.gov/MHMI/mmgd3.pdf. Last accessed 4/15/06
26. Agency for Toxic Substances and Disease Registry. Medical Management Guidelines. Blister Agents: Nitrogen Mustard (HN-1) ($C_6H_{13}Cl_2N$) Nitrogen Mustard (HN-2) ($C_5H_{11}Cl_2N$)

Nitrogen Mustard (HN-3) ($C_6H_{12}Cl_3N$) http://www.atsdr.cdc.gov/MHMI/mmg164.html. Last accessed 4/15/06

27. Rotenberg, JS. Cyanide as a Weapon of Terror. Pediatric Annals, 32(4):236–240, 2003

28. Sauer, SW, Keim, ME. Hydroxocobalamin: Improved Public Health Readiness for Cyanide Disasters. Annals of Emergency Medicine, 37(6):635–641, 2001

29. Centers for Disease Control and Prevention. Chemical Emergencies. Facts about Cyanide. http://www.bt.cdc.gov/agent/cyanide/basics/pdf/cyanide-facts.pdf. Last accessed 4/15/06

30. Brennan, RJ, Waeckerle, JF, Sharp, TW, Lillibridge, SR. Disaster Medicine. Chemical Warfare Agents: Emergency Medical and Emergency Public Health Issues. Annals of Emergency Medicine, 34(2):191–204, 1999

31. Agency for Toxic Substances and Disease Registry. Medical Management Guidelines for Hydrogen Cyanide. http://www.atsdr.cdc.gov/MHMI/mmg8.html, last accessed 4/15/06

32. Sauer, SW, Keim, ME. Hydroxycobalamin: Improved Public Health Readiness of Cyanide Disasters. Annals of Emergency Medicine, 37(6):635–641, 2001

33. Patocka, J, Fusek, J. Chemical Agents and Chemical Terrorism. Central European Journal of Public Health, 12(Suppl.):S75–S77, 2004

34. Borak, J, Diller, WF. Phosgene Exposure: Mechanisms of Injury and Treatment Strategies. Journal of Occupational and Environmental Medicine, 43(12):110–119, 2001

35. Doan, LG. Ricin: Mechanism of Toxicity, Clinical Manifestations and Vaccine Development. A Review. Journal of Toxicology: Clinical Toxicology, 42(2):201–208, 2004

36. Henghold II, WB. Other Biologic Toxin Bioweapons: Ricin, Staphylococcal Enterotoxin B and Trichothecene Mycotoxins. Dermatologic Clinics, 22:257–262, 2004

37. Dougherty, J. Moscow: Ricin Recipe Found on Chechen Fighter. CNN.com, January 13, 2003. http://www.cnn.com/2003/WORLD/europe/01/13/russia.ricin/index.html, last accessed 4/15/06

38. Anonymous. Ricin as a Weapon. CNN.com, October, 2003. http://www.cnn.com/2003/WORLD/europe/01/07/terror.poison.extremists/index.htmllast accessed 4/15/06

39. US Army Medical Research Institute of Infectious Diseases. Medical Management of Biological Casualties Handbook. Fort Detrick, Frederick, Maryland, Fourth Edition, February 2001

40. Centers for Disease Control and Prevention. Investigation of a Ricin-Containing Envelope at a Postal Facility – South Carolina, 2003. Morbidity and Mortality Weekly Report, 52(46):1129–1131, November 21, 2003

41. Marks, JD. Medical Aspects of Biologic Toxins. Anesthesiology Clinics of North America, 22:509–532, 2004

42. Rauber, A, Heard, J. Castor Bean Toxicity Re-Examined: A New Perspective. Vet Hum Toxicology, 27(6):498–502, 1985

43. Palatnick, W, Tenenbein, M. Hepatotoxicity from Castor Bean Ingestion in a Child. Journal of Toxicology: Clinical Toxicology, 38(1):67–69, 2000

44. Knight, B. Ricin a Potent Homicidal Poison. British Medical Journal, 3:350–351, 1979

45. Khan AS, Swerdlow, DL, Juranek, DD. Precautions Against Biological and Chemical Terrorism Directed at Food and Water Supplies. Public Health Reports, 116:3–14, 2001

46. Meinhardt, PL. Water and Bioterrorism: Preparing for the Potential Threat to US Water Supplies and Public Health. Annual Review of Public Health, 26:213–237, 2005

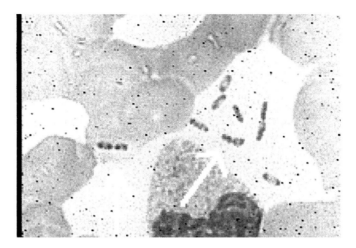

Fig. 2.4 Plague bacteria in blood (*arrows*). From Plague bacteria in blood. CDC Division of Vector-Borne Infectious Diseases (DVBID). http://www.cdc.gov/ncidod/dvbid/plague/p1.htm

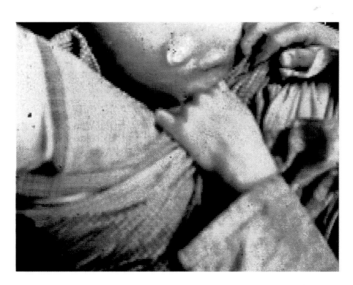

Fig. 2.5 Inguinal bubo on upper thigh of person with bubonic plague. From Inguinal bubo on upper thigh of person with bubonic plague. CDC Division of Vector-Borne Infectious Diseases (DVBID). http://www.cdc.gov/ncidod/dvbid/plague/p5.htm)

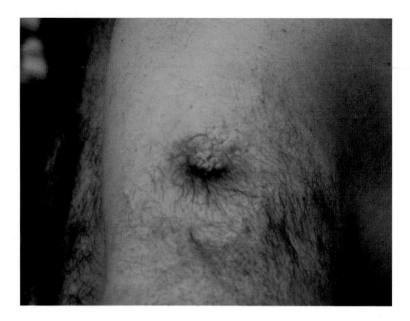

Fig. 2.7 Smallpox vaccination site

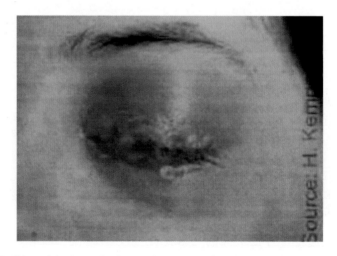

Fig. 2.8 Eyelid vaccinia due to inadvertent inoculation. From Kempe, H. Smallpox vaccination adverse reaction. CDC: Smallpox. http://www.bt.cdc.gov/training/smallpoxvaccine/reactions/adverse.html

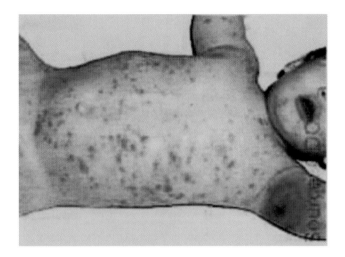

Fig. 2.9 Generalized vaccinia in an infant. From smallpox vaccination adverse reaction. CDC: Smallpox. http://www.bt.cdc.gov/training/smallpoxvaccine/reactions/adverse.html

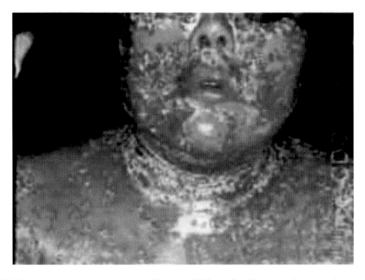

Fig. 2.10 Severe eczema vaccinatum in a 22 year old. From Smallpox vaccination adverse reaction. CDC: Smallpox. http://www.bt.cdc.gov/training/smallpoxvaccine/reactions/adverse.html

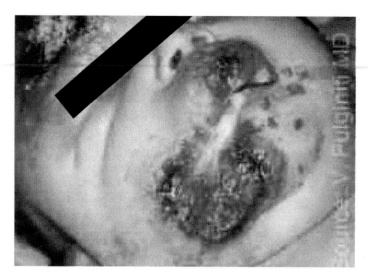

Fig. 2.11 Severe progressive vaccinia. From Fulginiti, V. Smallpox vaccination adverse reaction. CDC: Smallpox. http://www.bt.cdc.gov/training/smallpoxvaccine/reactions/adverse.html

FIGURE 2. Reported cases* of tularemia — United States, 1990-2000

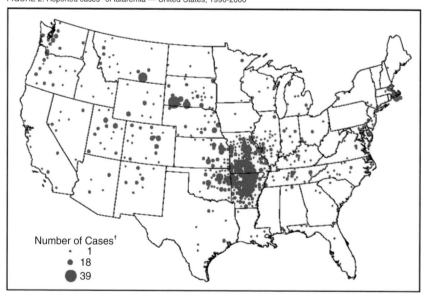

*Bases on 1,347 patients reporting country of residence in the lower continental United States. Alaska reported 10 Cases in four countries during 1990-2000.
† Circle size is proportional to the number of cases, ranging from 1-39.

Fig. 2.12 Reported cases of Tularemia, United States, 1990–2000. Based on 1,347 patients reporting county of residence in the lower continental United States. Alaska reported ten cases in four counties during 1990–2000. Circle size is proportional to the number of cases, ranging from 1 to 39. (From (40), public domain, Morbidity and Mortality Weekly Report 51, 9:181–185, 2002)

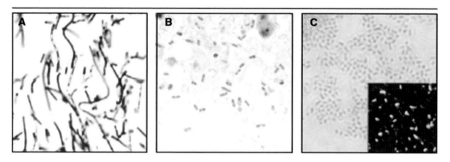

Fig. 2.14 Gram stain smears of the agents of anthrax (*Bacillus anthracis*) Plague (*Yersinia pestis*), and Tularemia (*Francisella tularensis*). *B anthracis* is a large (0.5–1.2 μm × 2.5–10.0 μm), chain-forming, gram-positive rod. *Y pestis* is a gram-negative, plump, non-spore-forming, bipolar-staining bacillus that is approximately 0.5–0.8 μm × 1–3 μm. *F tularensis* is a small (0.2 μm × 0.2–0.7 μm), pleomorphic, poorly staining, gram-negative coccobacillus (inset, direct immunofluorescence of smear of *F tularensis*; original magnification × 400. (From Dennis DT, et al. (43). Copyright© 2001 American Medical Association. All rights reserved.)

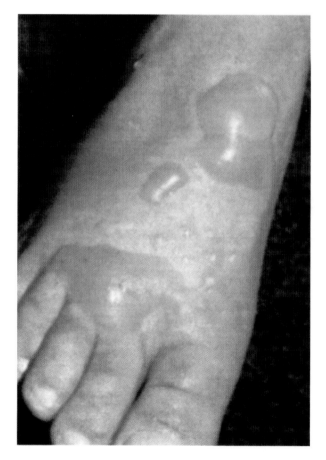

Fig. 3.1 Dorsum of right foot about 48 h after exposure to sulfur mustard vapor with characteristic blisters. (Courtesy of Professor Steen Christensen, Ronne, Denmark; Anitta Lild, photographer, Aarhus, Jutland.)

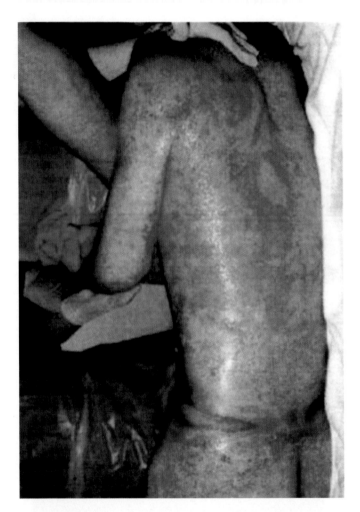

Fig. 3.2 Iranian soldier with mustard agent burns several weeks after exposure; injuries are beginning to heal. (Courtesy of Veijo Mehtonen, Karolinska University Hospital, Stockholm, Sweden)

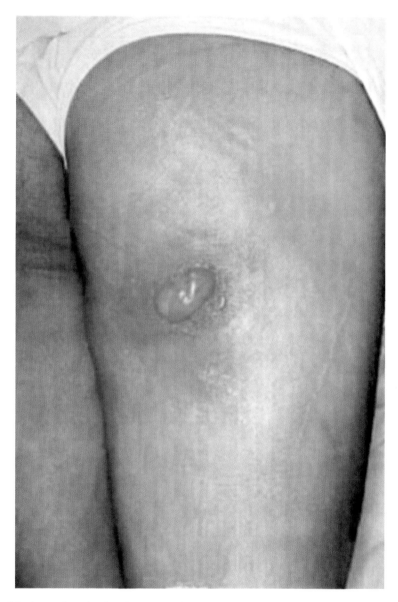

Fig. 4.1 Acute ulceration in a Peruvian patient who inadvertently placed a 26-Ci ^{192}Ir source in his back pocket, 3 days postexposure. The source remained in the pocket for approximately 6.5 h (From the medical basis for radiation accident preparedness, proceedings of the fourth international conference on accident preparedness, March 2001. Reproduced with permission of Routledge/Taylor & Francis Group, LLC. Also available at: http://www.bt.cdc.gov/radiation/criphysicianfactsheet.asp#B.)

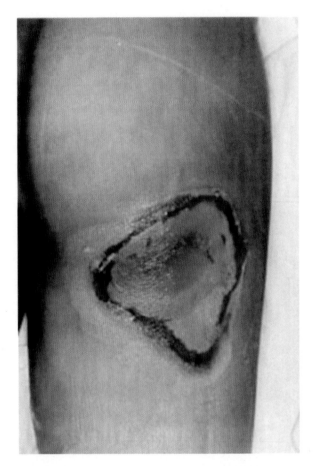

Fig. 4.2 Same patient, 10 days postexposure (from the medical basis for radiation accident preparedness, proceedings of the fourth international conference on accident preparedness, March 2001). Reproduced with permission of Routledge/Taylor & Francis Group, LLC. Also available at: (http://www.bt.cdc.gov/radiation/criphysicianfactsheet.asp#B, last accessed 5–11–06)

Chapter 4
Radiological Terrorism

Features of Radiological Terrorist Attacks

Radiological terrorism is the use of radioactive material to cause human casualties, environmental destruction and maximum disruption, panic and fear (1) in the general population for political purposes. Since the atomic bombing of Hiroshima in 1945, with 150,000 casualties and 75,000 fatalities (2), people have feared nuclear explosives more than any other weapons of mass destruction, because of the ability of these weapons to cause immediate devastation and trauma, and because radiation, undetected by human senses, can cause ongoing morbidity and mortality, including cancer, years after exposure (3).

Adding to this fear is the worldwide public awareness of the consequences of accidents involving radiation. From 1944 to 2002, in the United States, 243 radiation accidents occurred, causing 1,342 casualties meeting the criteria for significant radiation exposure (4). Worldwide, over the same period, 403 radiation accidents caused 133,617 casualties, with nearly 3,000 significant exposures and 120 deaths (4). In 1987, in Goiania, Brazil, an incident involving a medical source of radioactive Cesium (^{137}Cs) contaminated 200 people, 20 significantly, resulting in four deaths (4). The public is quite familiar with the 1986 Chernobyl reactor accident, which exposed over 116,500 people and caused at least 28 fatalities due to acute radiation sickness (4). Although these experiences have made the public aware and fearful of the potential harmful effects of radioactive material, they have also given us some knowledge in the evaluation and management of radiation victims.

Radioactive materials, used in industry and health care, are ubiquitous. Authorities have already confiscated radioactive materials from sellers in international black markets (5). Although detonating a nuclear bomb is the worst possible scenario, terrorists can use radioactive materials to fabricate other less lethal, but effective weapons. This chapter will discuss the five potential types and sources of radioactive weapons (1,3):

- Simple radiologic device (SRD): placement of an unshielded, high-level radioactive substance in a public place
- Radiological dispersal device (RDD), also known as a dirty bomb. These bombs use a conventional explosive to disperse radioactive material

A. L. Melnick (ed.), *Biological, Chemical, and Radiological Terrorism.*
© Springer 2008

- Sabotage of a commercial nuclear reactor
- Homemade nuclear weapon
- Nuclear weapon stolen from the military arsenal of a nuclear power

Simple Radiologic Devices

A SRD is the easiest type of weapon for terrorists to assemble. Surreptitiously, terrorists could place a device containing a high-energy radioactive source in one location, or they could simply spread the material by hand or aerosol in a highly populated area, such as an airport, train station or arena, to expose a maximum number of people (1). Similar to a biological attack, the impact of an attack using a SRD is likely to be covert and delayed. Like biological agents, radioactive exposures do not have an immediate impact due to an interval between exposure and the onset of illness. At lower exposure doses, the onset of clinical symptoms may occur after several weeks (4). Consequently, the most likely responders to SRD attacks will be family physicians and other health care providers, when patients present to primary care offices and emergency departments after developing symptoms. Following an SRD attack, the resulting symptoms and interval between exposure and symptom onset would be a function of the exposure dose, which, in turn, is a function of the radioactive source material, the distance from the exposed person to the source, the length of time exposed to the source and the level of shielding from the source (5).

Recent experience suggests that the use of a SRD, intentional or unintentional, is a plausible scenario. One potential SRD source is radioactive Cesium (^{137}Cs), which has many industrial and medical uses. Industry uses ^{137}Cs in highway construction in devices that measure the density of asphalt. In the Southeast United States, several of these devices have been missing or stolen, with their location unknown (1). The 1987 incident in Goiania, Brazil occurred after thieves stole a ^{137}Cs therapy source, still contained in its shielding, from a hospital, and sold it for scrap metal. Other involved individuals then broke up the source and shared it. None of the people involved was aware that the device was harmful, and authorities did not detect the incident for 15 days. By that time (1):

- Two hundred and forty-nine persons had been contaminated (out of 112,800 people screened)
- One hundred and twenty of those had external contamination on clothes and shoes
- One hundred and twenty-nine had external and internal contamination
- Twenty required hospitalization
- 14 developed bone marrow depression
- Eight required treatment with granulocyte-macrophage-colony stimulating factor
- Four died from hemorrhage and infection

(From Leikin JB, et al. (1) Reprinted with permission from Elsevier)

Stolen radioactive sources, specifically ^{60}Co (radioactive cobalt), have caused injuries elsewhere, including Juarez, Mexico, and Thailand. Within the United

States, thieves stole sixteen brachiotherapy sources of ^{137}Cs from a hospital in North Carolina and an industrial radiography source of ^{192}Ir (radioactive iridium) in Florida. Authorities have not recovered the materials (1).

Some elements used in SRDs have chemical as well as radiological toxicity. For example, cesium, an alkali metal, will explode if exposed to water. Cesium hydroxide, a strong base, is quite corrosive, and can attack glass. Clinicians and responders will need to be aware of the spectrum of risk posed by chemicals used in SRDs and other devices (1).

Radiologic Dispersal Devices

Radiologic dispersal devices (RRDs) would also be relatively easy for terrorists to assemble. RDDs, also known as "dirty bombs," are simply conventional explosives attached to radioactive materials (1,5,6). Common radioactive materials, such as ^{137}Cs, are potential sources for dirty bombs. Once detonated, the RDD can contaminate a large area, but because the material is widely dispersed, the level of contamination at any specific location would likely be small. People close to the site of the explosion, however, might suffer physical, potentially lethal injuries from the blast as well as greater radiation doses. For most victims, aside from blast injuries, external contamination with radiologic particles would be the primary problem. Health care providers responding to the victims should consider all exposed victims externally contaminated and at risk for skin injury from beta particles, described later in this chapter. In addition, all victims would require assessment for potential internal contamination through inhalation or absorption through wounds (5).

Based on computer modeling, detonation of a dirty bomb containing materials such as ^{137}Cs or ^{192}Ir would probably not have a large direct effect on the health of an exposed population. Aside from physical blast injuries, most people exposed would receive less than 100 mrem (millirem) of radiation exposure, which would provide a chronic disease risk of about 1/20,000, equivalent to smoking 100 cigarettes. Those few in the highest exposed group who received 5,000 mrem would suffer chronic risks equivalent to a long-term smoker's risk of cancer. Health care providers treating exposed patients could reduce the exposure levels by removing clothing and washing residual contamination off the skin. Of course, terrorists would probably not announce that the bomb they detonated contained radioactive material. Until authorities detected the radioactive source, other than the immediate blast effects, the radiological injuries could be covert and delayed, determined only when patients developing symptoms arrived at physician offices and emergency rooms after an incubation period.

Although the long-term health risks resulting from detonation of a RDD are relatively small, anxiety and fear associated with even low-level radioactive contamination could have significant economic and social consequences. Following the Goianai, Brazil incident, concerns over radioactive contamination led to a decrease in agricultural sales of 20% and a 15% decrease in the gross domestic product

(GDP) of Brazil's Goias State, with GDP levels not returning to preincident levels for 5 years (6).

Although assembling dirty bombs is not difficult, the process involves some risk. Commercial radioactive sources of substances such as ^{137}Cs and ^{192}Ir are powerful enough to present a hazard during assembly and transport of a device. To turn the material into an effective RDD, terrorists would have to remove the radioactive material from its shielding so it could be dispersed by the explosive. Exposure to such unshielded material for an hour at a distance of 1 m would provide enough radiation exposure to cause death without medical care. Although this type of exposure would not prevent many terrorists from assembling such a device, it would create problems for processing, handling and storing the device, and would make it easier for authorities to detect the source during processing and transport (6).

Nuclear Reactor Sabotage

Fortunately, for a couple of reasons, the likelihood of a terrorist attack on a nuclear reactor is quite low. Nuclear reactors operate under tight security and incorporate safety systems. In addition, the extensive shielding around reactors would require large amounts of explosives to create a breach. Even if terrorists could transport large amounts of explosives, they would have to breach a security cordon to reach the reactor. Alternatively, they could commandeer a jumbo jet plane to crash into a reactor or a nuclear pond of used cores, but they would have to breach security measures to do so. Computer modeling indicates that the construction of most reactors would sustain a 300 mph impact from a commercial aircraft, but not all scientists agree with these findings (1).

Even if terrorists succeeded in detonating an explosive at a reactor site, the health consequences would be limited. The reactor accident at the Three Mile Island, Pennsylvania nuclear power plant caused a small release of radiation, insufficient to cause any radiation injuries. Bypassing several safety systems caused the Chernobyl reactor incident, involving two explosions, fires and reactor core meltdown. This accident caused the following early phase health effects (1):

1. Two hundred and thirty-seven hospitalizations
2. One hundred and thirty-four cases of acute radiation syndrome (ARS)
3. Twenty-eight deaths within the first 3 months
4. Two deaths from the initial explosions
5. One death from congestive heart failure

(From Leikin JB, et al. (1) Reprinted with permission from Elsevier)

The two isotopes primarily responsible for the health effects were ^{137}Cs and ^{131}I (radioactive iodine). Given the extent of the accident, the effective response led to relatively few deaths (1). However, the significant widespread environmental contamination necessitated a permanent evacuation of 25,000 people.

Improvised Nuclear Devices and Stolen Nuclear Weapons

Detonation of an improvised or stolen nuclear weapon by terrorists is the worst-case radiological attack scenario (5). Although difficult to construct, due to requirements for sophisticated engineering and expertise, an improvised nuclear device could produce a yield similar to the Hiroshima bomb, with release or radiation, blast, thermal pulses, and radioactive fallout (1). At a minimum, a small nuclear detonation could cause damage equal or exceeding the September 11 attacks in New York City. Even if the nuclear detonation were unsuccessful, the conventional explosion associated with the device could cause significant environmental contamination with the nuclear weapons material, such as plutonium or uranium (1).

The high security associated with storage of nuclear weapons, at least in the western world, makes the probability of stealing a nuclear weapon remote. However, it is possible that 50–100 small nuclear weapons, with a 1 kiloton rating, are unaccounted for in the former Soviet Union (1). Terrorists could fashion these weapons into "suitcase bombs." If they were to detonate one such weapon, the blast range would reach 400 yards, thermal radiation would extend to the blast distance and nuclear radiation, including gamma particles and neutrons, would reach half a mile (1). If terrorists detonated the device in the air, the resulting electromagnetic pulse could damage solid-state equipment, including solid-state defibrillators, electrocardiograph machines, ventilators and other life-saving equipment. Radioactive fallout could cause high exposures for up to half a mile, requiring sheltering people for at least 2 weeks (1).

Certainly, the technical expertise to develop crude devices, including improvised nuclear devices, exists worldwide (4). Whereas terrorist attacks with SRDs and RDDs would cause a limited number of casualties, attacks with improvised or sophisticated nuclear weapons, if used in a populated area, have the potential for mass casualties and disruption. The Joint Commission on Accreditation of Healthcare Organizations has already directed hospitals to plan and prepare for a terrorist attack involving nuclear weapons, specifically asking them to (2):

– Incorporate contingency planning for loss of infrastructure and personnel
– Develop plans for relocating victims to operational hospitals
– Coordinate activities with appropriate local, state and federal agencies

Radiation Injury: Mechanism of Action

Ionizing radiation is electromagnetic energy or energetic particles emitted from a source (1). Ionizing radiation causes injury by depositing energy in tissue (5). The energy leads to formation of free radicals, which can damage DNA and other cellular structures and processes. The extent of injury and the risk of chronic health effects are proportional to the dose received and the rate of delivery. Cellular repair mechanisms can handle injuries caused by a given dose received slowly. The same dose, received more rapidly, can overwhelm cellular repair mechanisms, leading to cell death and malignant transformation (5). High exposures, received acutely, can kill some parenchymal cells. If the cells are not critical for survival, the clinical effect may be negligible. However, acute doses that kill large numbers of parenchymal cells or kill cells essential for organ function will cause clinical symptoms. Rapidly dividing cells, such as those of the gastrointestinal mucosa and the bone marrow, are most sensitive. At radiation doses below 100 rad (1.0 Gy), damage is limited, with most cells surviving, although some of the cells may undergo malignant transformation (5).

Depending on the incident, radioactive material cause radiation exposure in one or more (any combination) of three ways (1,2):

- *External radiation (irradiation)*: because radioactive material is not deposited on or in the body, decontamination is not necessary
- *External contamination*: In this scenario, radioactive material is present on external body surfaces; as with chemical contamination, responders should use caution to avoid contaminating other health care workers and facilities
- *Internal contamination*: Though inhalation, ingestion or transdermal absorption, radioactive material is deposited into body tissues

Types of Ionizing Radiation

There are several types of ionizing radiation, including alpha particles, beta particles, neutrons, gamma rays and X-rays. Alpha particles, containing two protons and two neutrons, contain a large amount of energy but cannot penetrate very far. While alpha particles can travel 2–3 cm in air, they can penetrate only microns into tissue. Clothing and even the outer, dead layers of skin will block alpha particles and prevent them from causing any injury to live tissue. Therefore, external contamination by alpha particles is not hazardous. On the other hand, alpha particles emitted from sources that have entered the body through ingestion, inhalation or wounds can cause significant damage to adjacent live tissue. Alpha particles are therefore a significant internal hazard (1,7). Radioisotopes with atomic numbers of 82 and higher, such as uranium or plutonium, are the major sources of alpha particles (4).

Beta particles are high-energy electrons. Compared to alpha particles, beta particles are less massive, can travel farther, up to 1 m in air, and penetrate deeper, up to a centimeter into exposed skin. A light material, such as aluminum or thick plastic, can block penetration. Clothing, including hospital protective clothing, will only partially block beta particle penetration. Depending on the radioactive isotope source, beta particles can have varying degrees of energy, measured in mega electron volts (MeV). Beta particles containing low levels of energy, 0.1 MeV, will penetrate 0.15 cm into tissue, whereas those with 5 MeV can penetrate 5 cm into live tissue. Beta particles left on the skin can cause severe burns to the skin and to the anterior compartment of the eye. Like alpha particles, beta particles are a significant internal hazard (1,4,7).

Neutrons, emitted from nuclear detonations, particle accelerators and nuclear weapon assembly facilities and not found in fallout, can penetrate deeply, causing extensive damage in two ways, either collision with other particles and/or neutron capture (1,4,7). Several elements, such as sodium, can "capture" neutrons. When exposed to neutron radiation, nonradioactive sodium (^{23}Na) can capture a neutron to become radioactive sodium (^{24}Na). In this way, exposed persons can become radioactive (1).

Gamma rays, high-energy rays with no mass and with short wavelengths, are very penetrating, traveling many meters in air and penetrating many centimeters into tissue. These characteristics make gamma rays capable of causing whole-body exposure (7). Lead, concrete or uranium shielding can markedly attenuate exposure, but cannot completely prevent penetration. These materials are usually not available on short notice, however. Clothing will not protect against gamma radiation, but it can prevent skin contamination by isotopes that emit gamma radiation. X-rays are similar to gamma rays but with a longer wavelength (1).

The human exposure measure for ionizing radiation is the radiation absorbed dose (rad), reflecting the mount of energy the ionizing radiation deposits in the body. The International System skin dose unit for radiation absorbed dose, the gray (Gy) is replacing the rad as a measure. 1 Gy, equivalent to $1 \, J \, kg^{-1}$ is equivalent to 100 rads; 10 mGy is equivalent to 1 rad. These measures are independent of the form or the radiation, and can reflect exposures that are single or multiple, or long or short duration (7). Exposure is proportion to dose and time of exposure, and inversely proportional to the square of the distance from the source (1).

Depending on the dose, dose rate and route of exposure, radiation can cause Acute Radiation Syndrome (ARS), cutaneous injury and scarring, chorioretinal damage (due to exposure to infrared energy), and increased long term risk for cancer, cataract formation (especially due to neutron irradiation), infertility and fetal abnormalities, such as growth retardation, fetal malformations, increased teratogenesis and fetal death (2).

Radiation injury causes two types of effects on biologic symptoms, stochastic and deterministic. Stochastic effects are "all or nothing" effects. At increasing doses, the probability of a stochastic effect increases, but once the stochastic effect occurs, further increases in exposure will not worsen the severity of the effect. A common stochastic effect is radiation-associated malignancy. In comparison, the severity of deterministic effects is proportional to the dose. Examples of deterministic effects include suppression of hematopoiesis, cataract formation and fertility impairment (4).

Nonradiation Hazards from Improvised Nuclear Devices and Nuclear Detonations

In addition to radiation exposure, and depending on the distance from the detonation, a nuclear explosion can expose people to two other types of energy, heat and blast. Heat accounts for approximately 35% of the energy released in a nuclear detonation. The bomb blast, or shock, accounts for approximately another 50%. Radiation energy accounts for only 15% of the energy from the detonation (2).

Heat and light cause thermal injuries, such as flash burns, flame burns and retinal burns. Temporary depletion of photopigment from the retinal receptors causes flash blindness. The blast wave causes physical injuries, such as fractures, lacerations, visceral ruptures, pulmonary hemorrhage and edema.

Radiation Injury: Clinical Presentation

Acute Radiation Syndrome

ARS, also known as radiation sickness, occurs after whole-body or significant partial-body exposure to more than 1 Gy at a relatively high dose rate (2). To cause ARS, the exposure must meet the following conditions (8):

– The absorbed dose must be large, generally greater than 0.7 Gy (70 rad), although patients may have mild symptoms at doses as low as 0.3 Gy (30 rad).
– The dose usually must be external. Ingested or inhaled radioactive materials have rarely caused ARS.
– The radiation must be penetrating, involving X-rays, gamma rays or neutrons.
– The whole body, or a significant portion of the body, must receive the dose. The most frequent radiological accidents cause local injury, frequently the hands, and do not cause ARS.
– The dose rate must be rapid, with the dose usually received within minutes. Doses split into fractions and delivered intermittently rarely cause ARS, compared to the same dose delivered at one time.

The most replicative cells, particularly spermatocytes, lymphohematopoietic cells and intestinal crypt cells are the most sensitive to the effects of ionizing radiation. The resulting clinical picture reflects damage to these cellular elements, and includes hematopoietic, gastrointestinal, cerebrovascular and cutaneous component syndromes. Each syndrome consists of four phases, prodromal, latent, manifest illness, and recovery or death. The time course and severity of the syndromes reflect the degree and rate of exposure (2). Table 4.1 illustrates the first three phases, including onset time, associated signs and symptoms, affected organ systems and prognosis (7).

Depending on the absorbed dose, patients will progress through the four phases at different rates, following a predictable clinical course. The prodromal phase usually begins within 48 h, but can occur as late as 6 days following exposure. Clinicians can estimate the dose a patient may have absorbed based on symptoms, system onset and laboratory studies. The presence and onset time of nausea and vomiting and the results of serial CBCs can help clinicians determine the severity of exposure. For example, significant lymphocytopenia developing in the first 6–48 h is a reliable indication that a patient will require prolonged, intense observation and treatment (5).

Table 4.1 Acute radiation syndrome

Phase	Feature	Dose range					
		0–100	100–200	200–600	600–800	800–3,000	>3,000
Prodromal	Nausea, vomiting	None	5–50%	50–100%	75–100%	90–100%	100%
	Time of onset		3–6h	2–4h	1–2h	<1h	Minutes
	Duration		<24h	<24h	<48h	<48h	N/A
	Lymphocyte count	No effect	Minimal decrease	<1,000 at 24h	<500 at 24h	Decreases within hours	Decreases within hours
	CNS function	No effect	No effect	Routine task performance cognitive impairment for 6–20h	Simple, routine task performance cognitive impairment for >24h	Rapid incapacitation / May have a lucid interval of several hours	
Latent	No symptoms	>2 weeks	7–15 days	0–7 days	0–2 days		None
Manifest illness	Signs, symptoms	None	Moderate leukopenia		Severe leukopenia, purpura, hemorrhage, pneumonia, hair loss after 300 rad	Diarrhea, fever, electrolyte imbalance	Convulsions, ataxia, tremor, lethargy
	Time of onset		>2 week		2 days–2 weeks		1–3 days
	Critical period		None		4–6 weeks; greatest potential for effective medical intervention	2–14 days	1–48h

(continued)

Table 4.1 (continued)

Phase	Feature	Dose range					
		0–100	100–200	200–600	600–800	800–3,000	>3,000
	Organ system	None			Hematopoietic, respiratory (mucosal) systems	GI tract mucosal systems	CNS
	Hospitalization	0%	<5%	90%	100%	100%	100%
	Duration of hospitalization		45–60 days	60–90 days	90+ days	Weeks to months	Days to weeks
	Mortality	None	Minimal	Low with aggressive therapy	High		Very high; significant neurologic symptoms indicate lethal dose

From Military Medical Operations Armed Forces Radiobiology Research Institute (7)

During the relatively brief latent phase, prodromal symptoms improve, and patients may appear recovered. Although patients may be asymptomatic, rapidly proliferating hematopoietic and gastrointestinal cells continue to die during the latent phase. The duration of the latent phase varies, depending on the radiation dose absorbed, the presence of any coexisting illness or injury and other patient characteristics (4). The manifest illness phase, characterized by moderate to severe immunosuppression, soon follows, with symptoms lasting up to weeks, depending on the absorbed dose. Clinical manifestations depend on several factors, including the organ system most involved (hematopoietic, gastrointestinal, vascular, neurological and cutaneous), the absorbed dose, and any associated coexisting illnesses or injuries (4).

Supralethal absorbed doses cause an accelerated progression, with patients experiencing all phases within hours rather than weeks, with death following within 2–12 days, depending on the dose (2). Radiation victims with associated physical trauma from blast effects are likely to have higher morbidity and mortality compared to uninjured patients, due to increased likelihood of complications such as hemorrhage, sepsis and delayed wound healing (4). Patients surviving the manifest illness phase enter the recovery phase, which can last from weeks to months.

Table 4.2 illustrates the four distinct syndromes involving the hematopoietic, gastrointestinal and cerebrovascular systems.

The Hematopoietic Syndrome

The hematopoietic syndrome results from whole body irradiation sufficient to suppress the production and function of formed blood elements. Although some bone marrow suppression can occur with doses as low as 0.7 Gy, the syndrome is seldom associated with absorbed doses less than 1 Gy (100 rads). Doses greater than 2–3 Gy suppress the ability for hematopoietic progenitor cells to divide. White blood cells, especially lymphocytes, are particularly sensitive to radiation injury. Depending on the absorbed dose, within weeks after exposure, patients can develop a hematologic crisis, with bone marrow hypoplasia or aplasia. Maximum bone marrow suppression generally occurs 2–4 weeks after exposure. Patients can develop pancytopenia, predisposing them to infection, particularly with Gram-negative bacteria. In addition to infection, hemorrhage and poor wound healing can also contribute to death (2,4,5).

Lymphocytopenia commonly occurs and tends to develop before other cytopenias (2). The predictability of lymphocytopenia following radiation exposure makes it somewhat useful as a prognostic indicator. An absolute lymphocyte count drop of 50% within the first 24h after exposure, followed by a more severe decline over the ensuing 48h, is characteristic of a lethal exposure (2). Some investigators have developed models using lymphocyte counts as measures of radiation exposure. However, associated injuries, such as burns and trauma, can also cause lymphocytopenia. Although some studies have validated the lymphocyte count predictive models, including models that account for coexisting injuries, clinicians should not rely solely on lymphocyte counts in establishing a prognosis or estimating absorbed dose (2).

Table 4.2 Syndromes associated with acute radiation exposure

Syndrome/Dose	Phase			
	Prodrome	Latent	Manifest illness	Recovery or death
Hematopoietic >0.7 Gy (>70 rads) (mild symptoms may occur as low as 0.3 Gy or 30 rads)	Lymphocytopenia Symptoms are anorexia, nausea and vomiting. Onset occurs 1 h to 2 days after exposure. Stage lasts for minutes to days	Although patients may be asymptomatic, rapidly proliferating cells continue to die; stage lasts 1–6 weeks	Symptoms are anorexia, fever and malaise Drop in all blood cell counts for several weeks; survival decreases with increasing dose; most deaths occur within a few months after exposure	In most cases, bone marrow cells begin to replicate; full recovery for a large % of individuals from a few weeks up to 2 years after exposure. Death may occur in some patients at 1.2 Gy (120 rads); the $LD_{50/60}{}^{a}$ is about 2.5–5 Gy (250–500 rads). Sepsis and hemorrhage are primary causes of death
Gastrointestinal >10 Gy (>1,000 rads) (some symptoms may occur as low as 6 Gy or 600 rads)	Abdominal pain, anorexia, nausea, vomiting and diarrhea. Onset occurs within a few hours after exposure; stage lasts about 2 days	Although patients may be asymptomatic, rapidly proliferating cells continue to die; stage lasts less than 1 week	Malaise, abdominal pain, nausea, vomiting, severe diarrhea, high fever, dehydration, electrolyte imbalance, gastrointestinal hemorrhage, anemia cardiovascular collapse, malnutrition, bowel obstruction, sepsis, renal failure	At doses greater than 12 Gy, mortality rate exceeds that of hematopoietic syndrome; death due to infection, dehydration and electrolyte imbalance within 2 weeks of exposure; the $LD_{100}{}^{b}$ is about 10 Gy (1,000 rads)

Cerebrovascular >50 Gy (5,000 rads) (some symptoms may occur as low as 20 Gy or 2000 rads)	Nausea, vomiting, watery diarrhea, burning sensation of skin, disorientation, fever, extreme nervousness, confusion, impairment of cognitive function prostration, hypotension, ataxia and convulsions; onset within minutes of exposure; stage lasts for minutes to hours	Lucid period up to 5–6h; patient may return to partial functionality	Watery diarrhea, convulsions, coma, respiratory distress, high fever, and cardiovascular collapse; differential diagnosis to consider is sepsis and septic shock; day	Death from cardiovascular collapse, cerebral edema, increased intracranial pressure and cerebral anoxia within 3 days in severe exposure. No recovery expected.

Adapted from http://www.bt.cdc.gov/radiation/arsphysicianfactsheet.asp, last accessed 9–11–05

[a]$LD_{50/60}$ dose necessary to kill 50% of the exposed population in 60 days

[b]LD_{100} dose necessary to kill 100% of the exposed population

Other cytopenias develop later depending on the absorbed dose and dose rate. After exposures less than 5 Gy, granulocyte counts may transiently increase before decreasing (2). The increase, known as an abortive rise, may be a prognostic indicator of a survivable exposure (2). Coexisting physical trauma and burns resulting from improvised nuclear devices complicate the treatment of patients with hematopoietic syndrome, and increase the mortality rate (2).

The Gastrointestinal Syndrome

As radiation exposure increases, patients are more likely to develop the gastrointestinal syndrome. Radiation doses grater than 5 Gy can destroy intestinal mucosal stem cells, resulting in loss of intestinal crypts and interruption of the intestinal mucosal barrier. Within hours after exposure, patients experience a rapid onset of gastrointestinal symptoms including abdominal pain, nausea, vomiting and diarrhea. Depending on the exposure, these symptoms can continue for 1–2 days, followed by a symptom-free latent period lasting up to a week. The recurrence of gastrointestinal symptoms, including vomiting, severe diarrhea and high fever, signals the end of the latent period. Systemic complications include electrolyte imbalance, dehydration, malabsorption with concomitant malnutrition, ileus resulting in bowel obstruction, gastrointestinal hemorrhage resulting in anemia, sepsis, acute renal failure and cardiovascular collapse (2,5). Beyond exposure doses of 12 Gy, the mortality rate from the gastrointestinal syndrome exceeds the mortality rate of the hematopoietic syndrome (2).

The Cerebrovascular Syndrome

Whole-body, ionizing radiation doses greater than or equal to 20–30 Gy (2,000–3,000 rad), cause hypotension and cerebral edema, contributing to the cerebrovascular syndrome. The prodromal phase, beginning almost immediately after exposure, includes nausea, vomiting, disorientation, confusion, prostration, hypotension, ataxia and convulsions. Patients presenting with fever, hypotension and major impairment of cognitive function have most likely experienced a supralethal dose of radiation, and are likely to die within several days. Physical examination may reveal papilledema, ataxia, and reduced or absent deep tendon and corneal reflexes. Patients may experience a latent, lucid period of up to several hours. Soon after, watery diarrhea, respiratory distress, hyperpyrexia and cardiovascular collapse follow. The differential diagnosis, which clinicians should consider, includes acute sepsis and septic shock. Within 2 days, patients are likely to die from circulatory complications of hypotension, cerebral edema, increased intracranial pressure and cerebral anoxia. Fortunately, events sufficient to cause this degree of exposure have rarely occurred, affecting only a few accident victims worldwide (5).

The Cutaneous Syndrome

Some skin damage frequently accompanies ARS. However, the cutaneous syndrome can also result from localized acute radiation exposure to the skin, usually from direct handling of radioactive sources or from contamination of the skin or clothes (2,8) (see Figs. 4.1 and 4.2) With localized exposure, even with high doses, the victim frequently survives, because the whole body usually does not receive the localized dose. However, if a patient with localized radiation induced cutaneous injury has also received whole body irradiation from an external source, the cutaneous damage increases the risk for death from the whole body exposure (2). Patients with the hematopoietic syndrome due to whole body irradiation will recover more slowly, if at all, from cutaneous injury due to bleeding, infection and poor wound healing (2).

Radiation damage to the basal cell layer can lead to inflammation, erythema and dry or moist desquamation. In addition, radiation can damage hair follicles, causing epilation. Within a few hours after exposure, exposed patients may develop a transient and inconsistent erythema associated with itching. These symptoms resolve, followed by a latent phase of more than a week. 12–20 days after exposure, patients present with intense erythema and desquamation or blistering. Ulceration may also be visible (5,8). Epidermal and sometimes, dermal loss characterizes the cutaneous injury from radiation exposure. Although the skin injury may cover a small area, the damage may extend deeply into soft tissue, affecting muscle and bone. Patients may develop significant local edema with the potential for a compartment syndrome (2).

Compared to thermal burns, radiation induced burns develop more than a week after exposure. Therefore, patients presenting with burn injuries immediately after exposure are suffering from thermal rather than radiation burns. Table 4.3 illustrates the relationship between exposure dose and cutaneous injury.

Radiation Injury: Diagnosis, Triage and Exposure Assessment

The diagnosis of ARS, especially after an unannounced attack with a SRD, may be difficult, because ARS does not appear as a unique disease. Like biologic agent exposures, radiation exposure may not have an immediate impact due to the interval between exposure and the onset of symptoms. Consequently, the most likely responders to future radiological attacks may be family physicians and other primary health care providers. For example, after exposure to a SRD, some exposed patients would arrive at their doctors' offices and local emergency rooms several days later, while others may have traveled, showing up at emergency rooms distant from their homes. Their prodromal symptoms might appear at first to be an ordinary gastrointestinal illness, with abdominal pain, nausea, vomiting and diarrhea. Following the prodrome, the exposed patients would enter the latent phase, feeling well and recovered from what appeared to be a brief gastrointestinal illness.

In the past, radiation accidents have frequently resulted in a delayed diagnosis. In a study of four radiation accidents due to lost sources (Mit Halfa, Egypt, May 2000,

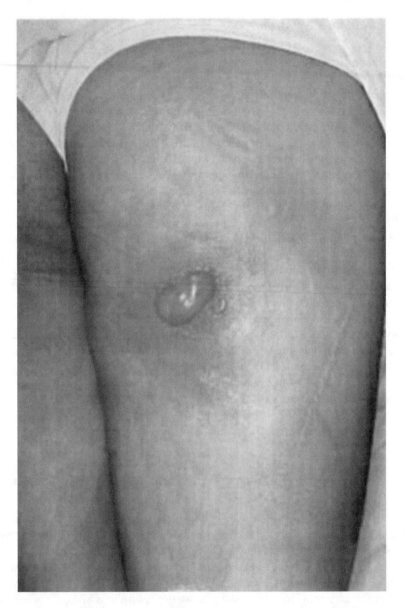

Fig. 4.1 (See color Plate) Acute ulceration in a Peruvian patient who inadvertently placed a 26-Ci ^{192}Ir source in his back pocket, 3 days postexposure. The source remained in the pocket for approximately 6.5 h (From the medical basis for radiation accident preparedness, proceedings of the fourth international conference on accident preparedness, March 2001. Reproduced with permission of Routledge/Taylor & Francis Group, LLC. Also available at: http://www.bt.cdc.gov/radiation/criphysicianfactsheet.asp#B.)

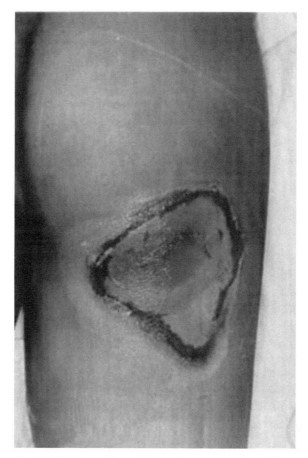

Fig. 4.2 (See color Plate) Same patient, 10 days postexposure (from the medical basis for radiation accident preparedness, proceedings of the fourth international conference on accident preparedness, March 2001). Reproduced with permission of Routledge/Taylor & Francis Group, LLC. Also available at: (http://www.bt.cdc.gov/radiation/criphysicianfactsheet.asp#B, last accessed 5–11–06)

Bangkok, Thailand, February 2000, Tammiku, Estonia, October 1994 and Goiania, Brazil, September 1987) a mean 22 days elapsed between exposure and diagnosis (5).

Nevertheless, astute clinicians can make a correct diagnosis by taking a thorough medical history. Clinicians should consider ARS in any patient with nausea and vomiting unexplained by other causes. Additional evidence pointing toward ARS includes bleeding, epilation, or white blood cell and platelet counts abnormally low a few days or weeks after any unexplained nausea and vomiting (8).

Because terrorists are unlikely to announce an attack with a simple radiological device or a RDD, there may be no warning that contaminated patients are arriving at an

Table 4.3 Cutaneous radiation injury

Grade	Skin dose[a]	Prodromal stage	Latent stage[b]	Manifest illness stage	Third wave of erythema[c]	Recovery	Late effects
I	>2 Gy (200 rads)	1–2 days postexposure or not seen	No injury evident for 2–5 weeks postexposure[b]	2–5 weeks postexposure, lasting 20–30 days: redness of skin, slight edema, possible increased pigmentation 6–7 weeks postexposure, dry desquamation	Not seen	Complete healing expected 28–40 days after dry desquamation (3–6 months postexposure)	Possible slight skin atrophy Possible skin cancer decades after exposure
II	>15 Gy (1500 rads)	6–24 h postexposure with immediate sensation of heat lasting 1–2 days	No injury evident for 1–3 weeks postexposure	1–3 weeks postexposure; redness of skin, sense of heat, edema, and skin may turn brown 5–6 weeks postexposure, edema of subcutaneous tissues and blisters with moist desquamation Possible epithelialization later	10–16 weeks postexposure, injury of blood vessels, edema, and increasing pain Epilation may subside, but new ulcers and necrotic changes are possible	Healing depends on size of injury and the possibility of more cycles of erythema	Possible skin atrophy or ulcer recurrence Possible telangiectasia (up to 10 years postexposure) Possible skin cancer decades after exposure

III	>40 Gy (4000 rads)	4–24 h postexposure, with immediate pain or tingling lasting 1–2 days	None or less than 2 weeks	1–2 weeks postexposure: redness of skin, sense of heat, slight edema, "possible" increased pigmentation. Followed by erosions and ulceration as well as severe pain	10–16 weeks postexposure: injury of blood vessels, edema, new ulcers, and increasing pain. Possible necrosis	Can involve ulcers that are extremely difficult to treat and that can require months to years to heal fully	Possible skin atrophy, depigmentation, constant ulcer recurrence, or deformity. Possible occlusion of small vessels with subsequent disturbances in the blood supply, destruction of the lymphatic network, regional lymphostasis, and increasing fibrosis and sclerosis of the connective tissue. Possible telangiectasia. Possible skin cancer decades after exposure

(continued)

Table 4.3 (continued)

Grade	Skin dose	Prodromal stage	Latent stage	Manifest illness stage	Third wave of erythema	Recovery	Late effects
IV	>550 Gy (55,000 rads)	Occurs minutes to hours postexposure, with immediate pain or tingling, accompanied by swelling	None	1–4 days post-exposure accompanied by blisters Early ischemia (tissue turns white, then dark blue or black with substantial pain) in most severe cases Tissue becomes necrotic within 2 weeks following exposure, accompanied by substantial pain	Does not occur due to necrosis of skin in the affected area	Recovery possible following amputation of severely affected areas and possible skin grafts	Continued plastic surgery may be required over several years Possible skin cancer decades after exposure

Source: Centers for Disease Control and Prevention, Cutaneous Radiation Injury: Fact Sheet for Physicians. June 29, 2005 http://www.bt.cdc.gov/radiation/criphysicianfactsheet.asp

[a] Absorbed dose to at least $10 \, cm^2$ of the basal cell layer of the skin

[b] Skin of the face, chest, and neck will have a shorter latent phase than the skin of the palms of the hands and the skin of the feet

[c] Especially with beta exposure

emergency room or office (1). Therefore, responders may not be aware of the existence, source of contamination or dose absorbed. Once clinicians suspect ARS, if possible, they should document the specific source, and the time of onset and severity of symptoms.

Triage

Appropriate triage is essential for evaluating and sorting out individuals who may need immediate treatment. Once health care responders suspect radiation exposure, they should (2,5,8):

- Provide first aid and resuscitation, including securing ABCs (airway, breathing and circulation) and beginning physiologic monitoring, such as vital signs, blood gases, electrolytes and urine output as appropriate.
- Minimize external radiation to rescue and treatment personnel. The Oak Ridge Associated Universities Web site (http://www.orau.gov/reacts/care.htm#Techniques, last accessed 5–11–06) contains detailed guidelines for protection of health care and rescue personnel (9). Strict isolation precautions, including gowns, masks, caps, double gloves and shoe covers are required when evaluating and treating contaminated patients. In addition, staff should change gloves frequently to avoid cross contaminating other patients and staff. Staff should use appropriate radiation detection devices to detect contaminants in the hospital to facilitate removal and decontamination. After use, health care staff should remove their protective equipment, placing the equipment in clearly labeled, sealed containers. All health care workers who have adhered to the Oak Ridge guidelines have avoided contamination from handling radiation accident victims (2).
- Stabilize the patient, medically and surgically, and provide definitive treatment of serious injuries, including major trauma, burns and respiratory injury if evident. Patients should receive necessary surgical interventions within 36 h and no later than 48 h after exposure; surgery after that time is contraindicated for 6 weeks or until evidence appears that the patient is immunocompetent and that incised tissue is capable of revascularizing (10).
- Besides obtaining blood samples to address trauma, obtain blood samples for complete blood counts helpful in estimating exposure dose, paying particular attention to the lymphocyte count and human leukocyte antigen typing before any initial transfusion.
- Assess the patient for contamination and decontaminate as necessary.

External Decontamination

Fortunately, skin or wound contamination rarely presents a life-threatening risk to either patients or health care personnel (5). The best possible scenario is decontamination in the field before transport; however, following an attack with a radiologic dispersion device (RDD), patients suffering trauma will most likely present to emergency departments before undergoing external contamination.

The first step in external decontamination is removal of outer clothing and shoes, which should reduce the level of contamination by 90% (5). A radiation detector, held at a constant distance from the skin and passed over the entire body, is useful in assessing any residual external contamination. Following the assessment, washing the skin and hair with soap and warm water, along with gentle brushing to remove contaminated particles is effective in removing any residual contamination. Health care responders should take care to avoid damaging the skin during the decontamination process. In addition, covering open wounds can help prevent additional internal contamination. Following the first attempt at decontamination, responders should repeat the assessment process with the radiation detector, at the same distance from the skin as they did initially. If any residual contamination is still present, response staff should repeat hair and skin washing and brushing and reassess with the radiation detector. The ultimate decontamination goal is to reduce the level of external contamination below two times the background radiation level, or until the repeated attempts fail to reduce the level by 10% or more (5).

Cleaning wounds to remove contamination is essential, because wounds promote internal contamination through absorption of radioactive materials directly into the circulatory and lymphatic systems (5). The technique used depends on the nature of each wound. Standard decontamination techniques, such as irrigation, are effective against abrasions. However, lacerations and puncture wounds can present challenges due to poor access to the contaminants. If irrigation is ineffective, some lacerations may require excision of contaminated tissue. Likewise, puncture wounds may be difficult to decontaminate with oral irrigators or water jets, although irrigation is worth trying. Wounds containing radioactive shrapnel are particularly problematic and require special care. Amputation has been necessary when removal of radioactive shrapnel from heavily contaminated extremities was unsuccessful (5).

Biodosimetry

After stabilization and external decontamination, patients require assessment for radiation injury based on dose, specific isotope involved and the presence of internal contamination. By performing individual biodosimetry, physicians can predict the subsequent clinical severity, survivability and treatment required, as well as triage patients with subclinical or no exposure (2). The three most useful items for estimating exposure doses in a mass casualty situation are:

- Time from exposure to onset of emesis
- Lymphocyte depletion kinetics
- Presence of chromosome dicentrics

Clinicians can crudely estimate the absorbed dose from the clinical presentation and peripheral leukocyte counts. The interval from exposure to emesis onset decreases with increasing doses. If the interval is less than 4 h, the effective whole body dose is probably at least 3.5 Gy. If the interval is under 1 h, the patient probably received a dose of 6.5 Gy or more. Patients with this level or exposure are likely to experience a complicated medical course with a high fatality rate (5).

Lymphocytes are the most radiosensitive of all blood elements, and their count numbers decline following first-order kinetics after high-level total body exposure (5,10). The rate of decline is related linearly to the total body exposure does, making lymphocyte count monitoring particularly helpful in dose estimation (11). Patients presenting within 8–12 h of exposure should have complete blood counts with leukocyte differential immediately after exposure, repeated every 2–3 h during the first 8 h after exposure, repeated every 4–6 h during the ensuing 2 days, and repeated twice per day for the following 3–6 days to monitor declines in lymphocyte counts (2,8). At a minimum, to estimate exposure dose, patients should have three (preferably six) blood counts with differential obtained within the first 4 days after exposure to calculate a slope for lymphocyte count decline (2). Figure 4.3, the Andrews Lymphocyte Nomogram, illustrates the relationship between the rate of lymphocyte depletion and the severity of injury (8).

If available, a qualified cytogenic laboratory can help estimate exposure dose by analyzing chromosome aberrations in peripheral blood lymphocytes. After exposure, lymphocytes can display several types of chromosome aberrations. Dicentrics, chromosomes with two centromeres, are biomarkers for exposure to ionizing radiation (7). Clinicians interested in evaluating chromosome dicentrics should request 10 mL of peripheral blood drawn 24 h after exposure, placing the sample in a lithium-heparin tube or an ethylenediaminetetraacetate (EDTA) tube (2,7). During transport to the lab, the samples require a cold pack to remain at 4°C, but not frozen. The laboratory will isolate the blood lymphocytes, stimulate them to grow in culture, arrest cell proliferation during the first metaphase, and observe metaphase

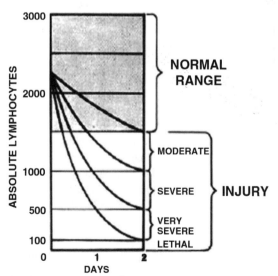

From Andrews GA, Auxier JA, Lushbaugh CC. *The Importance of Dosimetry to the Medical Management of Persons Exposed to High Levels of Radiation. In Personal Dosimetry for Radiation Accidents.* Vienna: International Atomic Energy Agency; 1965.

Fig. 4.3 Andrews lymphocyte nomogram (reprinted with permission)

spreads microscopically for enumeration of dicentrics. Using an established dose response curve, the laboratory will report the estimated dose the exposed patient received (7). Because of the necessary incubation times, results will not be available for 48–72 h after sample submission (2).

The Armed Forces Radiobiology Research Institute Web site (http://www.afrri. usuhs.mil, (2,7) last accessed 1–01–06) features a radiation casualty management software program, the biological assessment tool (BAT), that clinicians can use to estimate exposure dose (12). The software archives clinical information, including the extent of contamination, the presence of wounds and infection, and displays the diagnostic information in a concise format. The software includes an interactive map of the human body that allows users to document the location of a personnel dosimeter, radiation-induced erythema and radioactivity detected with an appropriate detection device. The Institute is also developing triage software for palm devices that will allow first responders to triage suspected radiation casualties based on initial, prodromal features.

Whether or not the BAT is available, using medical cards or flow charts, clinicians caring for exposed patients should document prodromal signs and symptoms as a function of time after exposure throughout the course of management (2). Documentation should include the body location of radioactivity, thermal and traumatic injuries, the degree of erythema and lymphocyte counts. Health care staff can enter these data into BAT or alternative tools at triage stations to facilitate estimation of exposure doses and appropriate triage.

Physicians caring for pregnant women exposed to radiation should attempt to estimate the fetal exposure. Although the uterus provides some protection, the human embryo and fetus are more sensitive to radiation exposure than adults are, and the health consequences for the fetus may be severe at doses too low to immediately affect the mother. Such health consequences can include growth retardation, malformations, impaired brain function and cancer (13).

Fetal exposure is a function of the external and internal maternal exposure. The external dose to the mother's abdomen provides a reasonable estimation of the external exposure to the fetus. Estimating the internal fetal dose is more complex. Any contaminant ingested or absorbed by the mother eventually entering the maternal blood stream may pass through the placenta to the fetus. Although the placenta provides some protection, most contaminants reaching the maternal circulation are detectable in the fetal circulation. Fetal concentrations depend on the specific contaminant and the stage of fetal development. For example, substances such as iodine, needed for fetal growth and development, reach higher concentrations in the fetus compared to the mother. In addition, any radioactive material that concentrates in the maternal tissues adjacent to the uterus, such as the bladder, can cause fetal exposure. Internal exposures to substances tending to concentrate in specific organs, such as iodine-131 and iodine-123 in the thyroid, iron-59 in the liver, gallium-67 in the spleen and strontium-90 and yttrium-90 in the bones, can cause exposure to their corresponding fetal organs.

Physicians can obtain assistance in estimating fetal dosages. Hospital health and medical physicists may be available to help. The National Council on Radiation

Protection and Measurements (NCRP) Report Number 28, Radionuclide Exposure of the Embryo/Fetus contains information useful for estimating fetal exposures. The report, available at http://www.ncrponline.org/ncrprpts.html (last accessed 1–29–06) contains fetal radiation dose estimates for 83 radionuclides (14). The report also contains information the mechanisms and consequences of prenatal radiation exposure.

Clinicians seeking additional help with fetal dose estimation can locate their state Radiation Control/Radiation Protection Contact through the Conference of Radiation Control Program Directors, Inc. (CRCPD) Web site at http://www.crcpd.org/map/map.asp (last accessed 1–29–06). In addition, the Health Physics Society (HPS) Web site contains a list of certified Health Physicists at http://www.hps1.org/aahp/members/members.htm (last accessed 1–29–06) who can help with fetal dose estimation.

After estimating fetal exposure, clinicians should consider the potential health effects on the fetus. Potential fetal health effects other than cancer are a function of gestational age and radiation dose (13). The information in Table 4.4 can help physicians advise their pregnant patients, but the table does not provide definitive recommendations. However, clinicians should consider these basic principles in providing advice to pregnant women exposed to radiation:

- The main health concern for significant exposures greater than 0.1 Gy early in the pregnancy (before 2 weeks of gestation) is death of the embryo. If the embryo survives the exposure, noncancer health consequences are unlikely, no matter how high the exposure dose. The reason for this is that the few cells contained in the embryo are progenitors for many other cells. Damage to one cell in the embryo will generally cause the death of the embryo. Surviving embryos successfully implanting in the uterus are unlikely to exhibit congenital abnormalities (13).
- Throughout gestation, radiation-induced noncancer health effects are undetectable for fetal doses below 0.05 Gy. Available research suggests that doses below 0.05 Gy represent no risk at any stage of development. However, research on rodents suggests that doses in the 0.05–0.10 Gy range may present a small risk of malformations or central nervous system abnormalities at some stages of gestation. Nevertheless, when providing advice regarding prenatal exposure, clinicians can consider 0.10–0.20 Gy as a practical threshold for congenital effects in the human embryo or fetus (13).
- Between 8 and 15 weeks of gestation, radiation can impair brain development, with atomic bomb survivor data revealing an average IQ loss of 25–31 points per Gy above 0.10 Gy. The risk for severe mental retardation increases by 40% per Gy at doses above 0.10 Gy (13).
- Between approximately 16 weeks gestation and birth, radiation-induced noncancer health effects are unlikely for fetal exposures below 0.50 Gy. Although some researchers believe that doses above 0.10 Gy between 16 and 25 weeks of gestation present a small risk for impaired brain function, most researchers believe that following 16 weeks gestation, 0.50–0.70 Gy doses represent the threshold for congenital effects (13).

Table 4.4 Potential health effects, other than cancer, of prenatal radiation exposure

Acute radiation dose[a] to the embryo/fetus	Time postconception				
	Blastogenesis (up to 2 weeks)	Organogenesis (2–7 weeks)	Fetogenesis		
			(8–15 weeks)	(16–25 weeks)	(26–38 weeks)
<0.05 Gy (5 rads)[b]	Noncancer health effects NOT detectable				
0.05–0.50 Gy (5–50 rads)	Incidence of failure to implant may increase slightly, but surviving embryos will probably have no significant (noncancer) health effects	Incidence of major malformations may increase slightly Growth retardation possible	Growth retardation possible Reduction in IQ possible (up to 15 points, depending on dose) Incidence of severe mental retardation up to 20%, depending on dose	Noncancer health effects unlikely	Noncancer health effects unlikely
>0.50 Gy (50 rads) The expectant mother may be experiencing ARS in this range, depending on her whole-body dose	Incidence of failure to implant will likely be large,[c] depending on dose, but surviving embryos will probably have no significant (noncancer) health effects	Incidence of miscarriage may increase, depending on dose	Incidence of miscarriage probably will increase, depending on dose	Incidence of miscarriage may increase, depending on dose	Incidence of miscarriage and neonatal death will probably increase depending on dose[d]

Substantial risk of major malformations such as neurological and motor deficiencies	Growth retardation likely	Growth retardation possible, depending on dose
Growth retardation likely	Reduction in IQ possible (>15 points, depending on dose)	Reduction in IQ possible, depending on dose
	Incidence of severe mental retardation >20%, depending on dose	Severe mental retardation possible, depending on dose
	Incidence of major malformations will probably increase	Incidence of major malformations may increase

Source: Centers for Disease Control and Prevention. Prenatal Radiation Exposure: A Fact Sheet for Physicians, March 23, 2005. http://www.bt.cdc.gov/radiation/pdf/prenatalphysician.pdf

Note: This table is intended only as a guide. The indicated doses and times postconception are approximations.

[a] Acute dose: dose delivered in a short time (usually minutes). Fractionated or chronic doses: doses delivered over time. For fractionated or chronic doses the health effects to the fetus may differ from what is depicted here

[b] Both the gray (Gy) and the rad are units of absorbed dose and reflect the amount of energy deposited into a mass of tissue (1 Gy = 100 rads). In this document, the absorbed dose is that dose received by the entire fetus (whole-body fetal dose). The referenced absorbed dose levels in this document are assumed to be from beta, gamma, or X-radiation. Neutron or proton radiation produces many of the health effects described herein at lower absorbed dose levels

[c] A fetal dose of 1 Gy (100 rads) will likely kill 50% of the embryos. The dose necessary to kill 100% of human embryos or fetuses before 18 weeks' gestation is about 5 Gy (500 rads)

[d] For adults, the LD50/60 (the dose necessary to kill 50% of the exposed population in 60 days) is about 3–5 Gy (300–500 rads) and the LD100 (the dose necessary to kill 100% of the exposed population) is around 10 Gy (1,000 rads)

- Although the central nervous system is less sensitive to radiation between 16 and 25 weeks gestation, higher doses at this stage can cause similar central nervous system impairment as do lower doses between 8 and 15 weeks. At doses above 0.70 Gy, the average IQ loss is about 13–21 points per Gy. In addition, above 0.70 Gy, the risk for severe mental retardation is about 9% per Gy (13).
- At 16–25 weeks, the fetal thyroid is active and susceptible to damage from radioactive iodine exposure. Maternal exposures will concentrate in the fetal thyroid at this stage of development (13).
- At 26 weeks and beyond, the fetus is less sensitive to noncancer effects from radiation exposure. However, large doses, above 1 Gy increase the risk for miscarriage, fetal death and neonatal death (13).
- In sufficient dosage, ionizing radiation can impair development occurring at the time of exposure. Data for pregnant atomic bomb survivors demonstrate permanent physical growth retardation at increasing exposures, especially above 1 Gy, and especially if the exposure occurs in the first trimester. The survivor data suggest a 3–4% reduction of height at age 18 for exposures greater than 1 Gy (13).

Table 4.5 describes the risk for childhood cancer from prenatal exposure and the lifetime cancer risk for exposure at age 10. Researchers do not know whether the carcinogenic effects of a given radiological exposure vary with gestation. The current wisdom is that carcinogenic effects are constant throughout pregnancy. However, available animal data suggest that exposure during the early stages of pregnancy, during blastogenesis and organogenesis, is less likely carcinogenic. The same data suggest that late in gestation, fetuses are strongly sensitive to carcinogenic effects of ionizing radiation (13).

Also unknown is the lifetime cancer risk following prenatal exposure to radiation. When advising pregnant women exposed to radiation, clinicians should consider that available data suggest that lifetime cancer risk from prenatal exposure is similar to, or slightly higher than, the cancer risk secondary to childhood exposure (Table 4.5).

Internal Decontamination

Clinicians suspecting internal contamination should request samples of urine, stool, vomit and wound secretions to determine the specific contaminant. Patients admitted with airways or endotracheal tubes are more likely to have internal contamination (9). Treatment of ingestion exposures with aluminum hydroxide or magnesium carbonate antacids can prevent or at least minimize internal contamination by reducing gastrointestinal absorption. Following ingestion of strontium isotopes, patients should receive aluminum-containing antacids. Gastric lavage administered within 1–2 h after ingestion can also help reduce internal contamination. Patients suffering from large ingestion doses should receive cathartics, including enemas, to decrease gastrointestinal transit time (5). For patients with significant inhalation exposures to insoluble radionuclides, pulmonary lavage may be considered but is seldom indicated (5).

Table 4.5 Estimated risk for cancer from prenatal radiation exposure

Radiation dose	Estimated childhood cancer incidence[a,b] (%)	Estimated[c] lifetime cancer incidence[d] (exposure at age 10) (%)
No radiation exposure above background	0.3	38
0.00–0.05 Gy (0–5 rads)	0.3–1	38–40
0.05–0.50 Gy (5–50 rads)	1–6	40–55
>0.50 Gy (50 rads)	>6	>55

From Centers for Disease Control and Prevention. Prenatal Radiation Exposure: A Fact Sheet for Physicians, March 23, 2005. http://www.bt.cdc.gov/radiation/pdf/prenatalphysician.pdf.

[a]Data published by the International Commission on Radiation Protection

[b]Childhood cancer mortality is roughly half of childhood cancer incidence

[c]The *lifetime cancer* risks from prenatal radiation exposure are not yet known. The lifetime risk estimates given are for Japanese males exposed at age 10 years from models published by the United Nations Scientific Committee on the Effects of Atomic males exposed at age 10 years from models published by the United Nations Scientific Committee on the Effects of Atomic Radiation

[d]Lifetime cancer mortality is roughly one-third of lifetime cancer incidence

Although potassium iodide does not protect the thyroid from external radiation, patients suffering from internal radioiodine contamination should receive potassium iodide to prevent or reduce thyroid uptake. To be effective, patients must receive the potassium iodide within a few hours after exposure (5,11). Compared to adults, children are more susceptible to the effects of radioiodine. Consequently, the Federal Drug Administration (15) and World Health Organization recommendations for administration of potassium iodide differ for children and adults. Table 4.6 contains the FDA recommendations for potassium iodide administration.

Adults older than 40 should receive potassium iodide only if the projected thyroid exposure is 5 Gy or greater. On the other hand, exposed neonates, infants and children should receive potassium iodide to avoid thyroid exposures as low as 10 mGy. Exposed pregnant women should receive potassium iodide to protect themselves as well as their fetus. Administration of potassium iodide to lactating women can reduce the level of radioiodine in milk, but their breast-feeding infants should still receive potassium iodide (15). Potential potassium iodide side effects include rashes, allergic reactions and gastrointestinal symptoms, and patients with underlying thyroid disease can develop iodine-induced thyroid dysfunction (5). Because the protective effect of potassium iodide lasts for only 24 h, patients with continued exposure through ingestion or inhalation should continue to receive daily doses until the significant exposure has ceased. Physicians should avoid repeat potassium iodide dosing in infants to reduce the risk of hypothyroidism during the critical stage of brain development. Likewise, physicians should avoid repeat dosing in pregnant and lactating women if possible. If repeat dosing is necessary, the

Table 4.6 FDA recommendations for potassium iodide administration

Threshold thyroid radioactive exposures and recommended doses of KI for different risk groups

	Predicted thyroid exposure (cGy)	KI dose (mg)	No. of 130 mg tablets	No. of 65 mg tablets
Adults over 40 years	≥500			
Adults over 18 through 40 years	≥10	130	1	2
Pregnant or lactating women	≥5			
Adoles over 12 through 18 years[a]	≥5	65	1/2	1
Children over 3 through 12 years[a]	≥5			
Over 1 month through 3 years	≥5	32	1/4	1/2
Birth through 1 month	≥5	16	1/8	1/4

From United States Food and Drug Administration, Center for Drug Evaluation and Research. Guidance: Potassium Iodide as a Thyroid Blocking Agent in Radiation Emergencies, http://www.fda.gov/cder/guidance/4825fnl.pdf.

[a]Adolescents approaching adult size (≥ 70 kg) should receive the full adult dose (130 mg)

neonate will require T4 and TSH monitoring with administration of thyroid hormone if hypothyroidism develops (15).

The FDA has approved the oral administration of Prussian Blue (ferric hexacyanoferrate) to treat internal contamination with cesium and thallium (16). Prussian Blue works by increasing fecal excretion of these elements. Patients require treatment only if the exposure dose of ^{137}Cs exceeds the annual limit (200 uCi from inhalation or 100 uCi from ingestion) (5). Clinicians should consult with a health physicist to determine whether exposure has exceeded the annual limit. Treatment for exposures between one and ten times the annual limit is controversial. However, exposures exceeding ten times the limit usually indicate the need for treatment. Once treatment has reduced the level of internal contamination below the annual limit, Prussian Blue treatment can stop. However, the clinician can use his or her discretion to discontinue treatment if residual levels remain above the annual limit after prolonged treatment (5).

The FDA recommends 3 g Prussian Blue three times daily for adolescents and adults and 1 g three times daily for children aged 2–12 years for a minimum of 30 days. Clinicians can adjust the dosage and length of treatment based on the level of internal contamination. The chief Prussian Blue side effect is constipation, and clinicians should use Prussian Blue carefully for patients with impaired gastrointestinal motility (5).

Patients suffering from internal contamination with the transuranic elements (plutonium, americium and curium) should receive treatment with the chelating agents, Ca-DTPA and Zn-DTPA. These agents react with the transuranic elements to form complexes amenable to urinary excretion. For adults, the FDA recommends a 1 g loading dose of Ca-DTPA administered intravenously as soon as feasible after exposure. Children younger than 12 years of age should receive 14 mg kg^{-1} Ca-DTPA intravenously. Because Ca-DTPA is teratogenic, pregnant women should receive Zn-DTPA instead if it is available. Maintenance treatment is 1 g Zn-DTPA for adults or 14 mg kg^{-1} Zn-DTPA for children given intravenously once per day for days, months or years, depending on the level of internal contamination. Administration of Ca-DTPA by nebulizer is also effective. Clinicians caring for patients receiving chelation treatment should monitor serum levels of trace minerals, such as zinc, magnesium and manganese, throughout the course of therapy (5).

Radiation Injury: Treatment

Following initial triage, stabilization, external decontamination, dose assessment and internal decontamination, clinicians should categorize patients into appropriate treatment groups based on general treatment guidelines (2). These guidelines should complement but not replace clinical judgment. Patients with low (<1 Gy) exposure doses do not require treatment for ARS. Those with very high (>10 Gy) doses require only supportive and comfort care because of the grave prognosis (2). Table 4.7 summarizes the recommended guidelines for patient categorization. Because the hematopoietic syndrome is responsible for most of the mortality below 10 Gy of exposure, treatment for radiation injury is directly chiefly at the hematopoietic syndrome. Treatment of the hematopoietic syndrome includes cytokine (colony-stimulating factors) therapy, transfusion and stem-cell transplantation. Short-term treatment with cytokines may be appropriate for relatively low exposure doses (≤3 Gy). Patients with higher exposure levels, for example, above 7 Gy, or those with concomitant traumatic injuries or burns, may require prolonged treatment with cytokines, blood component transfusions and stem cell transplantation (SCT) (5). In addition, patients with the hematopoietic syndrome may need antibiotics for prophylaxis or treatment of infections.

Treatment of the Hematopoietic Syndrome

Cytokine Therapy

Cytokine therapy works by enhancing the survival, amplification and differentiation of granulocyte progenitor cells. Currently, three recombinant cytokines, sargramostim (granulocyte macrophage colony stimulating factor), filgrastim (granulocyte colony stimulating factor) and pegfilgrastim (pegylated filgrastim) are licensed for treating chemotherapy-induced neutropenia (2,5). Although the FDA has not approved any of these agents for managing radiation-induced aplasia, the Radiation Studies Branch at the CDC has recently developed an investigational new drug protocol for their use in patients exposed to high doses of ionizing radiation (5).

Evidence for the effectiveness of these agents comes from their use in cancer patients, human radiation accident victims, and animal studies. Filgrastim and sargramostim have hastened neutrophil recovery 3–6 days in patients following

Table 4.7 Guidelines for treatment of radiologic victims[a]

Variable	Proposed radiation dose range for treatment with cytokines	Proposed radiation dose range for treatment with antibiotics[b]	Proposed radiation dose range for referral for SCT consideration
	←	Gy	→
Small-volume scenario (≤100 casualties)			
Healthy person, no other injuries	3–10[c]	2–10[d]	7–10 for allogeneic SCT; 4–10. If previous autograft stored or syngeneic donor available
Multiple injuries or burns	2–6[c]	2–6[d]	NA
Mass casualty scenario (>100 casualties)			
Healthy person, no other injuries	3–7[c]	2–7[d]	7–10 for allogeneic SCT[e]; 4–10 If previous autograft stored or syngeneic donor available
Multiple injuries or burns	2–6[e]	2–6[d,e]	NA

Source: Waselenko JK, et al. (2), Reprinted by permission of the American College of Physicians

[a]Consensus guidance for treatment is based on threshold whole-body or significant partial-body exposure does. Events due to a detonation of a RDD resulting in ≤100 casualties and those due to detonation of an improvised nuclear device resulting in >100 casualties have been considered. These guidelines are intended to supplement (and not substitute for) clinical findings based on examination of the patient. NA = not applicable; SCT = stern-cell transplantation

[b]Prophylactic antibiotics include a fluoroquinolone, acyclovir (if patient is seropositive for herpes simplex virus or has a medical history of this virus), and fluconazole when absolute neutrophil count is $<0.500 \times 10^9$ cells L^{-1}

[c]Consider initiating therapy at lower exposure dose in nonadolescent children and elderly persons. Initiate treatment with granulocyte colony-stimulating factor or granulocyte-macrophage colony-stimulating factor in victims who develop an absolute neutrophil count $<0.500 \times 10^9$ cells L^{-1} and are not already receiving colony stimulating factor

[d]Absolute neutrophil count $<0.500 \times 10^9$ cells L^{-1}. Antibiotic therapy should be continued until neutrophil recovery has occurred. Follow Infectious Diseases Society of America guidelines (17) for febrile neutropenia if fever develops while the patient is taking prophylactic medication

[e]If resources are available

myelotoxic therapies, including bone marrow and SCT. Neutrophil recovery time was similar whether patients received early or delayed filgrastim therapy after transplantation (5). In the Radiation Emergency Assistance Center Center/Training Site (REACT/TS) registry of radiation accident victims (http://www.orau.gov/reacts/registry.htm), patients receiving filgrastim and sargramostim have had faster neutrophil recovery following radiation accidents. However, there was variation in the administration of these agents, making it difficult to draw conclusions about the clinical effectiveness of these agents following radiation exposure. For example, many of the patients in the registry received both agents, patients received therapy at various intervals after exposure, and some patients received interleukin-3 (2,5). In contrast to the human studies, several studies involving rhesus macaques have demonstrated a shortening of the period of severe neutropenia following administration of colony stimulating factors within 1–2 days post-60-Cobalt irradiation (5).

Table 4.8 contains the Strategic National Stockpile Radiation Working Group recommendations for cytokine treatment following exposure to ionizing radiation (2). Once biodosimetry reveals that a patient has suffered from whole-body or significant partial-body exposure greater than 3 Gy (>2 Gy for patients with multiple injuries or burns), or if clinical signs and symptoms reveal a level three or four degree of hematotoxicity (see Table 4.9), clinicians should immediately begin cytokine therapy. Later, the clinician can adjust cytokine dosage based on other information, such as chromosome dicentrics. Although lab studies may reveal an

Table 4.8 Recommended doses of cytokines

Cytokine	Adults	Children	Pregnant women[a]	Precautions
G-CSF or filgrastim	Subcutaneous administration of 5 µg kg^{-1} of body weight per day, continued until ANC >1.0 × 10^9 cells L^{-1}	Subcutaneous administration of 5 µg kg^{-1} per day, continued until ANC >1.0 × 10^9 cells L^{-1}	Class C (same as adults)	Sickle-cell hemoglobinopathies, significant coronary artery disease, ARDS; consider discontinuation if pulmonary infiltrates develop at neutrophil recovery
Pegylated G-CSF or pegfilgrastim	One subcutaneous dose, 6 mg	For adolescents >45 kg: one subcutaneous dose, 6 mg	Class C (same as adults)	Sickle-cell hemoglobinopathles, significant coronary artery disease, ARDS
GM-CSF or sargramostim	Subcutaneous administration of 250 µg m^{-2} per day, continued until ANC >1.0 × 10^9 cells L^{-1}	Subcutaneous administration of 250 µg m^{-2} per day, continued until ANC >1.0 × 10^9 cells L^{-1}	Class C (same as adults)	Sickle-cell hemoglobinopathles, significant coronary artery disease, ARDS; consider discontinuation if pulmonary infiltrates develop at neutrophil recovery

Source: Waselenko et al. (2), Reprinted by permission of The American College of Physicians. *ANC* absolute neutrophil count, *ARDS* acute respiratory distress syndrome, *G-CSF* granulocyte colony-stimulating factor, *GM-CSF* granulocyte-inacrophage colony-stimulating factor

[a] Experts in biodosimetry must be consulted. Any pregnant patient with exposure to radiation should be evaluated by a health physicist and matemal-feral specialist for an assessment of risk to the fetus. Class C refers to US Food and Drug Administration Pregnancy Category C, which indicates that studies have shown animal, teratogenic, or embryocidal effects, but there are no adequate controlled studies in women; or no studies are available in animals or pregnant women

Table 4.9 Levels of hematopoietic toxicity[a]

Symptom or sign	Degree 1	Degree 2	Degree 3	Degree 4
Lymphocyte changes[b]	$\geq 1.5 \times 10^9$ cells L^{-1}	$1–1.5 \times 10^9$ cells L^{-1}	$0.5–1 \times 10^9$ cells L^{-1}	$<0.5 \times 10^9$ cells L^{-1}
Granulocyte changes[c]	$\geq 2 \times 10^9$ cells L^{-1}	$1–2 \times 10^9$ cells L^{-1}	$0.5–1 \times 10^9$ cells L^{-1}	$<0.5 \times 10^9$ cells L^{-1}
Thrombocyte changes[d]	$\geq 100 \times 10^9$ cells L^{-1}	$50–100 \times 10^9$ cells L^{-1}	$20–50 \times 10^9$ cells L^{-1}	$<20 \times 10^9$ cells L^{-1}
Blood loss	Petechiae, easy brulsing, normal hemoglobin level	Mild blood loss with <10% decrease in hemoglobin level	Gross blood loss with 10–20% decrease in hemoglobin level	Spontaneous bleeding or blood loss with >20% decrease in hemoglobin level

Source: Waselenko et al. (2), by permission of the American College of Physicians.

[a]Modified from Dainiak N (24)

[b]Reference value, $1.4–3.5 \times 10^9$ cells L^{-1}

[c]Reference value, $4–9 \times 10^9$ cells L^{-1}

[d]Reference value, $1.40–400 \times 10^9$ cells L^{-1}

initial granulocytosis followed by neutropenia, the patient should receive cytokine therapy continuously. Once the absolute neutrophil count rebounds from its nadir and reaches 1.0×10^9 cells L^{-1}, it is appropriate to discontinue cytokine treatment. However, monitoring should continue, and clinicians should resume cytokine treatment if the neutrophil count declines significantly ($< 0.5 \times 10^9$ cells L^{-1}) after discontinuation of initial cytokine treatment.

Children younger than 12, adults over 60 and patients of any age with multiple injuries or burns are generally more susceptible to radiation injury. Therefore, these patients should receive cytokine therapy at lower levels (>2 Gy) of whole or partial-body exposure. Patients with exposures above 6–7 Gy involved in an accident with over 100 casualties will generally have a poor prognosis for survival. In such events involving mass casualties, given the level of resources available, it may make sense to withhold cytokine treatment from these patients, especially if they also suffer from significant traumatic injuries or burns. Given that cytokines are expensive and critical resources requiring administration for long periods, physicians may have to make difficult triage decisions regarding their use. For example, it may be prudent to give cytokine treatment preferably to patients without additional injuries because of their greater chance for survival, such as adults under 60 with 3–7 Gy exposures and children and adults ≥ 60 with 2–7 Gy exposures. Cytokine doses are equivalent to those given to patients with chemotherapy related neutropenia (2).

In addition to cytokines, patients with anemia may benefit from receiving epoetin and darbepoetin, even though studies have not established their effectiveness following radiation accidents (2). The response to these agents takes up to 3–6 weeks, and patients may require supplementation with iron (2).

Transfusion

Patients with severe bone marrow dysfunction will require cellular component transfusions, such as packed red blood cells and platelets. Hospitals and health care providers caring for victims of radiological events will have time to mobilize potential blood donors, because bone marrow suppression generally occurs 2–4 weeks following exposure. Of course, trauma patients may require immediate transfusion due to blood loss. Because bone marrow suppression is associated with immunosuppression, the cellular components must undergo leukoreduction and irradiation (25 Gy) to prevent transfusion-associated graft-versus-host disease in the recipients. Clinicians caring for transfused patients may have trouble differentiating graft-versus-host complications from direct radiation-induced organ damage. Symptoms of both may include fever, pancytopenia, rashes, desquamation, diarrhea, and liver function abnormalities. In addition to preventing graft-versus-host disease, leukoreduction of the cell components before transfusion reduces the frequency of febrile nonhemolytic reactions, reduces the immunosuppressive effects of the transfusion and provides protection against platelet alloimmunization and cytomegalovirus infections (2).

Stem Cell Transplantation

Most of the data related to the effectiveness of SCT are from its use in patients with hematological malignant conditions. For these conditions, matched related and unrelated allogeneic SCT have been life saving and potentially curative (2). Experience is limited and less positive for SCT in treating patients with radiation-induced bone marrow aplasia following radiation accidents. Although radiation accident victims have experienced transient engraftment, their outcomes have been dismal secondary to associated burns, trauma and radiation damage to other organs. A review of 29 cases involving SCT treatment of radiation accident victims revealed that all patients with burns died and only three of the 29 victims survived beyond 1 year. The review did not indicate whether the SCT affected survival (2). SCT of two patients following a 1999 radiation accident in Japan had similar results, with both patients experiencing donor-cell engraftment before going on to die of radiation-induced organ damage or infection (2).

Given our experience with SCT following radiation exposure, clinicians should consider SCT following exposures of 7–10 Gy in patients without accompanying burns or other major organ toxicity and if a suitable donor is available (see Table 4.7). Patients demonstrating residual hematopoiesis (granulocyte counts above 0.50 × 10^9 cells L^{-1} and platelet counts exceeding 100 × 10^9 cells L^{-1} 6 days after exposure) may not be candidates for SCT. Nevertheless, clinicians should consider stem cell infusions for patients with exposures above 4 Gy when (rarely) a syngeneic donor or previously harvested autologous bone marrow is available (2).

Infection treatment and prophylaxis: Victims of radiological attacks are at risk for infection due to disruption of the skin or mucosal barriers and due immune suppression from a reduction in lymphohematopoietic cells (2). Studies in irradiated dogs have revealed a reduction in mortality following antibiotic administration. During the neutropenic phase, control of infections is especially important. Patients who are not neutropenic should receive antibiotics directed at specific foci of infection caused by the most likely pathogens. On the other hand, neutropenic patients may benefit from prophylaxis with fluoroquinolones. Patients with severe neutropenia (absolute neutrophil count $<0.500 \times 10^9$ cells L^{-1}) should receive prophylaxis with broad-spectrum antibiotics while the neutropenia lasts. Prophylaxis may include (2):

– A fluoroquinolone with streptococcal coverage or a fluoroquinolone without streptococcal coverage plus penicillin (or a penicillin congener)
– An antiviral agent (acyclovir or one of its congeners)
– An antifungal agent (such as fluconazole)

In murine studies, quinolones have been effective in controlling endogenous gram-negative systemic infections following radiation. Quinolones are also effective in preventing endogenous Klebsiella and Pseudomonas infections. In addition, penicillin supplementation has prevented treatment failures in cancer patients with treatment-induced neutropenia (2).

Patients should receive antibiotics until the neutrophil count improves ($>0.500 \times 10^9$ cells L^{-1}) or until they develop neutropenic fever or some other indication that the antibiotics are not effective. Patients developing specific focal infections while neutropenic should receive antibiotics directed at the cause of the infection. Clinicians should withdraw quinolone treatment for patients developing a fever while receiving the fluoroquinolone and should instead treat for a gram-negative infection such as Pseudomonas aeruginosa, which can be rapidly fatal in a neutropenic patient (2). If available, primary care physicians may want to consult with an infectious disease specialist familiar with the recommendations of the Infectious Diseases Society of America. Because animal studies have revealed that altering the anaerobic gut flora may worsen outcomes, patients should not receive gut prophylaxis unless they have a clinical indication, such as an abdominal wound or *Clostridium difficile* enterocolitis (2).

Immunosuppressed radiation victims with positive serology for herpes simplex viruses are at risk for reactivation of HSV infection, with resulting clinical picture that mimics radiation stomatitis. These patients should receive prophylaxis with acyclovir or one of its congeners. If serology results are not available, patients with a history of oral or genital herpes infection should receive acyclovir prophylaxis. Patients who develop severe mucositis require assessment for HSV reactivation (2).

Studies in patients undergoing allogeneic bone marrow transplantation have revealed that oral fluconazole, $400 \, mg \, d^{-1}$, is effective in reducing the severity of invasive fungal infections and subsequent mortality. The evidence of fluconazole effectiveness is less clear in patients with bone marrow suppression secondary to chemotherapy.

Immunosuppressed radiation victims may also be at risk for reactivation of cytomegalovirus (CMV) and *Pneumocystis carinii* pneumonia. In a limited casualty situation, if resources are available, clinicians should obtain CMV serology. In addition, patients should have a sensitive assay (antigen assessment or polymerase chain reaction test) every 2 weeks for 30 days postexposure, while those with documented previous CMV exposure should have the assay repeated until 100 days postexposure (2). Patients developing lymphopenia should have a CD4 cell count considered at 30 days postexposure. Those with a CD4 count below 0.2000×10^9 cells L^{-1} are at risk for *Pneumocystis carinii* pneumonia. Physicians should withhold trimethoprim-sulfa prophylaxis until the leukocyte count is above 3.0×10^9 cells L^{-1} or until the absolute neutrophil count is above 1.5×10^9 cells L^{-1}. Atovaquone, dapsone and aerosolized pentamidine are alternative prophylactic agents. Patients should continue prophylactic treatment until the CD4 count reaches or exceeds 0.2000×10^9 cells L^{-1}, which may occur over several months (2).

Supportive and Comfort Care

Supportive and comfort care include administration of antiemetic agents, antidiarrheal agents, fluids, electrolytes, analgesia and topical burn creams. Radiation victims developing multiorgan failure within hours of exposure should receive only expectant care (treatment for comfort with psychosocial support) because they were undoubtedly received an exposure greater than 10 Gy and their prognosis is grave.

On the other hand, patients developing multiorgan failure several days to weeks after exposure should receive routine critical care because they have likely received a moderate exposure and have a reasonable chance of survival. Significant burns, hypovolemia and hypotension require early resuscitation with fluids. Additional critical care may include endotracheal intubation, anticonvulsant agents, anxiolytic agents and sedatives as necessary (2).

Radiation victims should not receive prophylaxis for nausea and vomiting for a couple of reasons. First, the time from exposure to onset of these symptoms is a useful component of exposure assessment. Secondly, the short onset time for clinically significant exposures makes prophylaxis for vomiting impractical. At low exposure doses, the duration of vomiting varies from about 48 to 72 h, making prolonged antiemetic therapy unnecessary. Prophylaxis for gastrointestinal ulceration is an additional component of supportive care. Physicians should avoid instrumentation of the gastrointestinal tract, since the mucosa is friable and likely to slough and bleed following instrumentation.

Radiation victims exposed to doses greater than 10–12 Gy have virtually no chance for survival, and are therefore not candidates for definitive care. These patients should receive comfort measures rather than aggressive definitive treatment. Comfort measures should include analgesia, antiemetic agents and antidiarrheal agents. In addition, these patients, their families and their friends would benefit from psychological support and spiritual care.

References

1. Leikin, JB, McFee, RB, Walter, FG, Edsall, K. A Primer for Nuclear Terrorism. Disease-a-Month, 49(8):485–516, 2003
2. Waselenko, JK, MacVittie, TJ, Blakely, WF, et al. Medical Management of the ARS: Recommendations of the Strategic National Stockpile Radiation Working Group. Annals of Internal Medicine, 140(12):1037–1051, 2004
3. Federation of American Scientists. Special Weapons Primer. Weapons of Mass Destruction. http://www.fas.org/nuke/intro/nuke/intro.htm, last accessed 9–04–05
4. Hogan, DE, Kellison, T. Nuclear Terrorism. The American Journal of the Medical Sciences, 323(6):341–349, 2002
5. Koenig, KL, Goans, RE, Hatchett, RJ, et al. Medical Treatment of Radiological Casualties: Current Concepts. Annals of Emergency Medicine, 45(6):643–652, 2005
6. Ring, JP. Radiation Risks and Dirty Bombs. Health Physics 86(2 Suppl.):S42–S47, 2004
7. Military Medical Operations Armed Forces Radiobiology Research Institute. Medical Management of Radiological Casualties Handbook. Second Edition. Bethesda, Maryland 20889–5603 http://www.afrri.usuhs.mil April 2003
8. Centers for Disease Control and Prevention. ARS: A Fact Sheet for Physicians, http://www.bt.cdc.gov/radiation/pdf/arsphysicianfactsheet.pdf, last accessed 9–11–05
9. Oak Ridge Associated Universities, Oak Ridge Institute for Science and Education. Guidance for Radiation Accident Management, Managing Radiation Emergencies, Guidance for Hospital Medical Management. Radiation Emergency Assistance Center Center/Training Site (REAC/TS), http://www.orau.gov/reacts, last accessed 1–01–06
10. Walker, RI, Cerveny, RJ (Eds.). Textbook of Military Medicine Medical Consequences of Nuclear Warfare. Falls Church, VA: Office of the Surgeon General, 1989. Available at http://www.afrri.usuhs.mil
11. Goans, RE, Holloweay, EC, Berger, ME, Ricks, RCF. Early Dose Assessment in Criticality Accidents. Health Physics, 81(4):446–449, 2001
12. Military Medical Operations Armed Forces Radiobiology Research Institute. Biodosimetry Assessment Tool (BAT) Software Application. http://www.afrri.usuhs.mil/www/outreach/biodostools.htm#BATregister, last accessed 12/31/05
13. Centers for Disease Control and Prevention. Prenatal Radiation Exposure: A Fact Sheet for Physicians, March 23, 2005. http://www.bt.cdc.gov/radiation/pdf/prenatalphysician.pdf, last accessed 1–29–06
14. National Council on Radiation Protection and Measurements. NCRP Report No. 128: Radionuclide Exposure of the Embryo/Fetus. Bethesda, Maryland: NCRP, 1998, http://www.ncrponline.org/ncrprpts.html (last accessed 1–29–06)
15. United States Food and Drug Administration, Center for Drug Evaluation and Research. Guidance: Potassium Iodide as a Thyroid Blocking Agent in Radiation Emergencies, http://www.fda.gov/cder/guidance/4825fnl.pdf, last accessed 1–01–06
16. United States Food and Drug Administration, Center for Drug Evaluation and Research. Guidance for Industry on Prussian Blue for Treatment of Internal Contamination with Thallium or Radioactive Cesium, Availability. Federal Register/Vol. 68, No. 23/Tuesday, February 4, 2003/Notices, http://www.fda.gov/OHRMS/DOCKETS/98fr/03–2597.pdf, last accessed 1–01–06
17. Hughes, WT, Armstrong, DN, Bodey, GP, et al. Guidelines for the use of Antimicrobial Agents in Neutropenic patients with Cancer. Clinical Infectious Diseases, 34:730–751, 2002.

Chapter 5
Mental Health and Terrorism

The intentional use or threatened use of biological, chemical and radiological agents has proven effective in coercing and intimidating populations. One review of available literature on biological, chemical and radiological terrorism identified several terrorist aims (1):

- Create mass anxiety, fear and panic
- Create mass feelings of helplessness, hopelessness and demoralization
- Destroy the public's assumptions about their own personal security
- Disrupt the infrastructure
- Demonstrate how civil authorities are incapable of protecting the public and the Environment (Adapted from Alexanderet al. (1), with permission from the Royal College of Physicians.)

Biological, chemical and radiological terrorist attacks are especially terrifying because they may occur unannounced and undetected, because the attacks can occur in places people generally consider safe, and because the injuries they cause may be unusual and prolonged (2). As a result, the use of these weapons is likely to cause mass fear and anxiety, making it likely that mental health casualties will greatly outnumber physical casualties. Risk communication research has identified criteria for exposures associated with prolonged mental health effects. Biological, chemical and radiological attacks fulfill all of these criteria in that they cause exposures that are:

- Involuntary
- Man-made
- Unfamiliar
- Threatening to children
- Capable of causing long term effects that threaten future generations

Based on historical observations, mass sociogenic illness might follow a real or threatened terrorist event involving chemical, biological or radiologic materials (3). Shortly after the September 11, 2001 terrorist attack on the World Trade Center, minor events were sufficient to cause mass anxiety. On September 29, 18 days after the World Trade Center attack, paint fumes at a middle school in Washington State,

A. L. Melnick (ed.), *Biological, Chemical, and Radiological Terrorism.*
© Springer 2008

3,000 miles from New York, created a terrorism scare. As a result, 16 students and one teacher went to a local hospital for evaluation (3). A few days later, on October 3, 1,000 students in Manila, Philippines, overwhelmed local clinics complaining of upper respiratory symptoms following a rumor about bioterrorism (3). Within another week, 35 people suddenly developed nausea, headaches and sore throats after a man sprayed an unknown substance into a subway station in Maryland. Evaluation of the substance revealed window-cleaning solution (3).

Soon after these events, the deluge of patient calls to family physicians following the anthrax attacks in October 2001, mostly from the unexposed yet anxious patients, illustrated the critical role primary care physicians play in responding to patient anxieties regarding terrorism, real and imagined. This chapter discusses the epidemiology of mental health conditions subsequent to terrorist events, followed by treatment and prevention recommendations for primary care physicians.

Epidemiology

The October 2001 anthrax events revealed that terrorist attacks do not have to cause many casualties to create mass anxiety and disruption (1,4). Other than that experience, however, we have little historic data to tell us how the public will react following a large-scale biologic, chemical or radiological attack (1). Most available information comes from studies of public reactions to natural disasters, "conventional" terrorist events, such as the Sarin attack in Tokyo and the September 11 attack, and nuclear accidents (1,5,6). Additional information is available from studies of soldier's reactions to military campaigns involving toxic agents (1).

Besides the paucity of historic data, another difficulty associated with mental health studies of disaster victims is the lack of standardization of criteria used for case definitions of mental health disorders following mass trauma, such as post-traumatic stress disorder (PTSD) (6,7). Diagnostic criteria for PTSD, as noted in the fourth edition of the diagnostic and statistical manual (DSM-IV), should go beyond specified combinations of symptoms to include requirements for symptom duration and the patient's ability to function (6,7). Specifically, for a PTSD diagnosis, the patient must have symptoms for more than 1 month, and the symptoms must cause clinically significant distress or impair the patient's ability to function (6,7). In addition, the symptoms must occur after the traumatic event and could not have existed before the event. Unfortunately, many studies have used questionnaires that fail to distinguish new symptoms following traumatic events from previous prevalent symptoms such as sleeplessness that many people have at various times (6). The consequence is that many studies tend to inflate the prevalence of PTSD.

In addition to problems with study design and study instruments, the DSM-IV diagnostic criteria themselves lack specificity, making case definitions difficult in epidemiologic studies of mass trauma victims. For example, the DSM-IV criteria for PTSD define exposure vaguely as "the person experienced, witnessed, or was confronted with" the event (6,7). Fortunately, the accompanying explanatory text adds details about exposure. To meet the case definition, the patient must develop characteristic symptoms following "exposure to an extreme traumatic stressor involving direct personal experience of an event that involves actual or threatened death or serious injury, or other threat to one's physical integrity; or witnessing an event of a similar nature or learning that a loved one experienced such an event (6,7)." Although this definition allows family members of those directly exposed to a traumatic event to be candidates for PTSD, it is still unclear whether those witnessing traumatic events on television at a remote location could be candidates for the disorder.

The DSM-IV introduced a new diagnosis, Acute stress disorder (ASD) (7). In recognizing this new disorder, the American Psychiatric Association was attempting to identify trauma victims at risk for developing PTSD (8). Unfortunately, experience with trauma victims has not confirmed the usefulness of ASD in predicting PTSD. Although approximately 3/4 of patients developing ASD within 1 month of a traumatic event go on to develop PTSD, most patients with PTSD have not previously met the criteria for ASD (8).

Given that mental health studies of trauma victims suffer from difficulties with case definition, exposure definition and study design, past events still offer some insight into mental health risks associated with terrorist events. During the 1991 Persian Gulf War, 18 missile attacks involving 39 surface-to-surface Scud Missiles hit Israel. Many Israelis living near the attack sites suffered stress due to the uncertainty regarding when an attack might occur, the location of the attack and whether the warhead contained chemical weapons. As a result, over 40% of nearly 800 hospitalizations were due to psychological symptoms, and nearly 30% of the casualties had mistakenly injected themselves with atropine (9).

Studies following two recent terrorist attacks in the United States, the April 1995 Oklahoma City Federal Building bombing and the September 11 World Trade Center attack in New York City, have shed some additional light on the mental health outcomes following terrorist events.

Until the September 11 attacks, the Oklahoma City bombing was the most severe terrorist attack in United States history. In that attack, 19 children and 148 adults died, and 684 persons suffered injuries. Property damage, valued at $625 million, included demolition or significant damage to over 800 building structures. Following the tragedy, the Oklahoma State Health Department developed a registry of nearly 1,100 survivors directly exposed to the blast based on proximity to the federal building. Interviews with a sample of 182 of these survivors, most of whom suffered injuries from the blast, revealed that nearly half met the criteria for one or more psychiatric disorders with over one-third qualifying for a PTSD diagnosis related to the bombing (based on DSM-III criteria) (10). Several factors similar to those found in previous studies of disaster victims predicted postdisaster PTSD, including:

- Degree of exposure, based on the number of injuries
- Female sex (compared to men, women were more than twice as likely to have PTSD, major depression and anxiety disorder. In addition, women were more likely to qualify for any postdisaster mental health diagnosis)

- Psychopathology present before the disaster
- Secondary exposure through harm to intimate contacts, such as injury and death (10)

Two studies conducted after the September 11 World Trade Center attacks looked at psychological symptoms soon after the event. One study, a national, random-digit dialing survey of over 500 adults conducted 3–5 days after the attack, revealed that nearly half were bothered "quite a bit" or "extremely" by at least one of five selected symptoms from a PTSD Checklist (11,12). Over a third reported that their children had one or more stress symptoms (12). Another study of over 1,000 adults living in Manhattan identified through random digit dialing revealed that 7.5% had symptoms consistent with PTSD and 9.7% had symptoms consistent with major depression 5–9 weeks after the September 11 attacks (12). Those living closest to the attack site were nearly three times as likely to have PTSD symptoms compared to those living further away (13).

The National Study of American's Reactions to September 11 (N-SARS) was a web-based, cross-sectional study of a national sample of adults conducted 1–2 months after the attacks. The sample of over 2,000 included respondents drawn from 1,196 households in New York City, 369 households in Washington DC, 776 households from other major metropolitan areas and 790 households from the rest of the nation. Measures included symptoms of PTSD (PTSD Checklist) and other clinically significant psychological distress (14). The study revealed that the prevalence of probable PTSD, based on the PTSD checklist score, was associated with proximity to the World Trade Center attack site, with a prevalence of 11.2% in New York City compared to a 4.3% national prevalence. In addition, the prevalence of probable PTSD was significantly associated with the number of hours participants watched television coverage of the event on September 11 and the following few days, as well as the number of different traumatic events participants observed on television (14). Having been in the World Trade Center or surrounding buildings at the time of attack and the number of hours of TV coverage watched each day were also significantly associated with PTSD symptoms (14).

Certainly, this cross-sectional study does not prove that watching mass traumatic events on television increases the risk for PTSD. It is possible that participants already experiencing symptoms were more likely to watch television coverage of the events. In addition, the current DSM-IV criteria are not clear whether television viewing of traumatic events constitutes indirect exposure (6,7) and the PTSD checklist score is not equivalent with a clinical diagnosis of PTSD. However, physicians assessing patients for possible PTSD might consider the amount of exposure to television coverage as a correlate of distress. In other words, patients watching large amounts of television coverage may be more likely to be suffering from distress, including PTSD (14).

An additional finding from the national survey was that 61% of New York City adults and nearly 50% of the rest of the national sample reported at least one child in the household having been upset following the attacks. Although the adult participant's own reactions may have biased these results, and although the reported symptoms may not have been clinically significant, physicians, other health care providers and others interacting with children, such as parents and teachers, should be diligent about assessing the level of distress in children following natural or man made disasters (14).

The Nationwide Longitudinal Study of Psychological Responses to September 11 examined the nationwide psychological response to the World Trade Center attack from 9 days to 6 months after the attack (15). Nearly 3,000 participants completed a web-based survey within 9–23 days following the attack. A sub-sample of nearly 1,000 of the original participants, all living outside of New York City, completed a second survey 2 months after the attacks, and nearly 800 completed a third survey approximately 6 months after the attacks. Six months after the attack, individuals without any direct exposure to the attacks continued to experience some psychological effects. After 6 months, PTSD symptoms, while declining, remained elevated, and more than 1/3 participants continued to have anxiety that future terrorist attacks could affect themselves or their loved ones (15). At 6 months, after adjustment for preexisting mental health conditions, demographics and time, two factors, the severity of loss and the use of several coping behaviors, predicted higher levels of distress. Coping strategies predicting higher levels of distress included denial, self-distraction, self-blame, seeking social support and disengagement from coping efforts. On the other hand, participants actively engaged in other coping behaviors reported significantly lower levels of distress 6 months after the attacks (15). There was no association between substance abuse and distress.

Another study, a random digit dial telephone survey of nearly 1,000 adults in Manhattan, revealed an increased use of tobacco, alcohol and marijuana 5–8 weeks after the September 11 World Trade Center attacks. Participants with increased smoking or marijuana use were more likely to experience PTSD symptoms and depression, and those with increased alcohol use were more likely to suffer from depression only (16).

A review of over 160 studies of disaster victims, including the Oklahoma bombing study, revealed that at least a third of those surviving suffered from clinically significant distress (6,17,18). Most survivors experiencing long-term impairments due to stress developed their symptoms immediately after the traumatic event. Delayed symptom onset was rare (17,18). The review found that poor mental health outcomes following disasters were more likely in females, middle-aged adults and ethnic minorities. Other patient characteristics associated with poor mental health outcomes included low socioeconomic status, previous psychiatric history and little previous disaster exposure. Additional risk factors associated with poor mental health outcomes included family issues, such as childcare responsibilities for adult females, parental distress for children, and significant distress by other family members.

Besides individual and family characteristics, exposure severity and resource loss have been associated with poor mental health outcomes (6,17,18). On the other hand, studies of children and adults exposed to traumatic events such as war, domestic violence and natural disasters revealed several individual factors associated with a lower risk of adverse mental health outcomes. These factors include good intellectual functioning, effective self-regulation of emotions and attachment behaviors, positive self-concept, optimism, altruism, an ability to turn helplessness into hopefulness and an active coping style in confronting stressors (8).

Diagnosis of Mental Health Symptoms Following Terrorist Attacks

Based on what we know from available epidemiologic studies, the psychological effects resulting from a manmade or natural disaster will not be limited to those directly exposed or physically injured. Clinicians will not be able to predict their patients' psychological response based on personal loss or proximity to the disaster. Although most people exposed to large-scale traumatic events will not develop a diagnosable psychiatric illness, many will experience sleep disturbances, difficulty concentrating and feeling emotionally upset (4). The presence of such health symptoms alone following a terrorist attack does not constitute pathology. Rather than considering these symptoms as reflecting mental health disorders, clinicians caring for these patients should understand that such symptoms might represent a normal response to an extremely abnormal event (15,19). Compared to everyday practice, in which most primary care physicians treat patients they identify as ill, following a disaster, physicians caring for patients with mental health symptoms will need to shift their focus to health rather than disease (19).

After a biological, chemical or radiological attack, patients may present with a variety of mental health responses, including distress responses, behavioral changes, psychosomatic symptoms, including medically unexplained symptoms, psychological symptoms and psychiatric illness, such as PTSD (20). Categories of common mental health responses include (20,21):

- Physical symptoms and signs, such as fatigue, nausea, fine motor tremors, tics, paresthesias, profuse diaphoresis, dizziness, nausea, diarrhea, tachypnea, tachycardia, and a choking or smothering sensation
- Emotional symptoms, such as anxiety, grief, irritability, feeling overwhelmed and a sense of vulnerability
- Cognitive changes, such as memory loss, anomia, difficulty making decisions, decreased attention span, difficulty concentrating, distractibility, difficulty with math calculations, inability to distinguish trivial problems from major problems
- Behavioral changes, such as insomnia, acting out, social withdrawal, crying easily, use of "gallows" humor, hyper-vigilance, ritualistic behavior
- Increased use of substances, including increased smoking, increased use of alcohol and other drugs (16); increased substance use may also accompany PTSD and depression (16)
- Spiritual effects, such as crisis of faith, anger at God, anger displacement toward those in authority, questioning basic religious beliefs

- Long-term behavioral effects, including nightmares, intrusive thoughts, uncontrolled affect, difficulties with relationships, difficulties with jobs and/or school, decreased libido and changes in appetite

Children

Children respond to disasters based on their developmental stage, their level of exposure and the response of others around them (22). Physical injury, proximity to the disaster, witnessing injury and death of family members or other loved ones, the extent and duration of disruption of daily activities, parental reactions and family disruption all contribute to how children respond. Relevant developmental factors include cognitive, physical, educational and social development and experience. In addition, the emotional state of children and their families before the disaster help predict their response after. Therefore, primary care physicians who have provided continuous care for families, including emotional support, are well suited to help families, including children, to adjust following a disaster (22).

Children tend to display five primary responses secondary to loss, exposure to trauma and disruption of routine for about a month following a disaster (23):

- Increased dependency on caregivers
- Nightmares
- Developmental regression
- Specific fears related to reminders of the disaster
- Play and reenactments of the disaster

Toddlers often respond to the upheaval in their lives by becoming more dependent on caregivers, developing sleep abnormalities and regressing developmentally. Regressive behavior in school aged children and younger children may include enuresis, encopresis, thumb sucking, loss of acquired speech, increased clinging, whining and fear of the dark (23). These normal responses will usually respond to reassurance and will not require referral for counseling unless they persist (23). Repetitive play behavior, such as reenacting the disaster, can serve as a normal means of coping for toddlers and preschoolers following a disaster (23).

Older school aged children and preadolescents might also regress, talk and play about the trauma, display hostility to others, including family and friends, and lose interest in activities they previously enjoyed (22,23). Like their younger counterparts, adolescents may also lose interest in previously enjoyed activities. Regressive features in older children and adolescents may include competing for parental attention, a reduction in responsible behaviors and increased dependency (23). In addition, adolescents may have trouble sleeping, display fatigue and begin abusing illicit drugs (22). Young children and adolescents may both develop anxiety, depression, headaches, decreased appetite, guilt, and PTSD symptoms, including nightmares, avoidance of reminders of the traumatic event and irritability (22). In general, boys take longer to recover and are more likely to express hostile behaviors, whereas girls become more distressed, verbal about their feelings and ask more questions (23).

Somatic complaints, such as headaches, abdominal pain and chest pain frequently occur in children and adolescents and usually resolve without treatment (23). Hostile behaviors in toddlers and preschoolers may include hitting, biting and pinching, whereas school age children may engage in fighting or have difficulty getting along with their peers. Adolescents may express hostility and anger through excessive rebellion and delinquent behaviors (23).

The American Academy of Pediatrics has developed a booklet containing information and tools for primary care physicians useful for assessing and treating children following disasters (23). The booklet suggests that physicians can rapidly assess the extent a disaster has affected a child or adolescent by inquiring specifically about:

– Changes in sleep patterns
– Apathetic behavior and decreased motivation
– Regressive behavior, such as enuresis, encopresis and biting
– Changes in relationships with family members and peers, such as increased clinging, dependency or withdrawal
– Change in school grades
– Fears and worries

Available at http://www.mentalhealth.samhsa.gov/publications/allpubs/SMA95–3022/default.asp, the booklet includes information about screening scales primary care physicians might find useful in assessing children for behavior problems and PTSD.

Anxiety and Somatization Disorders

One difficulty in assessment is that clinicians may confuse distress symptoms with symptoms due to physical injury from direct exposure to biological, chemical or radiological agents (24). Following an attack, many exposed and unexposed patients might present to physician offices and emergency departments with a variety of symptoms, such as tachypnea, tachycardia, tremors and other nonspecific signs and symptoms. Clinicians caring for patients without pathognomic signs and symptoms of physical injury will have difficulty with triage, potentially subjecting unexposed patients to unnecessary treatment, while potentially delaying treatment for those exposed.

Symptoms secondary to nerve agent exposure may be especially difficult to differentiate from stress-associated somatic symptoms. Disaster somatization reaction (DSD), an alternative nosological term to "mass hysteria," "psychogenic illness," "worried well," "vicarious victims" and "contagious fear," classifies the response in patients who interpret their anxiety symptoms as due to direct exposure or infection, or who develop symptoms similar to those identified with exposure or infection (25).

Table 5.1 Disaster somatization disorder symptoms compared to symptoms secondary to nerve agent exposure or atropine antidote administration

DSR versus nerve agent exposure versus autoinjection (5,15)

	Disaster somatization reaction	Severe exposure	Mild exposure	Atropine antidote
Symptoms	No exposure; sympathetic autonomic nervous system predominance	Muscarinic predominance	Nicotinic predominance	No exposure; antimuscarinic predominance
Onset	Variable	Seconds to minutes	Minutes to hours	Minutes
General effects	Anxiety, insomnia	Loss of consciousness	Anxiety, insomnia	Fatigue, dry skin perspiration
Respiratory effects	Trouble breathing, tightness in chest	Dyspnea, bronchorrhea, respiratory arrest	Rhinorrhea	–
Cardiac effects	Sinus tachycardia	Dysrhythmias	–	Tachycardia
Ocular effects	Pupillary dilatation, eye irritation	Miosis, blurred vision, eye pain, conjunctival injection	If transdermal exposure, no change in pupil size	Midriasis, blurred vision
Musculoskeletal effects	Weakness	Fasciculations, weakness, flaccid paralysis	Fasciculations, and weakness	–
Gastrointestinal effects	Nausea, vomiting	Vomiting, diarrhea	Nausea	Constipation, vomiting
Central nervous system effects	Lightheadedness, headache	Convulsions	Lightheadedness, headache	Confusion, dizziness
Ear, nose, and throat effects	Dry mouth	Copious secretions, stridor due to laryngeal paralysis	Sialorrhea, weakness of the tongue	Dry mouth

Source: Diamond et al. (25), Reprinted by permission of Psychiatric Annals and SLACK, Inc.

Table 5.1 illustrates the difficulty differentiating between nerve agent exposure, symptoms secondary to atropine antidote administration and DSD symptoms. Patients with nerve agent exposures may present with minimal physical findings but with significant mental status changes, leading to a misdiagnosis of anxiety reaction or other psychiatric disorder. On the other hand, as the news of the terrorist attack spreads, patients without exposure may develop symptoms such as "twitching," stomach upset and headache, perceive that they are exposed, and seek immediate medical attention. On presentation, because their exposure status may be unclear, these patients will require decontamination, potentially causing bottlenecks and increased panic (25). In addition, some of these patients may receive unnecessary atropine, causing additional symptoms and confusion.

Similarly, following a radiological attack, patients unexposed to radiation may present with autonomic arousal symptoms and signs secondary to stress, including tachypnea, tachycardia, nausea and diarrhea. These findings may also appear in patients as a direct consequence of radiation exposure (26). Like a nerve agent attack, once the news about vomiting in radiological attack victims spreads, many unexposed people who believe they are in the radioactive plume path may develop disaster somatic reactions such as nausea and vomiting. As more people in the affected community develop these symptoms, the level of anxiety in the general population could increase (25). Confusion about the need to evacuate versus shelter in place may create additional anxiety in those unexposed (25).

Posttraumatic Stress Disorder

A diagnosis of PTSD in adults and children requires the presence of several conditions (7,23,27):

- The patient must have been exposed to an extreme stressor or traumatic event to which s/he responded with fear, helplessness and horror
- The patient must have three distinct types of symptoms, for at least a month, including:

  • Reexperiencing the event: undesired recall of the incident through distressing images, nightmares or flashbacks
  • Avoidance of reminders of the event, including avoidance of persons, places or thoughts associated with the incident
  • Physiological manifestations of hyperarousal symptoms for at least 1 month, such as insomnia, irritability, impaired concentration, hyper-vigilance and increased startle reactions (10,27)

Table 5.2 contains the complete DSM-IV criteria for PTSD (7). ASD, another anxiety disorder, shares several features with PTSD. Both occur following exposure to a traumatic event, and both include reexperiencing the event, avoidance of reminders of the event and increased arousal. However, unlike PTSD, symptoms of ASD are transient, lasting a maximum of 4 weeks (range 2 days to 4 weeks) and they must have an onset within 4 weeks of the traumatic event (7,28). In addition, a diagnosis of ASD requires fewer symptoms in each category. Compared to PTSD, ASD has more dissociative symptoms, such as diminished awareness of surroundings (e.g., patients may describe feeling "in a daze") and ASD patients are more likely to have temporary amnesia about the event (7,28). As mentioned earlier, although approximately 3/4 of patients developing ASD go on to develop PTSD, most patients with PTSD have not previously met the criteria for ASD (8).

Table 5.2   Diagnostic criteria for 309.81 posttraumatic stress disorder

A. The person has been exposed to a traumatic event in which both of the following were present:
   (1) The person experienced, witnessed, or was confronted with an event or events that involved actual or threatened death or serious injury, or a threat to the physical integrity of self or others
   (2) The person's response involved intense fear, helplessness, or horror. Note: In children, this may be expressed instead by disorganized or agitated behavior
B. The traumatic event is persistently reexperienced in one (or more) of the following ways:
   (1) Recurrent and intrusive distressing recollections of the event, including images, thoughts, or perceptions. Note: In young children, repetitive play may occur in which themes or aspects of the trauma are expressed
   (2) Recurrent distressing dreams of the event. Note: In children, there may be frightening dreams without recognizable content
   (3) Acting or feeling as if the traumatic event were recurring (includes a sense of reliving the experience, illusions, hallucinations, and dissociative flashback episodes, including those that occur on awakening or when intoxicated). Note: In young children, trauma-specific reenactment may occur
   (4) Intense psychological distress at exposure to internal or external cues that symbolize or resemble an aspect of the traumatic event
   (5) Physiological reactivity on exposure to internal or external cues that symbolize or resemble an aspect of the traumatic event
C. Persistent avoidance of stimuli associated with the trauma and numbing of general responsiveness (not present before the trauma), as indicated by three (or more) of the following:
   (1) Efforts to avoid thoughts, feelings, or conversations associated with the trauma
   (2) Efforts to avoid activities, places, or people that arouse recollections of the trauma
   (3) Inability to recall an important aspect of the trauma
   (4) Markedly diminished interest or participation in significant activities
   (5) Feeling of detachment or estrangement from others
   (6) Restricted range of affect (e.g., unable to have loving feelings)
   (7) Sense of a foreshortened future (e.g., does not expect to have a career, marriage, children, or a normal life span)
D. Persistent symptoms of increased arousal (not present before the trauma), as indicated by two (or more) of the following:
   (1) Difficulty falling or staying asleep
   (2) Irritability or outbursts of anger
   (3) Difficulty concentrating
   (4) hyper-vigilance
   (5) Exaggerated startle response
E. Duration of the disturbance (symptoms in Criteria B, C, and D) is more than 1 month
F. The disturbance causes clinically significant distress or impairment in social, occupational, or other important areas of functioning
Specify if:
Acute: if duration of symptoms is less than 3 months
Chronic: if duration of symptoms is 3 months or more
Specify if:
With Delayed Onset: if onset of symptoms is at least 6 months after the stressor

From (7), by permission of the American Psychiatric Association.

Although primary care physicians can readily identify PTSD symptoms, the diagnosis may be difficult, because PTSD symptoms have substantial overlap with symptoms of depression and other anxiety disorders and because patients may not readily report traumatic exposures. Many patients with PTSD will present with physical complaints including musculoskeletal, gastrointestinal and neurologic symptoms (29). In addition, it is unclear whether experiencing a traumatic event on television or at a remote site constitutes exposure sufficient for the diagnosis (6). Physicians might easily miss making the diagnosis unless they ask specific questions about exposure to the event. Asking questions and active listening tend to break down diagnostic and treatment barriers by acknowledging exposure to the event as a legitimate explanation for the symptoms (27). Given the overlap between PTSD symptoms with other disorders, primary physicians encountering patients with the following characteristics should ask them about exposure to a traumatic event and the presence of PTSD symptoms (27,29):

– Nonspecific symptoms such as palpitations, dyspnea, tremor, and insomnia
– Depression
– Mood swings
– Avoidance behaviors
– Nonadherence to treatment
– Increased tobacco, alcohol or other drug use

Given the DSM-IV criteria, evaluating a patient in one office visit will not be sufficient to diagnose PTSD. Continuity of care is essential in determining whether patients have PTSD. Most distress symptoms are transient. To make the diagnosis, primary care physicians should document an accumulation of symptoms, a lack of improvement or a deterioration of the patient's condition and the persistence or development of a functional disability during several office visits over 3–4 weeks (30).

Treatment of Mental Health Conditions Following Terrorist Attacks

Emergent Treatment

Many of the psychological consequences of a disaster are preventable immediately after the event, at the time of triage and early treatment. Rapid identification of the nature of the biological, chemical or radiological agent and the extent of exposure can help differentiate somatization symptoms from symptoms due to physical injury (31). Delirium secondary to infections from exposure to biological agents may respond to treatment with antipsychotic and anxiolytic agents (31). However, clinicians must be aware that antipsychotic medications and antibiotics metabolized through the cytochrome p-450 system may interfere with each other and that antipsychotic medication side effects, such as agitation or somnolence, may be difficult to distinguish from an infectious encephalopathy (31). Phenothiazines used to treat emesis or psychotic symptoms can cause pseudoparkinsonism, akathisia or other neurologic symptoms that are difficult to interpret in a mass-disaster situation. It is also unknown whether antipsychotic treatment contributes to a greater likelihood of PTSD (31). Therefore, to minimize confusion and avoid unnecessary complication, clinicians should use a conservative approach when using psychotropic medications to control behavior immediately postdisaster (31).

If possible, creating a quiet, safe location removed from high-activity triage areas, where health care staff can still observe symptoms, may help facilitate recovery (31) and reduce behavioral disturbances in patients with transient symptoms. An appropriate and safe location also serves to minimize exposure to dead and injured victims and other disturbing images (19).

Counseling and Education

Counseling and education are essential treatment components for patients traumatized by natural or manmade disasters. Although clinicians are often reticent to ask patients about distressing events, providing patients with an opportunity to talk about their traumatic experience can be very helpful. On the other hand, many patients with persistent distress fail to report their symptoms to their physicians, and they may even feel uncomfortable talking with family members about their distress (32). This inability to talk with friends and loved ones about disaster related thoughts and emotions can lead to a perceived lack of support and increased distress symptoms (32). Primary care clinicians can help by asking their patients about their reactions to a recent terrorist attack or disaster and by providing support and brief counseling even when patients visit for other problems (32). Through counseling and education, primary care clinicians can offer patients a feeling of safety and support, help them understand their physical and emotional injuries and help them understand the recovery process (27).

Unfortunately, following the September 11 attacks, even though most distressed individuals had difficulty with daily activities, one study revealed that only 11% reported obtaining information or counseling from healthcare providers (32). In addition, only half of the patients receiving prescription medications to cope had received education or counseling from healthcare providers. These findings indicated that primary care clinicians should consider providing additional support beyond psychotropic medications.

Clues that patients are distressed include requests for anxiolytic medications and increased use of alcohol, tobacco and other drugs (16). When encountering patients who request anxiolytic medications, primary care clinicians should be able to provide brief counseling and educational materials in the office, as well as information about how to find additional educational materials through appropriate sites on the Internet (28,30,32). For example, the National Alliance for the Mentally Ill (NAMI) Web site at http://www.NAMI.org (last accessed 3–05–06) has outstanding resources and directions to local support groups for patients with anxiety disorders (28). Following a disaster, primary care clinicians can also monitor patients for symptoms related to abuse of alcohol, tobacco and other drugs and intervene appropriately by providing information, brief counseling and treatment referral as indicated.

By answering questions, addressing concerns and by letting patients know they are not helpless, primary care clinicians can easily reassure patients and reduce the trauma that many families have already experienced. Table 5.3 contains a list of suggested answers for questions patients were likely to ask in the aftermath of the October 2001 anthrax attacks (33). Clinicians should consider consulting with their local public health officials (see Chap. 6) for updates and additional information useful for addressing patient concerns.

In addition to educating their distressed patients, primary care clinicians can help them understand that their symptoms represent a normal psychological and biological response to overwhelming stress, and that they are not weak nor suffering from character flaws (27). By listening uncritically to their patients, and by letting their patients understand that they are not alone, primary care clinicians can build a therapeutic alliance with patients that can help them through recovery (27).

One of the barriers for obtaining counseling may be a fear that disclosure of stress or anxiety could lead to adverse consequences, such as loss of employment. For example, law enforcement officers might be concerned that by requesting assistance they may be lose their right to carry a weapon, or an elected official may be concerned that requesting counseling could affect election results (27). Primary care clinicians are in a unique position to reassure patients that "normal people" can benefit from counseling and other therapeutic interventions after a disaster and that such treatments are completely confidential (27).

Counseling Children and Their Parents

Primary care clinicians can help children by letting listening to them and letting them know that their fears and grief are normal reactions to a disaster (23). In addition, primary care clinicians can inform parents about available community services and can help parents understand that what they and their children are experiencing is normal (23). Parents should know not to interfere with their child's repetitious trauma-associated talk or play unless it is dangerous (23). On the other hand, parents should encourage their children to ask questions, and they should talk with their children about the disaster while giving age-appropriate information. Parents should consider limiting television viewing of the terrorist events for younger children, but should watch such events together with older children while discussing what they are seeing. Clinicians should talk to verbal children without their caregivers present, because they may hear a different perception compared to those of parents, guardians and teachers (23). During these discussions, primary care clinicians can emphasize the child's bravery, courage, strengths and ability to

Table 5.3 Common patient questions related to anthrax and suggested answers

Question	Answer
What is my risk of getting anthrax from the mail?	The current risk of anthrax from exposure to an envelope or other object containing anthrax is low, because transmission from secondary aerosolization of anthrax spores is unlikely. Primary aerosolization results from the initial release of anthrax, whereas secondary aerosolization is due to the agitation (from wind or human activities) of particles that have settled after the primary release. The particles that have settled tend to be large and require large amounts of energy to be resuspended in air. Therefore, residue on mail or packages is unlikely to cause any additional infections
How do I know if an item of mail is suspicious?	Share the FBI criteria with patients (see page 21)
How should I handle a suspicious envelope or package?	Do not shake or empty the contents of a suspicious package or envelope
	Do not carry the package or envelope, show it to others, or allow others to examine it
	Put the package or envelope on a stable surface; do not sniff, touch, taste, or look closely at it or any contents that may have spilled
	Alert others in the area about the suspicious package or envelope
	Leave the area, close any doors, and take actions to prevent others from entering the area
	If possible, shut off the ventilation system
	Wash hands with soap and water to prevent spreading potentially infectious material to face or skin. Seek additional instructions for exposed or potentially exposed persons
	If at work, notify a supervisor, a security officer, or a law enforcement official
	If at home, contact your local law enforcement agency
	If possible, create a list of persons who were in the room or area when this suspicious letter or package was recognized and a list of persons who also may have handled this package or letter. Give the list to both the local public health authorities and law enforcement officials
Should my family purchase gas masks?	Gas masks are generally ineffective against communicable disease. In addition, they provide protection against chemicals only when properly fitted and tested. For complete protection, people would have to wear them 24 h d^{-1}, 7 days per week, because we cannot predict the time and location of a terrorist attack. Therefore, we do not recommend purchasing gas masks
Should my family be vaccinated for bioterrorist-used germs?	At this time, the risk of vaccine complications and the cost of vaccinating the entire population outweigh the benefits of vaccinating everyone in the United States. In addition, only the CDC and the military have the vaccines – they are not available in physicians' offices or at local health departments. In the case of a terrorist attack, public health authorities and physicians will quickly identify people at risk of exposure, and make vaccines and preventive antibiotics available to them

(continued)

Table 5.3 (continued)

Question	Answer
Should my family stockpile antibiotics just in case?	There are several reasons why public health authorities and most physicians recommend against stockpiling antibiotics. Specific antibiotics are effective only against specific infections, and we cannot predict which agents terrorists will use. People must take the antibiotics at the proper time after exposure for them to be effective, which means that they must know when they have been exposed. Antibiotics taken inappropriately can lead to resistant bacteria, which can put the entire community at risk. The CDC has stockpiled large amounts of antibiotics, and we will make these available immediately to exposed people within 12 h of the recognition of an attack
Should I get a laboratory test for anthrax?	No, and here is why:
	Nasal swabs and blood tests are inaccurate
	You can be exposed and still have a negative test
	On the other hand, a positive test DOES NOT mean you have inhaled enough germs to get sick
	Therefore, decisions on whether to give preventive antibiotics must be based upon risk assessment rather than testing results
	Testing is done only as part of the public health investigation into a confirmed or highly probable exposure
	The decision to test is a public health and law enforcement decision
	The public health lab will do the testing only in case of a credible threat
Is our water supply safe from terrorism?	Yes. In general, routine water treatment (chlorine, filtering) in our public water systems would take care of biological agents terrorists might place in the system, just as they handle natural germs. If terrorists were to add chemical agents, the water would so dilute the chemicals that they would pose little threat
What can my family do to protect itself?	The best thing for families to do: develop a disaster plan just as they would for natural disasters. The disaster plan should include an emergency communications plan, a meeting place, and a disaster supplies kit. Parents should check with their children's school to get a copy of the emergency plan of the school. More information is obtainable at the local Red Cross chapter or at the Red Cross Web site: http://www.redcross.org/services/disaster/keepsafe/unexpected.html

Source: From Melnick (33). Reprinted with permission.

cope with adversity, while reassuring them about steps their parents and the community are taking to keep them safe. In addition, encouraging children to express their fears through drawing and play might be helpful (23).

The main problem children of all ages face following a disaster is disruption of their lives, whether through injury, death or destruction of their home, their school or their community. In turn, this causes a loss of reliability, cohesion and predictability (23).

Therefore, clinicians can help parents by counseling parents to create and maintain a predictable schedule for their children. Routine bed times, night-lights and stuffed animals for younger children, and help with homework schedules and assigned chores for older children can be helpful, and parents should choose talking, routine family mealtimes, compassion and reassurance over punishment. Clinicians can also reassure parents that somatic complaints, such as headaches, abdominal pain and chest pain, commonly observed postdisaster, are not due to serious physical illness and will usually resolve with time (23). If the symptoms continue, primary care clinicians should refer these children to a mental health professional.

Setting limits on unacceptable behaviors may be sufficient for young children displaying hostile behaviors, such as hitting, biting or pinching (toddlers) or fighting and not getting along with other children (school aged children). On the other hand, setting limits for adolescents involved in rebellious and delinquent activity will not suffice. Instead, positive activities such as rebuilding the community, helping younger children or the elderly may help channel adolescent hostility in a positive manner (23). Adolescents may also respond to group activities and discussions through organizations such as the Boy or Girl Scouts or school clubs. Primary care clinicians can play a community role by advising such clubs and by leading discussions, in which adolescents can express their fears, grief and anxieties (23).

Primary care clinicians should consider mental health referral for the child and family if the child the following conditions (23):

- Regressive behaviors lasting longer than a few weeks
- Persisting somatic symptoms that interfere with the child's life
- PTSD, anxiety, or depression
- Children with psychopathology present before the disaster
- Children with suicidal ideation
- Children with other risky behaviors

Children and adolescents using alcohol and/or illicit drugs will need referral for evaluation and treatment.

Psychological Treatment

In most individuals, some degree of distress after a disorder is normal and resolves without treatment, and education and counseling may be all that is necessary to reassure them. Therefore, primary care clinicians should avoid indiscriminate pharmacologic treatment and mental health referral for all patients experiencing distress following a disorder (30). However, patients suffering extreme distress, such as those with dissociative symptoms or insomnia, are candidates for symptomatic treatment.

The goal of psychological treatment is to help patients confront their fears and emotional responses to the traumatic event while not becoming overwhelmed (27). The general theme of psychological treatment involves techniques to reduce distress associated with memories of the traumatic event while suppressing the associated physiological reactions (27). However, most of the evidence for the various forms of available psychological interventions, such as exposure therapy, individual and group trauma-focused behavioral cognitive therapy, stress management/relaxation and psychodynamic psychotherapy is anecdotal (30).

Exposure therapy involves helping patients address painful memories and feelings (27) through imaging. Examples of exposure therapy include having patients listen repeatedly to detailed audio tape recreations of the traumatic events or exposing patients to cues associated with the traumatic event, such as stepwise reexposure to automobile travel following an accident (34). Cognitive therapy involves having patients identify and process distorted thinking patterns and beliefs regarding themselves, the traumatic event and the world (27,34). For example, the therapist will ask patients to challenge their thinking by weighing available evidence and by responding to specific questions (34). Psychodynamic psychotherapy involves having patients integrate the traumatic event into their life experience, including understanding how it affects their relationships (27,34).

At present, there is reasonable evidence that psychological treatment can reduce traumatic stress symptoms in patients with PTSD. Specifically, individual trauma focused cognitive behavioral therapy (TFCBT) has the best evidence regarding effectiveness. Although there is less evidence, group TFCBT may also be effective (34). Some studies have shown that short courses of cognitive behavioral therapy (CBT) begun soon after the traumatic event have led to lower rates of PTSD 3–6 months later (30). There is also limited evidence that stress management/relaxation, which involves nontrauma focused cognitive behavioral techniques, is effective in treating PTSD symptoms (34).

Pharmacologic Treatment

Patients who continue to have severe symptoms after 3–4 weeks and who have not improved or have deteriorated after two or more serial assessments are candidates for psychotherapy, medication or a combination of both (30). Expert consensus recommends pharmacologic treatment for patients with persistent symptoms, such as depressed mood, hyperarousal, reexperiences, avoidance, dissociation and disrupted sleep, causing social, interpersonal and/or occupational impairment (30).

Medications can help alleviate these PTSD symptoms, and primary care clinicians should consider them a component of care for traumatized patients (27,35). Randomized clinical trials have demonstrated the effectiveness of selective serotonin-reuptake inhibitors (SSRIs) in reducing PTSD symptom severity, reducing comorbid mental health disorders, such as depression and panic disorder, improving function and improving quality of life (27,30,35). These agents were have been more effective than placebo in ameliorating the three PTSD symptom clusters, including reexperiencing, avoidance/numbing and hyperarousal (35). Because most of the randomized clinical trials contributing to the evidence base involved SSRIs, and because expert consensus (29) supports their use, these agents remain the first line choice of medication for treating PTSD (35). On the other hand, available evidence indicates that benzodiazepines, monoamine oxidase inhibitors (MAOIs), antipsychotic agents, lamotrigine and inositol are not effective and therefore not indicated for patients with PTSD (30,35). Primary care clinicians can initiate SSRI treatment with a low dose, increasing the dosage gradually to reach the most effective yet tolerated dose (30). Table 5.4 lists the recommended doses for initiating and maintaining PTSD patients on SSRIs.

Patients should receive a 2–3 month initial course of treatment, with close monitoring for improvement in PTSD symptoms such as reexperiencing (flashbacks, nightmares), hyperarousal (insomnia and startle responses) and avoidance (30). Patients showing no improvement after 8 weeks of maximal doses are candidates for treatment with a different SSRI or with either venlafaxine or mirtazapine (30). Those with partial responses may need more time to respond to the first line SSRI (30).

Because available evidence indicates that patients with chronic PTSD can relapse when discontinuing medications, primary care clinicians should consider long-term treatment for their patients with chronic PTSD. Expert consensus recommends continuing pharmacologic treatment for at least 1 year in patients with PTSD symptoms lasting three months or longer. In addition, these patients require regular follow-up to ensure compliance and reduce the possibility of relapse. Limited evidence suggests that CBT and SSRIs are likely to have complementary effects and that combination therapy may be more effective than either alone. For other patients, one modality may be effective for symptoms that do not respond to the other. Therefore, primary care clinicians treating patients for chronic PTSD should consider referring them for CBT whether or not pharmacologic treatment is working (35).

Table 5.4 Recommended doses of selective serotonin reuptake inhibitors (SSRIs) for treating posttraumatic stress disorder

SSRI	Initial dose (mg d^{-1})	Usual dose (mg d^{-1})	Maximum dose (based on package insert) (mg d^{-1})
Paroxetine IR (immediate release)	10–20	20–50	50
Paroxetine CR (controlled release)	12.5–25	25–75	75
Sertraline	25–50	50–150	200
Fluoxetine	10–20	20–50	80
Fluvoxamine	50	100–250	300
Citalopram	20	20–40	60

Source: Adapted with permission from Foa (36), Copyright 1999, and Ballenger (30), Copyright 2004, Physicians Postgraduate Press.

Expert consensus recommends that primary care clinicians should ensure that patients with PTSD begin treatment with CBT and/or SSRIs within 3–4 weeks of symptom onset (30). Treatment with both modalities is probably more effective than either treatment alone. Primary care clinicians are probably best suited to treat and follow patients with PTSD, because they have the skills to diagnose and treat the disorder, because patients have greater access to primary care clinicians compared to psychiatrists and because patients may be reluctant to see mental health professionals (27). Patients not responding to an adequate course of medications, exhibiting significant side effects, developing suicidal thoughts and behavior or exhibiting significant psychiatric comorbidity should receive a referral to specialized psychiatric care (30).

Prevention

Some advocates have suggested debriefing as a means to prevent the development of PTSD or other anxiety disorders following a disaster or terrorist attack. The goal of debriefing, also known as critical incident debriefing or psychological debriefing, is to reduce or prevent psychological morbidity following a traumatic event (37). The military developed debriefing as a method to maintain group morale and reduce distress for soldiers following combat. Later, in the 1980s, debriefing advocates transferred debriefing principles used following combat to treating stress following trauma in civilian situations.

The theory behind debriefing is that encouraging recollection, ventilation or reworking of the traumatic event will promote emotional processing or catharsis in exposed individuals. By doing so, its advocates believe it can reduce psychological distress and prevent the development of anxiety disorders such as PTSD. Voluntary debriefing has gained wide popularity in many civilian settings, domestically and internationally, reflected in its use for police officers following shootings, families of children undergoing bone marrow transplants, rescue workers in natural disasters, jurors involved in murder trials, train drivers who have run over people and many other settings (37). Sometimes, involvement in debriefing has been mandatory. For example, the United Kingdom has required debriefing for some police officers exposed to traumatic events (37). Debriefing can be administered in individual or group settings.

Available evidence indicates that debriefing is not effective in preventing PTSD and that it may even cause adverse effects. Eleven randomized control trials meeting the standards of Cochrane reviews evaluated the effectiveness of single sessions of individual debriefing within 1 month of traumatic events (8,37). In all cases, debriefing did not prevent PTSD, and in some cases, it had adverse results in that comparison subjects not receiving debriefing had fewer symptoms at follow-up (8). In addition, available evidence indicates that debriefing does not prevent other adverse outcomes, such as depression or anxiety (37).

There are several reasons why debriefing may have adverse effects (8):

– Instead of promoting healing, encouraging victims to revisit the traumatic event shortly after exposure might interfere with the natural process in which the brain consolidates the distressing memories and allows them to disappear gradually (8).
– Early focus on acute posttraumatic symptoms may cause participants to feel that there is something wrong with them.
– Premature adrenergic activation by having participants relive the event may facilitate the encoding of traumatic memories, thereby increasing the risk for PTSD.

At present, expert consensus recommends that patients exposed to traumatic events, such as terrorist attacks, should not receive individual debriefing sessions. In addition, there is no evidence that group debriefing is effective, nor is there any evidence that debriefing is effective for children (37). It is possible that there is no effective prevention for PTSD, other than preventing the traumatic event itself. Rather than referring patients for debriefing or participating in group debriefing, primary care clinicians should focus their efforts on identifying patients suffering from psychiatric disorders, such as depression, ASD and PTSD following traumatic events. These patients require early interventions, such as short courses of CBT, which have led to lower rates of PTSD after 3–6 months (30).

References

1. Alexander, DA, Klein, S. Biochemical Terrorism: Too Awful to Contemplate, Too Serious to Ignore. British Journal of Psychiatry, 183(6):491–497, 2003
2. Hyams KC, Murphy FM, Wessely, S. Responding to Chemical, Biological or Nuclear Terrorism: The Indirect and Long-Term Health Effects May Present the Greatest Challenge. Journal of Health Politics, Policy and Law, 27(2):273–191, 2002
3. Wessely, S, Hyams, KC, Bartholomew, R. Psychological Implications of Chemical and Biological Weapons. British Medical Journal, 323:878–879, 2001
4. LaPorte, RE, Ronan, A, Sauer, F, Saad, R, Shubnikov. Bioterrorism and the Epidemiology of Fear. The Lancet Infectious Diseases, 2:326, 2002
5. Polatin, PB, Yound, M, Mayer, M, Gatchel, R. Bioterrorism, Stress and Pain. The Importance of an Anticipatory Community Preparedness Intervention. Journal of Psychosomatic Research, 58:311–316, 2005
6. North, CS, Pfefferbaum, B. Research on the Mental Health Effects of Terrorism. Journal of the American Medical Association, 288(5):633–636, 2002
7. American Psychiatric Association. Diagnostic and Statistical Manual of Mental Disorders, 4th ed. Text Revision, Washington, DC, 2000
8. Friedman, MJ, Hamblen, JL, Foa, EB, Charney, DS. Fighting the Psychological War on Terrorism. Commentary on "A National Longitudinal Study on the Psychological Consequences of the September 11, 2001 Terrorist Attacks: Reactions, Impairment and Help Seeking." Psychiatry, 67(2):123–136, 2004
9. Bleich, A, Dycian, A, Koslowsky, M, Solomon, Z, Wiener, M. Psychiatric Implications of Missile Attacks on a Civilian Population. Israeli Lessons from the Persian Gulf War. JAMA, 268(5):613–5, 1992
10. North, CS, Nixon, SJ, Sharaiat, S, Mallonee, S, McMillen, JC, Spitznagel, EL, Smith, EM. Psychiatric Disorders Among Survivors of the Oklahoma City Bombing. Journal of the American Medical Association, 282(8):755–762, 1999

11. Blanchard, EB, Jones-Alexander, J, Buckley, TC, Forneris, CA. Psychometric Properties of the PTSD Checklist (PCL). Behaviour Research and Therapy, 34, 669–673, 1996
12. Schuster, MA, Stein, Jaycox, LH, et al. A National Survey of Stress Reactions After the September 11, 2001 Terrorist Attacks. New England Journal of Medicine, 345:1507–1512, 2001
13. Galea, S, Ahern, J, Resnick, H, et al. Psychological Sequelae of the September 11 Terrorist Attacks in New York City. New England Journal of Medicine, 346:982–987, 2002
14. Schlenger, WE, Caddell, JM, Ebert, L, et al. Psychological Reactions to Terrorist Attacks. Findings from the National Study of Americans' Reactions to September 11. JAMA, 288(5):581–588, 2002
15. Silver, RC, Holman, EA, McIntosh, DN, Poulin, M, Gil-Rivas, V. Nationwide Longitudinal Study of Psychological Responses to September 11. JAMA, 288(10):1235–1244, 2002
16. Vlahov, D, Galea, S, Resnick, H, Ahern, J, Boscarino, JA, Bucuvalas, M, Gold, J, Kilpatrick, D. Increased Use of Cigarettes, Alcohol and Marijuana Among Manhattan, New York, Residents After the September 11th Terrorist Attacks. American Journal of Epidemiology, 155(11):988–996, 2002
17. Norris, F, Friedman, M, Watson, P, Byrne, C, Diaz, E, Kaniasty, K. 60,000 Disaster Victims Speak. Part I. An Empirical Review of the Empirical Literature, 1981–2001, Psychiatry, 65(3):207–239, 2002
18. Norris, F, Friedman, M, Watson, P. 60,000 Disaster Victims Speak. Part II. Summary and Implications of the Disaster Mental Health Research. Psychiatry, 65(3):240–260, 2002
19. Norwood, AE, Ursano, RJ, Fullerton, CS. Disaster Psychiatry: Principles and Practice. Psychiatric Quarterly, 71(3):207–226, 2000
20. Compton, MT, Kotwicki, R, Kaslow, NJ, Reissman, DB, Wetterhall, SF. Incorporating Mental Health into Bioterrorism Response Planning. Public Health Reports, 120(Suppl. 1): 16–19, 2005
21. Flynn, BW, Norwood, AE. Defining Normal Psychological Reactions to Disaster. Psychiatric Annals, 34(8):597–603, 2004
22. Wolraich, ML, et al. American Academy of Pediatrics, Committee on Psychosocial Aspects of Child and Family Health. How Pediatricians Can Respond to the Psychosocial Implications of Disasters. Pediatrics, 103(2):521–523, 1999
23. Work Group on Disasters, American Academy of Pediatrics. Psychosocial Issues for Children and Families in Disasters: A Guide for the Primary Care Physician. http://www.mentalhealth. samhsa.gov/publications/allpubs/SMA95–3022/default.asp, last accessed 3/11.06
24. DiGiovanni, C. Domestic Terrorism with Chemical or Biological Agents: Psychiatric Aspects. American Journal of Psychiatry, 156(10):1500–1505, 1999
25. Diamond, DS, Pastor, LH, McIntosh, RG. Medical Management of Terrorism-Related Behavioral Syndromes. Psychiatric Annals, 34(9):689–695, 2004
26. Koenig, KL, Goans, RE, Hatchett, RJ, et al. Medical Treatment of Radiological Casualties: Current Concepts. Annals of Emergency Medicine, 45(6):643–652, 2005
27. Yehuda, R. Post-Traumatic Stress Disorder. New England Journal of Medicine, 346(2):108–114, 2002
28. Lange, JT, Lange, CL, Cabaltica, RBG. Priamry Care Treatment of Post-Traumatic Stress Disorder. American Family Physician, 62(5):1035–1040, 2000
29. Lecrubier, Y. Posttraumatic Stress Disorder in Primary Care: A Hidden Diagnosis. Journal of Clinical Psychiatry, 65(Suppl. 1):49–54, 2004
30. Ballenger, JC, Davidson, JRT, Lecrubier, Y, Nutt, DJ, Marshall, RD, Nemeroff, CB, Shalev, AY, Yehuda, R. Consensus Statement Update on Posttraumatic Stress Disorder From the International Consensus Group on Depression and Anxiety. Journal of Clinical Psychiatry, 65(Suppl. 1):55–62, 2004
31. Benedek, DM, Holloway, HD, Becker, SM Emergency Mental Health Management in Bioterrorism Events. Emergency Medicine Clinics of North America, 20:393–407, 2002

32. Stein, BD, Elliott, MN, Jaycox, LH, Collins, RL, Berry, SH, Klein, DJ, Schuster, MA. A National Longitudinal Study of the Psychological Consequences of September 11, 2001 Terrorist Attacks: Reactions, Impairment and Help Seeking. Psychiatry, 67(2):105–117
33. Melnick, AL. The Family Physician's Role in Responding to Biological and Chemical Terrorism. In Taylor, RB, et al (Eds.), Family Medicine. Principles and Practice, 6th ed., Springer, New York, 2003
34. Bisson, J, Andrew, M. Psychological Treatment of Post-Traumatic Stress Disorder (PTSD) (Review). The Cochrane Database of Systematic Reviews, Issue 3, Wiley, New York, 2005
35. Stein, DJ, Ipser, JC, Seedat. Pharmacology for Post Traumatic Stress Disorder (PTSD) (Review). The Cochrane Database of Systematic Reviews, Issue 1, Wiley, New York, 2006
36. Foa, EB, Davidson, JRT, Frances A (Eds.). Treatment of Posttraumatic Stress Disorder (Expert Consensus Guideline Series). Journal of Clinical Psychiatry, 60 (Suppl. 16):1–76, 1999
37. Rose, S, Bisson, J Churchill, R, Wessely, S. Psychological Debriefing for Preventing Post Traumatic Stress Disorder (PTSD) (Review). The Cochrane Database of Systematic Reviews, Issue 2, 2002

Chapter 6
The Primary Care Physician's Role in Supporting the Public Health Response to Biological, Chemical, and Radiological Terrorism

In October 2001, when the first anthrax patients sought medical care, none of them had a history suggesting exposure to anthrax. Given the rarity of anthrax, many other causes more likely explained their early, nonspecific symptoms. The diversity of anthrax victims, which included an infant, revealed that biological terrorism could affect anyone, regardless of age, gender, health status, occupation, or socioeconomic status (1). The anthrax events also taught us that alert clinicians who recognize a potential terrorist-caused illness, obtain the appropriate laboratory tests, and notify public health officials, play a critical role in protecting their communities as well as their individual patients (1). Early warnings to local health officials, who work closely with law enforcement, can be successful in preventing additional casualties.

This book has discussed some of the common agents and presentations of terrorist caused illness. The previous chapters discussed the role of primary care physicians in evaluating and treating individuals and families exposed to biological, chemical, and radiological attacks. Clearly, primary care physicians are on the front lines of detecting and responding to people affected by terrorist attacks and other disasters. This chapter discusses how primary care physicians and other clinicians can work with the public health system in early detection and community wide prevention and treatment of biological, chemical, and radiological disasters. Potential roles for primary care physicians include participating in surveillance activities, reporting suspected cases to public health officials, and responding to the surge of affected patients following manmade or natural disasters.

Surveillance and Reporting

Public health officials use surveillance, the ongoing, systematic collection, analysis and interpretation of health-related data, to recognize and respond to disease outbreaks to reduce morbidity and mortality (2). Disease reporting is an essential component of surveillance and outbreak detection. Once patients begin trickling in to physician offices and emergency departments, astute clinicians who recognize and report potential cases can enhance the speed at which public health authorities

A. L. Melnick (ed.), *Biological, Chemical, and Radiological Terrorism.*
© Springer 2008

analyze, recognize, and respond to a mass exposure event. The first five chapters of this book provided clinical information useful in identifying potential cases. Besides being able to recognize a clinical condition that may have public health significance, clinicians must know how to report such cases promptly to public health officials (3).

Within the United States, state governments have the constitutional authority to mandate clinicians, other healthcare providers and laboratories to report specific diseases and other specific health conditions (4). In assuming their authority, states have enacted legislation specifying which health conditions are reportable, often known as notifiable conditions, and delegating the responsibility for receiving reports to either state or local public health agencies. In addition, all states and territories participate in a national surveillance system by voluntarily reporting either aggregate or case-specific data to the Centers for Disease Control and Prevention (CDC).

At times, physician values have conflicted with mandatory reporting requirements. While public health is concerned with protecting the entire population, most clinicians believe their primary duty is serving their individual patients. Some clinicians have regarded requirements to notify public health officials using patient names and other sensitive information as a breach of confidentiality, whereas public health authorities have justified these reporting requirements by invoking the principles of using science and collective responsibility in protecting the public (4). The US Supreme Court has upheld public health reporting requirements in rulings on cases alleging that such requirements violate individual privacy (4). Clinicians should be aware that the Health Insurance Portability and Accountability Act (HIPAA) Privacy Rule, described later in this chapter, allows them to report conditions of public health significance to public health officials.

Even with mandatory reporting requirements, a comprehensive review of the literature revealed that the frequency clinicians report varies from 9 to 99% in the United States, with the variation related chiefly to the disease or condition reported (5). AIDS, sexually transmitted diseases and tuberculosis, all unlikely to be associated with a terrorist attack, have higher reporting rates compared to other communicable illnesses. Besides confidentiality concerns, other reasons for incomplete clinician reporting include lack of awareness of the legal mandate to report, lack of knowledge of which diseases are notifiable, lack of knowledge regarding how and where to report, an assumption that someone else will report the case and inadequate incentives for reporting or inadequate penalties for not reporting (5).

The quality and timeliness of disease reporting depends on an effective two-way communication between clinicians and public health officials (2). The clinician role involves reporting cases and clusters of notifiable and unusual diseases to health officials. Clinicians can overcome some of the barriers to reporting by obtaining contact information for their local and state public health officials and by keeping the information in a handy location. Large practices may want to consider setting up a system to detect increased numbers of patient visits for similar and unusual conditions. Clinicians should also consider assigning one of their staff as a point person for reporting potential cases to the local health department.

In communicating with clinicians, public health officials have several roles:

- Consulting on case diagnosis and management
- Issuing alerts to inform clinicians
- Providing surveillance summaries so community clinicians understand the extent of the outbreak and current control measures
- Making clinical and public health recommendations
- Informing clinicians about public health policies

Most public health officials will be eager to share information about reporting disease requirements, including the specific diseases and conditions that are reportable. For example, Oregon has an attractive handy poster with notifiable diseases and contact information, including an after-hours phone number that clinicians can hang in their offices (see Fig. 6.1). The Oregon Web site contains reporting forms and local health department fax numbers. Other states have similar tools for clinicians.

Several Internet sites may be helpful for clinicians who cannot find local and state public health contact information. The CDC Web site has a link to state health departments at http://www.cdc.gov/doc.do/id/0900f3ec80226c7a (last accessed 3–18–06). Alternatively, the Association of State and Territorial Health Officials has a directory of state public health agencies at http://www.statepublichealth.org/index.php (last accessed 3–18–06), and the National Association of County and City Health Officials (NACCHO) has a directory of local health departments at http://lhadirectory.naccho.org/phdir/(last accessed 3–18–06).

HIPAA Privacy Rules and Physician Reporting

Given clinician concerns regarding patient privacy, the CDC has produced a document that summarizes the HIPAA Privacy Rule regarding reporting information to public health authorities (6). Although the HIPAA Privacy Rule does not require reporting, it allows healthcare organizations and clinicians to report protected health information (PHI) to public health officials. PHI includes individually identifiable health information transmissible electronically or in any other form. The three types of individually identifiable health information concern (6):

- The past, present, or future physical or mental health or condition of an individual
- The provision of health care to an individual
- Payment for the provision of individual healthcare if the information identifies or provides a reasonable basis to believe someone can use it to identify the individual

All state laws require reporting of specific communicable diseases and unusual disease occurrences. The US Department of Health and Human Services (DHHS) recognizes the importance of sharing PHI to accomplish essential public health objectives (6). Therefore, the HIPAA Privacy rule expressly permits clinicians and hospitals to share PHI for public health purposes (6). Specifically, HIPAA allows "covered entities," "without individual authorization, to disclose PHI to a public

Public Health Reporting
...for clinicians

By law,[1] Oregon clinicians must report diagnoses (confirmed or suspected) of the following infections, diseases, and conditions. Both clinical and lab-confirmed cases are reportable. The parallel system of lab reporting does not obviate the clinician's obligation to report. Some conditions (e.g., Uncommon Illnesses of Public Health Significance, animal bites, HUS, PID, pesticide poisoning, disease outbreaks) are rarely if ever identified by labs. In short, we depend upon clinicians to report.

Reports should be made to the patient's local health department[2] and should include at least the patient's name, home address, phone number, date of birth, sex, the diagnosis, and the date of symptom onset. Most reports should be made within one (health department) working day of the diagnosis, but there are a number of exceptions (noted with asterisks, infra).

Disease reporting enables appropriate public health follow-up for your patients, helps identify outbreaks, provides a better understanding of morbidity patterns, and may even save lives. If local health department staff are unavailable, a state epidemiologist is always on call (503/731-4024; after hours, 503/731-4030).

SPECIFIC ETIOLOGIES

Anthrax***
Botulism***
Brucellosis
Campylobacteriosis
Chancroid
Chlamydia infection[3]
Cryptosporidiosis
Cyclospora infection
Diphtheria***
Escherichia coli (Shiga-toxigenic)[4]
Giardiasis
Gonorrhea
Haemophilus influenzae**
Hantavirus*
Hepatitis A
Hepatitis B
Hepatitis C (new infections)[5]
Hepatitis D (delta)
HIV infection and AIDS[6]
Legionellosis
Leptospirosis*
Listeriosis
Lyme disease
Malaria
Measles (rubeola)**
Meningococcal disease**
Plague***
Polio**
Rabies**
Rubella**
Pertussis

Q fever
Salmonellosis (including typhoid)
Shigellosis
Syphilis
Taenia solium/Cysticercosis*
Tetanus*
Trichinosis
Tuberculosis
Tularemia
Vibrio infection**
Yersiniosis

OTHER CONDITIONS

Animal bites
any Arthropod-borne infection[7]
HUS
Lead poisoning*
Marine intoxications***[8]
any Outbreak of disease***[9]
Pesticide poisoning**
PID (acute, non-gonococcal)*
any Uncommon illness of
    potential public health
    significance***[10]

TIMING OF REPORTS

*** Immediately—day or night
** Within 24 hours
* Within 1 week
If unspecified, report within
    1 working day

FOOTNOTES

1 ORS 433.004; OAR 333-018-0000 to 333-018-0015.
2 Refer to http://www.oshd.org/acd/dispt.htm for a list of local health departments and more details about what to report.
3 STDs, trachoma, TWAR, psittacosis—all of 'em—even if they're renamed Chlamydophila.
4 E. coli O157:H7 is the exemplar of this group.
5 Report only diagnoses of probable recent infection (e.g., post-transplant infections, persons with conversion of paired sera). Most cases are old or indeterminate; these are not reportable.
6 HIV/AIDS reports can be made directly to the state's HIV office (fax, 503/731-4425).
7 Including any of the scores of viral, bacterial, and parasitic infections typically spread by ticks, mosquitos, fleas, and their ilk (e.g., Lyme disease, malaria, ehrlichiosis, relapsing fever, typhus, babesiosis, dengue, yellow fever, Oroya fever, Colorado tick fever, West Nile fever, RMSF, SLE, WEE, EEE, filariasis, tsutsugamushi, Congo-Crimean hemorrhagic fever,...).
8 Paralytic shellfish poisoning, scombroid, domoic acid intoxication, ciguatera, etc.
9 Outbreaks are ≥2 cases from separate households associated with a suspected common source.
10 Don't make us list every exotic disease in the world. Ask yourself 'Might there be public health implications from a case of possible Ebola, smallpox, melioidosis, or whatever?' If the answer is 'yes'—or even 'maybe'—then pick up the phone. There are no penalties for overreporting.

Oregon Department of Human Services
Office of Disease Prevention and Epidemiology · 503/731-4024 (phone) · 503/731-4798 (fax) · www.oshd.org/acd DHS

Fig. 6.1 Conditions Notifiable by State Law in Oregon. (from: http://oregon.gov/DHS/ph/acd/reporting/mdposter.pdf, public domain)

health authority legally authorized to collect or receive the information for the purposes of preventing or controlling disease, injury, or disability including, but not limited to (6):

– Reporting of disease, injury, and vital events (e.g., birth or death)
– Conducting public health surveillance, investigations and interventions"

Without individual authorization, covered entities may also disclose PHI to any person "who may have been exposed to a communicable disease or may be at risk for contracting or spreading a disease or condition, when legally authorized to notify the person as necessary to conduct a public health intervention or investigation."

"Covered entities" include (6):

– "Health plans," defined as "individual or group plans that provide or pay the cost of medical care that includes the diagnosis, cure, mitigation, treatment, or prevention of disease. Health plans include private entities, such as health insurers and managed care organization and government organizations, such as Medicaid, Medicare, and the Veterans Health Administration."
– "Healthcare clearinghouses," defined as "public or private entities, including billing services, repricing companies, or community health information systems, that process nonstandard data or transactions received from another entity into standard transactions or data elements, or vice versa."
– "Health care providers," defined as "a provider of healthcare services and any other person or organization that furnishes, bills, or is paid for health care in the normal course of business. Healthcare providers, such as physicians, hospitals, and clinics, are covered entities if they transmit health information in electronic form in connection with a transaction for which a HIPAA standard has been adopted by DHHS."

The HIPAA Privacy Rule defines public health authorities as "agencies or authorities of the United States, states, territories, political subdivisions of states or territories, American Indian tribes, or an individual or entity acting under a grant of authority form such agencies and responsible for public health matters as part of an official mandate (6)." Public health authorities include (6):

– Federal public health agencies, such as the CDC, National Institutes of Health (NIH), Health Resources and Services Administration (HRSA), Substance Abuse and Mental Health Services Administration (SAMHSA), Food and Drug Administration (FDA), or the Occupational Safety and Health Administration
– Tribal Health Agencies
– State public health agencies, such as public health departments, divisions, or bureaus
– State public health agency registries, such as cancer and immunization registries, and state vital statistics programs
– Local public health agencies, such as county or city public health departments or multicounty health districts
– Anyone performing public health functions under a grant of authority from a public health agency

The Privacy Rule permits clinicians, as covered entities, to disclose protected health information (PHI) without authorization to public health authorities for the purpose of preventing or controlling disease. This includes reporting diseases and participating in public health surveillance, investigations, and interventions (6). Even if state law does not require reporting information related to a specific disease, the HIPAA Privacy Rule allows clinicians to report PHI to an authorized public health authority for the purpose of preventing or controlling disease or injury. For example, when conducting a disease investigation to protect the community, local public health officials might need additional information related to people affected by the disease. In some cases, they may need to contact victims to determine the etiology, identify their potentially exposed contacts and intervene to prevent the spread of the disease. The HIPAA Privacy Rule allows clinicians to share such PHI to help public health officials protect the broader community.

When clinicians receive requests for PHI from a public health official, they should be able to verify the health official's official status and identity in one of three ways (6):

- Health officials making requests in person should present official credentials, badges, or other proof of government status
- Requests in writing should appear on official government letterhead
- Requests from persons acting in behalf of public health officials should supply a written statement on official government agency letterhead stating that the person is acting under authority of the government agency

Although the Privacy Rule allows reporting for public health purposes, clinicians must still comply with certain HIPAA Privacy Rule requirements when disclosing PHI to public health authorities. One of the requirements is that they must provide their patients, when requested, an accounting of their disclosure to public health authorities. Typically, clinicians can accomplish this by providing the requesting patient an accounting of each disclosure by date, the PHI reported, the recipient agency and the purpose of the report. However, for multiple disclosures to the same public health agency over the same accounting period, the HIPAA Privacy Rule allows a simplified means of accounting. In these cases, the reporting clinician, clinic, hospital, or other health care provider need only identify the public health agency, the purpose of the disclosures and the PHI routinely disclosed when reporting. Rather than tracking the date of each disclosure, the clinician or other health care provider can merely include the date of the first and last disclosure during the accounting period and a description of the frequency of the disclosures. This means that clinicians need not annotate each patient's medical record whenever making routine public health reports (6).

Syndromic Surveillance

One of the challenges for rapid outbreak detection is that patients with many of the illnesses described in previous chapters, especially infections, will present with ill-defined syndromes or unexplained deaths (7). The first sign of a terrorist attack may be an increased number of visits to physician offices and emergency departments by patients with common symptoms, such as respiratory complaints. Given the varying degree of exposure and the lengthy incubation period of some of these illnesses, the first wave of patients may be small and geographically dispersed. Even the most astute clinicians seeing individuals in their offices may have difficulty recognizing and reporting an unusual disease pattern. Syndromic surveillance attempts to overcome this limitation by systemically and electronically monitoring and reporting illness syndromes and events, such as emergency department diagnoses or purchases of prescriptions or over the counter medications that reflect the prodromes of potential terrorist-caused illnesses (8).

By 2003, the New York City Health Department was monitoring more than 50,000 events daily, including 86% of all emergency department visits in New York City through coverage of 70% of all hospital emergency departments (9).

Syndromic surveillance has several advantages for rapid assessment of terrorist-caused illness. By using routinely collected medical record information available in many emergency departments and increasingly in physician offices, it can assess a large number of visits for illness episodes sometimes days before diagnostic tests have identified a specific etiologic agent (10). Syndromic surveillance systems have several characteristics and requirements (11):

- Existing data sources, preferably electronically stored, such as electronic ambulatory medical records, emergency department data, pharmacy records, school absentee data and other data sets covering large populations
- Designation of specific events for identification, which could include groups of symptoms or behaviors, for example, ICD-9 groupings or the sales volume of supplies related to potential syndromes, such over the counter medications, facial tissues, or orange juice
- A system for acquiring, integrating, and incorporating data with a wide range of architectures from multiple sources
- Data format standards, and translation agents that transform data from existing formats into standardized formats
- Data analysis methodologies that identify unusual temporal or spatial patterns of illness: to identify these patterns, the system must have at least a year of historical data for comparison. The historical data must include models that identify normal temporal (e.g., seasonal) variations as well as changes in population density, hospital market areas and health care referral relationships (11)
- Linkages/transmission to public health authorities for investigation and response

A report describing the Harvard Pilgrim Health Care monitoring system illustrates how a relatively simple syndromic surveillance system used in one organization might work (12). The system grouped ICD-9 codes recorded during patient encounters into syndrome categories, such as neurologic, upper gastrointestinal, lower gastrointestinal, upper respiratory, lower respiratory, influenza-like illness (fever > 37.8°C plus cough and/or sore throat in the absence of a known cause), dermatologic and sepsis/fever (12). If a patient presented with symptoms spanning two categories, the system counted the visit under both categories independently. The system produced a daily surveillance summary report that identified large numbers of episodes within the Harvard Pilgrim ambulatory care system, including a list and maps of residence of patients with respiratory and gastrointestinal symptoms (12). For each syndrome, statistical modeling compared the daily counts at the census tract level and the entire surveillance area with daily counts observed in each census tract and entire surveillance area over a 4-year period. Results revealed that the ambulatory care episodes for lower respiratory illness were closely associated with hospital admissions, with the admission data appearing to lag behind the ambulatory care data (11).

Syndromic surveillance in ambulatory settings can thus track common infections, such as influenza and potentially identify new, emerging infections. Detection of an increased frequency of common syndromes, such as respiratory illness, especially during an unusual time of year, can trigger additional diagnostic testing essential in identifying an etiology (10). Other advantages of syndromic surveillance include a high sensitivity, because the automated reporting system does not require individual physicians to recognize and report a specific etiology, and low cost, because automated electronic medical record systems are already available in many emergency departments and physician offices (10,12). In addition, diagnostic code data available in other automated settings, such as claims databases and nurse triage lines, can increase the range of and sensitivity of the surveillance system (12).

For these systems to work effectively, they must be timely, accurate, complete, and capable of distinguishing terrorist caused illness from background disease occurrences (10). Unfortunately, syndromic surveillance systems suffer from several disadvantages in these areas. Syndromic systems may have difficulty detecting terrorist-caused outbreaks too small to trigger statistical alarms (8) or occurring during the time of year when naturally occurring illness increases (8). Depending on the agent and its incubation period, some patients will not seek care until hospitalization is necessary, and neither emergency department data nor other ambulatory data will be available for analysis. In general, the shorter the incubation period, the less likely prodromal events, such as purchase of medications or ambulatory visits for nonspecific symptoms would trigger a syndromic surveillance system alarm (8). In addition, for severely ill patients, the time from arrival at the emergency presentation until admission may be very short. In some of these cases, such as pneumonic plague or anthrax, in which one case constitutes an outbreak, diagnostic test results may be available sooner than the syndromic surveillance system is capable of processing and analyzing the data (8). Regarding accuracy, an additional limitation is that the validity and reliability of physician diagnosis using ICD-9 or ICD-10 codes is unknown and not readily amenable to measurement (10). Clinicians practicing at different sites or different clinicians at the same site may code the same illness or syndrome differently (13).

Spatial data may present additional problems with accuracy. First, the only address available in a database may be home address, although the relevant exposure may have occurred elsewhere. Second, poor quality of the address data may preclude the accurate identification of specific patient location. Third, the use of different scales of analysis, such as census tract, zip code, or metropolitan area can lead to different interpretations when analyzing the data (11).

Administrative challenges pose a limitation to the completeness of any integrated system. Creating integrated systems that extend beyond the boundaries of a single health maintenance organization to area hospitals, emergency departments, and ambulatory settings will require administrative contracts, effective working relationships between information technology groups at each site and agreements on data elements, data architecture and standards, coding practices, security and policy issues (13). All of these elements must be in place before development and implementation of any effective, integrated syndromic surveillance system (13).

Patient confidentiality concerns may also limit the development of syndromic surveillance systems. Any automated reporting system will require confidentiality safeguards, such as the use of aggregated information (12). However, even with aggregated data, sorting by characteristics such as race, age, and zip code could still lead to identification of individuals. Therefore, surveillance systems will need standards restricting the display of aggregated data when numbers of events or population sizes are small (14). On the other hand, public health authorities may still need to be able to re-identify individuals to follow-up on cases (11).

A combination of state statutes and federal regulations, specifically HIPAA, described earlier in this chapter, govern the legal status of automated and manual disease reporting systems. In some states, revision of state rules may be necessary before implanting automated surveillance systems. After implementation of a Washington State syndromic surveillance pilot, state officials revised reporting regulations to require mandatory reporting by clinicians and hospitals of cases and case clusters compatible with potential bioterrorist pathogens (13). In general, HIPAA regulations permit clinicians and hospitals to transmit information to public health authorities if the transmission meets criteria for public health activity.

Given continued questions of timeliness, accuracy, confidentiality, and given the administrative hurdles facing development of complete, integrated syndromic surveillance systems, it is unlikely that automated syndromic surveillance systems will replace traditional clinician and laboratory initiated reporting systems within the next few years. Studies of the performance of syndromic surveillance systems are difficult due to the low frequency of large outbreaks of most diseases (11). Even if syndromic surveillance systems eventually demonstrate some utility, it is likely that they will complement, rather than replace, traditional clinician, and laboratory reporting.

For example, once the system identifies a spatial or temporal cluster of syndromic symptoms, public health officials will still need to work with clinicians and other healthcare providers to differentiate natural illness from terrorist-caused illness. The necessary detailed investigation will involve personal contact, either by phone or in person, with individual cases regarding their medical condition, any unusual illness manifestations or specific exposures (11). In addition, identification of cases will still require the appropriate laboratory and radiological studies on individuals with syndromic symptoms.

Responding to the Patient Surge Following a Terrorist Attack

Following the 2001 anthrax attacks, public health authorities advised over 10,000 persons to take postexposure prophylactic medications for up to 60 days (1,15). An additional 20,000 patients started prophylactic treatment until the epidemiologic investigation revealed that they were not exposed. Authorities established medication distribution sites, also known as points of dispensing, or PODs, in Florida, Washington DC, and the New York/New Jersey metropolitan area where potentially exposed patients received triage and prophylaxis. Hoaxes and false alarms affected thousands of others. In addition, thousands of co-workers, family members and friends contacted public health officials and primary care physicians with concerns that they were at risk. Across the United States, additional hoaxes and false alarms resulted in thousands of calls to public health officials and physicians (1). Ultimately, only 22 people developed anthrax, resulting in five deaths. In comparison, a more widespread attack with an aerosolized weapon could expose a much larger population, resulting in greater numbers of people requiring triage and prophylaxis. The health manpower requirements for high volume triage, mass prophylaxis and treatment would stretch and possibly overwhelm existing resources, especially if other health care business were to proceed as usual.

Primary care physicians will need to plan for changes in their office staffing and patient demand following a terrorist attack. The CDC has developed a pandemic influenza checklist for primary care offices that physicians may also find useful in planning for other large disease outbreaks, including manmade disasters. The entire checklist is available at (16) http://www.pandemicflu.gov/plan/medical.html (last accessed 3–19–06). Practices should consider creating planning committees to develop preparedness plans for the practice. Depending on the practice, the committees can range from two to several staff members, with representatives form administration, medical staff, nursing, reception, laboratory, and others as appropriate and assigning one person as overall preparedness planning coordinator. In addition to planning, office practices should consider conducting periodic exercises of the plan components. Specific issues practice preparedness planning committees should address include:

– Plans for triage and management of a patient surge during a real or imagined terrorist attack: Triage might include using e-mail or phone contact with patients to determine which patients need an office visit, thereby limiting visits to those that are medically necessary (16). Clinicians will need to decide whether to cancel nonessential medical visits, such as annual physicals and/or design separate blocks of time for potentially exposed patients. If possible, the practice should create a database of contact information for patients with regularly scheduled visits, making it easy for the practice to notify them for rescheduling or assigning them to another location for care, especially if the practice closes. Given the potential strain on hospitals, clinicians should work with their hospitals to develop plans and criteria for the disposition of additional patients, including hospitalization, home health care services or self-care at home. In some areas, local public health departments will work with hospitals to set up medical care points, alternative sites to hospitals and emergency departments, for triage and care of potentially affected patients.
– Plans for managing staff and supply shortages: During a large outbreak, staff may be absent due to illness in themselves or concern for their family members.

Clinicians should encourage their office staff to develop family care plans for their children and disabled family members, especially if conditions or imposed measures make commuting difficult or impossible. Family plans should include stockpiling at least a week's supply of food, water, medical supplies and other consumable necessities. Office practices should determine the number and type of staffing needed to maintain services and develop a plan for closing the practice or recruiting temporary personnel during a severe staffing shortage. Given the stress of caring for affected patients, some staff may need access to mental health counseling and faith-based resources (16). Clinician practices can avoid supply shortages during a large patient influx by estimating consumable resource needs, such as masks, gloves, hand hygiene products and medical supplies, and stockpiling appropriately. In addition, practices should have a contingency plan containing detailed procedures for acquiring supplies through normal and alternative channels when emergency supplies become exhausted (16).

– Plans for communication: Practices should create a list of points of contact for coordinating patient care, including all service providers they may need to communicate with during a mass disaster. Depending on the practice, the list might include contacts for local hospitals, long-term care facilities, social service agencies, mental health providers, emergency medical services, laboratories, and other relevant community organizations, such as the Red Cross. In addition, practices should list the names, titles and contact information for appropriate state and local public health department contacts and maintain the lists in an easily accessible location. Practices might want to consider designating one "point person" to communicate with the local public health department, hospitals, the media and others to ensure the provision of consistent messages (16). The point person can also be responsible for monitoring advisories and other communications from local, federal, and state public health authorities (16).

– Plans for infection control: Given that symptomatic patients may have a communicable disease, all practices should have an infection control plan in place and staff should have training in infection control. These plans are also essential for natural communicable disease outbreaks, such as influenza (16). The CDC has useful information for implementing respiratory hygiene and cough etiquette at http://www.cdc.gov/flu/professionals/infectioncontrol/resphygiene.htm (last accessed 3–25–06). If possible, practices should designate specific waiting room locations for patients with respiratory symptoms. Signage in appropriate languages can instruct symptomatic patients on respiratory hygiene and cough etiquette, such as using tissues to cover coughs and washing hands frequently. Practices should be prepared to distribute masks in pediatric and adult sizes to symptomatic patients who can wear them and provide facial tissues, waste receptacles and hand hygiene materials in waiting rooms and exam rooms (16). The CDC has information on Standard and Droplet precautions at http://www. cdc.gov/ncidod/dhqp/gl_isolation_standard.html (last accessed 3–25–06) and http://www.cdc.gov/ncidod/dhqp/gl_isolation_droplet.html (last accessed 3–25–06) that practices can use to develop office policies for their staff (16). Policies should include protection for staff who encounter patients initially, such as front desk and triage staff (16). In addition, practices should have plans for protecting immunocompromised and pregnant staff at risk of complications. Such protection could include reassignment away from patient care duties or paid administrative leave (16).

Beyond the Office: Volunteering to Help

Following Hurricane Katrina in 2005, many physicians volunteered for deployment to the gulf coast to care for victims. Unfortunately, public health authorities were often unable to put them to work due to their lack of training and the lack of infrastructure necessary to coordinate their efforts (17). Similarly, following the September 11, 2001 attacks, many clinicians, at their own personal risk, showed up at the disaster scenes, volunteering their time and skills to support the public health response. Although their intentions were good, their uncoordinated appearance at the disaster scenes caused problems for emergency managers and frustration for all involved (18) for several reasons:

– Credentialing was a problem. Overworked emergency managers did not know how to verify and account for credentials of unaffiliated volunteers, including volunteers from outside communities, especially given the stressed emergency management system
– Liability protection for volunteers was unresolved. For example, emergency managers and volunteers did not know who would provide legal protection for volunteer clinicians, especially those arriving from other areas of the country
– There was no mechanism providing treatment and compensation for injuries sustained by volunteers, including those who were working in hazardous environments
– Emergency management did not have a system in place to manage and supervise volunteers
– Emergency management agencies, already stressed by accounting for their own personnel, did not have resources to address issues such as housing, feeding, and protecting the volunteers

Consequently, emergency management had to turn away many highly skilled volunteers who could have been helpful (18). An important lesson from these events is that physicians can be most effective if they are well trained in disaster medicine, understand the importance of reestablishing the necessary infrastructure, and if they arrive as part of a coordinated, organized response. Another lesson from these events is that the public health and emergency response system will need clinicians and other healthcare volunteers following large outbreaks. The federal, state, and local public health system extended its resources operating point of dispensing (POD) sites to give prophylactic antibiotics to 30,000 people following the anthrax attacks. Without volunteer health professionals, a larger attack would overwhelm our public health response system (18). Two ways physicians can become part of an organized disaster response team include becoming members of the Medical Reserve Corps or Disaster Medical Assistance Teams (DMATs) (17).

The Medical Reserve Corps

In July 2002, the federal government founded the Medical Reserve Corps (MRC) as part of a larger attempt to encourage volunteerism among Americans. The MRC, sponsored by the Office of the Surgeon General and housed within the Department of Health and Human Services, is a component of the Citizen Corps, a national network of volunteers working to ensure hometown security (17–19). The Citizen Corps, housed in the Department of Homeland Security, is the umbrella organization for Community Emergency Response Teams (CERT), Neighborhood Watch, Volunteers in Police Service (VIPS) and Fire Corps, in addition to the MRC. In turn, the Citizen Corps and associated agencies, including the AmeriCorps, Senior Corps and the Peace Corps are components of the larger effort, the USA Freedom Corps, whose mission is to promote volunteerism and service. More information on the Freedom Corps and the Citizen Corps is available at http://www.usafreedomcorps.gov/and http://www.usafreedomcorps.gov/about_usafc/programs/citizencorps.asp.

The MRC mission is "to establish teams of local volunteer medical and public health professionals who can contribute their skills and expertise throughout the year and during times of community need (19)." Although the MRC is a federal program, individual units are community-based, supplementing existing local emergency and public health resources. The MRC Program office facilitates the development of additional local MRC units by providing a clearinghouse for information sharing and by providing forums to identify best practices and lessons learned (18). The purpose of the MRC program is to organize local teams of volunteers to prepare for and respond to emergencies, including natural and manmade disasters (an all-hazard approach), by proactively addressing identified barriers to volunteerism such as preidentification, registration, credentialing, training, liability, and activation.

The MRC program now includes more than 30,000 volunteers working in over 200 units throughout the United States. Organizations housing MRC units include local public health departments, boards of health, medical societies, emergency management agencies, and nongovernmental organizations within communities ranging from small rural counties to large cities (18). MRC units supplement existing public health and emergency management agencies. Besides participating in disaster response, MRC members volunteer to help with public health activities throughout the year, such as administering childhood immunizations and flu vaccinations or providing clinical and social services for homeless populations. The Surgeon General's office encourages MRC units to help with national priorities for public health, including disease prevention, improving health literacy, eliminating health disparities, and enhancing public health preparedness (18).

Given their broad range of community activities, MRC units recruit volunteers with varied backgrounds, including practicing and retired physicians, nurses, pharmacists, dentists, veterinarians, mental health professionals, paramedics, and epidemiologists (18,19). Nonmedical volunteers, such as interpreters, chaplains, office workers, legal advisors, and others offer support services.

Local MRC units have developed community-based solutions for some of the identified barriers to volunteerism, such as lack of training, credentialing and liability. By enrolling volunteers in the locally appropriate training programs and preferentially conducting the training with their response partners, MRC units ensure integration of their volunteers into the local response system (18). Training for clinician volunteers might address issues such as (18):

- Working with emergency response and public health systems
- Understanding emergency events
- Understanding activation procedures for MRC units
- The National Incident Management System, including how to work within an Incident Command structure

(From Hoard ML, et al. (18). Reprinted with permission fro Elsevier)

MRC volunteers also get opportunities to participate in exercises, such as working in point of dispensing (PODs) sites as part of a strategic national stockpile exercise.

Credentialing relates to professional qualifications such as licensure, education, including continuing education, professional training, board certification, and hospital privileges (18). At a minimum, MRC units address credentialing by verifying that all licensed health professional volunteer members have current, unencumbered licenses. Some MRC units have taken the additional step of conducting a full credentialing of their members. The Health Resources and Services Administration (HRSA), within the US Department of Health and Human Services, has established a new program, the Emergency System for the Advanced Registration of Volunteer Healthcare Personnel (ESAR-VHP). The goal of this program is to develop a national system of state-based registries of medical and public health volunteers, which would allow states to preidentify and credential MRC volunteers. Communities could then use MRC units to activate and deploy the volunteers on the registry, ensuring a cohesive, coordinated response (18). MRC units are also working their communities and states to address liability protection for volunteers. Clinicians interested in volunteering can find out where the nearest local MRC unit is by checking the MRC Web site at http://www.medicalreservecorps.gov (19). If a local unit does not exist, the MRC site provides information on how to get one started.

Disaster Medical Assistance Teams

Disaster Medical Assistance Teams (DMATs) are components of the National Disaster Medical System within the US Department of Homeland Security. Each DMAT, containing professional and para-professional medical personnel supported by logistical and administrative staff, provides medical care during disasters (17,20). Each DMAT must have a sponsoring organization, such as a hospital, public health agency, safety agency or nonprofit public or private organization that signs a Memorandum of Agreement (MOA) with the Department of Homeland Security (20). The sponsoring organization organizes the team, recruits members, arranges training, and coordinates dispatch (20). In addition to "standard" DMATs, specialized DMATs deal with specific conditions such as crush injuries, burns and mental health emergencies (20). The purpose of DMATs is to supplement local medical care until mobilization of other federal or contract resources or until the situation resolves (20).

As noted on the DMAT Web site, DMATs "deploy to disaster sites with sufficient supplies and equipment to sustain themselves for 72h while providing medical care at a fixed or temporary medical site." In a disaster involving mass casualties, DMAT responsibilities include triage, providing medical care and preparing patients for evacuation (20). During other events, DMATs may provide primary healthcare and may supplement overwhelmed local health care staff. Rarely, when authorities evacuate disaster victims to a remote location for medical care, DMATs may support patient reception and disposition to hospitals (20). In October 2001, 100 members from five DMATs participated in providing mass prophylaxis for thousands of New York City postal service workers potentially exposed to anthrax (21).

DMAT members must maintain the appropriate certification and licensure within their specific professional discipline. When activated, DMAT members become Federal employees, with all States recognizing their licensure and certification. In addition, DMAT members receive pay while serving as part time federal employees and they receive liability protection through the Federal Tort Claims Act (20). Although DMATs serve primarily as a local community resource available to support local, regional and state needs, as a national resource they are subject to federalization and deployment elsewhere (20).

Clinicians interested in joining a DMAT, must fill out a federal job application form available through the DMAT Internet site (20). After filling out the forms, applicants should mail them to the team leader for administrative officer in their local area. The Web links page on the DMAT Internet site contains a listing of response team Internet sites. Alternatively, clinicians interested in finding a team in their area can e-mail the National Disaster Medical System at ndms@usa.net (20). After completing the application, applicants must interview with the team before acceptance as a team member (17). If a local team does not exist, the DMAT Internet site contains information on starting a DMAT (20).

Primary Care Role in Responding to Biological, Chemical, and Radiological Terrorism

This book has identified key roles for primary care clinicians in protecting the health of their communities:

- Addressing patient concerns about their risks of terrorist-caused illness
- Participation in surveillance to detect an attack, including reporting potential exposures and any unusual cases or clusters of cases to local and state public health officials
- Working with public health officials to identify patients at risk of exposure and providing preventive treatment
- Working with public health officials to identify patients with terrorist-caused disease and providing effective treatment
- Educating patients and the community on the risks of biological, chemical, and radiological terrorism, including how to protect themselves and their families
- Detecting symptoms of psychological trauma following terrorist events, and providing compassionate counseling and treatment to address these symptoms

In several ways, family physicians are particularly well suited to respond to terrorism. First, family physicians are widely dispersed, in rural and urban areas, making them accessible for patients wherever manmade or natural catastrophic events might occur. Second, family physicians provide continuity care, essential for the appropriate care of patients and families with ongoing physical and emotional outcomes from violent events. Third, family physicians provide comprehensive care, and can take care of most of the health problems, including emotional issues, facing victims of terrorism. Fourth, family physicians understand how to coordinate care for patients, and can refer victims of mass disasters to other appropriate services as necessary. Most importantly, family physicians understand how to provide care in the context of family and community (22). As the events of September/October 2001 demonstrated, terrorism affects entire communities, whether or not individuals directly experience physical outcomes from the attacks. Family physicians, who understand how their patients and families interact with their community, can help identify and treat problems at the community level. Although horrible, past terrorist events illustrate the pivotal role that family physicians play, working in partnership with public health officials to protect and promote the health of families and communities.

References

1. Gerberding, JL, Hughes, JM, Koplan, JP. Bioterrorism Preparedness and Response. Clinicians and Public Health Agencies as Essential Partners. JAMA, 287(7):898–900, 2002
2. Centers for Disease Control and Prevention. Framework for Evaluating Public Health Surveillance Systems for Early Detection of Outbreaks. Morbidity and Mortality Weekly Report 53(RR05):1–11, May 7, 2004
3. Cherry, CL, Kainer, MA, Ruff, TA. Biological Weapons Preparedness: The Role of Physicians. Internal Medicine Journal, 33:242–253, 2003
4. Gostin LO. Public Health Law: Power, Duty and Restraint. Turning Point. Collaborating for a New Century in Public Health. University of Washington, Turning Point National Program Office, December 1999. Available at http://www.turningpointprogram.org/Pages/pdfs/publications/gostin.pdf, last accessed 3–18–06

5. Doyle, TJ, Glynn, MK, Groseclose, SL. Completeness of Notifiable Infectious Disease Reporting in the United States: An Analytical Literature Review. American Journal of Epidemiology, 155(9):866–874, 2002
6. Centers for Disease Control and Prevention. HIPAA Privacy Rule and Public Health. Guidance from the CDC and the U.S. Department of Health and Human Services. Morbidity and Mortality Weekly Report (MMWR), 52(Supp. 1):1–12, May 2, 2003. Also at http://www.cdc.gov/mmwr/preview/mmwrhtml/su5201a1.htm (last accessed 3–18–06)
7. Buehler, JW, Berkelman, RL, Hartley, DM, Peters, CJ. Syndromic Surveillance and Bioterrorism-Related Epidemics. Emerging Infectious Diseases, 9(10):1197–1204, 2003
8. Lewis, MD, Pavlin, JA, Mansfield, JL, O'Brien, S, Boomsma, LG, Elbert, YE, Kelley, PW. Disease Outbreak Detection System Using Syndromic Data in the Greater Washington DC Area. American Journal of Preventive Medicine, 23(3):180–186, 2002
9. New York City, Department of Health and Mental Hygiene. Key Agency Impact–2003. http://www.nyc.gov/html/doh/downloads/pdf/public/accomplish_2003.pdf, last accessed 3–12–06
10. Lazarus, R, Kleinman, KP, Dashevsky, I, DeMaria, A, Platt, R. Using Automated Medical Records for the Rapid Identification of Illness Syndromes (Syndromic Surveillance): The Example of Lower Respiratory Infection. BMC Public Health, 2001. http://www.biomedcentral.com/1471–2458/1/9, last accessed 3–12–06
11. Mandl KD, Overhage JM, Wagner MM, et al. Implementing Syndromic Surveillance: A Practical Guide Informed by the Early Experience. Journal of the American Medical Informatics Association, 11(2):141–150, 2004
12. Lazarus, R, Kleinman, KP, Dashevsky, I, Adams, C, Kludt, P, DeMaria, A, Platt, R. Use of Automated Ambulatory-Care Encounter Records for Detection of Acute Illness Clusters, Including Potential Bioterrorism Events. Emerging Infectious Diseases, 8(8):753–760, 2002
13. Lober, WB, Trigg, LJ, Karras, BT, Bliss, D, Ciliberti, J, Stewart, L, Duchin, JS. Syndromic Surveillance Using Automated Collection of Computerized Discharge Diagnoses. Journal or Urban Health, 80(2, Suppl. 1):i97–i106, 2003
14. Melnick, A. Introduction to Geographic Information Systems in Public Health, Jones and Bartlett Publishers, 2002
15. Hupert, N, Mushlin, AI, Callahan, MA. Modeling the Public Health Response to Bioterrorism: Using Discrete Event Simulation to Design Antibiotic Distribution Centers. Medical Decision Making 22(Suppl.):S17–S25, 2002
16. Centers for Disease Control and Prevention. Medical Offices and Clinics Pandemic Influenza Planning Checklist, Version 2.2, http://www.pandemicflu.gov/plan/medical.html, March 6, 2006 (last accessed 3–19–06)
17. Campos-Outcalt, D. Disaster Medical Response: Maximizing Your Effectiveness. The Journal of Family Practice, 55(2):113–116, 2006
18. Hoard, ML and Tosatto, RJ. Medical Reserve Corps: Strengthening Public Health and Improving Preparedness. Disaster Management and Response 3(2):48–52, 2005
19. United States Department of Health and Human Services, Office of the Surgeon General. Medical Reserve Corps Resource Site. http://www.medicalreservecorps.gov/page.cfm?pageID = 5 (last accessed 3–26–06)
20. United States Department of Homeland Security, National Disaster Medical Systems. DMAT. http://www.oep-ndms.dhhs.gov/dmat.html (last accessed 3–26–06)
21. Partridge, R, Alexander, J, Lawrence, T, and Suner, S. Medical Counterbioterrorism: The Response to Provide Anthrax Prophylaxis to New York City US Postal Service Employees. Annals of Emergency Medicine, 41(4):441–446, 2003
22. Saultz, JW (Ed.). Textbook of Family Medicine. New York: McGraw-Hill. 2000

Index